NHA CCMA Study Guide

2025-2026

Complete Review + 720 Questions and Detailed Answer Explanations for the Certified Clinical Medical Assistant Exam (4 Full-Length Exams)

Table of Contents

Chapter 1: Foundational Knowledge and Basic Science

Healthcare Systems and Settings

Medical Assistants and Their Role in Clinical Practice

Medical assistants (MA) are healthcare professionals who assist physicians primarily in outpatient settings. MAs are flexible healthcare team members trained in various clinical and administrative roles. They frequently work in clinics and medical offices (outpatient settings).

Clinical Duties

- Interview the patient and document relevant information (medical history).
- Prepare examination and treatment areas.
- Assist during examinations.
- Conduct basic laboratory and other diagnostic tests.
- Administer first aid.
- Provide wound care.
- Perform cardiopulmonary resuscitation.
- Educate patients.
- Dispose of waste.

Administrative Duties

- Manage appointments, correspondence, and office supplies.
- Conduct medical transcription.
- Arrange hospital admissions.
- Perform billing and bookkeeping tasks.
- Manage patient records.

Medical Providers and Allied Health Personnel

Medical provider: A licensed healthcare professional who provides services like diagnosis and treatment. They work in primary, nursing, and specialty care, as well as pharmacy.

Physician: A professional who practices medicine as a medical doctor (MD) or a doctor of osteopathic medicine (DO). Physicians have many specialties, which include anesthesiology, cardiology, dermatology, endocrinology, gastroenterology, general surgery, hematology, nephrology, neurology, obstetrics/gynecology, oncology, and pediatrics.

Nurse practitioner (NP): A nurse with clinical education and training. They can work as primary care providers and prescribe medication. NPs may require a physician's supervision in certain states.

Physician assistant (PA): A licensed professional who provides patient care under the supervision of a physician. They may prescribe medication.

Licensed practical nurse (LPN): A licensed nurse who provides basic nursing care.

Registered nurse (RN): A licensed nurse who completed a nursing program and a state board examination.

Licensing vs. Certification

A certification is a third-party verification awarded to a professional after they prove their ability to perform a specific job or skill. Whereas a federal, state, or local government agency grants a license that permits a professional to practice a regulated occupation or profession in a specific location.

MAs are not required to have a certification in most states. However, many employers prefer applicants with national-level certifications. The following is a list of credentials for medical assistants and the organizations that confer them.

- CCMA (Certified Clinical Medical Assistant) awarded by the National Healthcareer Association.
- CMA (Certified Medical Assistant) awarded by the Certifying Board of the American Association of Medical Assistants.
- RMA (Registered Medical Assistant) awarded by American Medical Technologists.
- NCMA (National Certified Medical Assistant) awarded by the National Center for Competency Testing.

To maintain the CCMA credential, an MA must receive ten continuing education units (CEUs) and recertify every two years.

Types of Health Organizations and Delivery Models

Inpatient care: Patient care that requires admission into a healthcare facility. Issues that may require inpatient care include serious injuries or illnesses and complex surgical procedures.

Outpatient care: Patient care that does not require admission into a healthcare facility. Situations handled in an outpatient setting include consultations, follow-ups, and many medical urgencies.

Managed care organization: A healthcare company that seeks to lower costs without compromising quality.

Accountable care organization: An organization of voluntary healthcare providers and hospitals that coordinate care for Medicare patients.

Patient-centered medical home: A model of care that prioritizes access and continuity of care, planning and management of care, and patient/caregiver engagement.

Hospice care: A medical service that focuses on end-of-life care.

Home healthcare: Medical care that can be provided at home.

Community health clinics: A model of care that provides affordable healthcare services for everyone, especially low-income or uninsured patients.

Concierge medicine: A model of care where patients pay a monthly or annual fee to a physician for continuous access to primary care.

Mobile health unit: A customizable mobile unit that provides various healthcare services, such as screenings, immunizations, and basic laboratory services.

Technology-Based Methods for Providing Healthcare and Health Information

Telehealth (telemedicine) uses technology-based methods to facilitate care and transfer health-related information to benefit patients. It can be accomplished with various devices that many people have in their homes (e.g., computers, smartphones, tablets). Healthcare providers and institutions can provide

- Virtual visits.
- Patient portals.
- Wearable technology.
- Remote monitoring and self-monitoring.
- Personal health apps.
- Electronic personal health records.
- Provider-to-provider communication.

Payment Models in Healthcare

Payment models correspond with specific healthcare services. These methods include

- Fee-for-service (payment per service).
- Capitation (payment per beneficiary).
- Bundled payments (payment per episode).
- Payment per day or visit.
- Payment per time period.
- Cost reimbursement (payment per dollar of cost).
- Percentage of charges (payment per dollar of charges).
- Contact capitation (payment per recipient).

General vs. Specialty Healthcare and Services

General (primary) care and specialty care are two forms of healthcare that work together continuously.

Primary care is the first line of defense in the healthcare system. It involves general practitioners, family physicians, pediatricians, nurses, medical assistants, and other healthcare providers.

Specialty care includes all the healthcare providers with advanced and specialized training in different areas of medicine like cardiology, pulmonology, neurology, gastroenterology, and dermatology.

Ancillary Services

Ancillary services are supplementary resources that complement medical care. They are divided into three categories.

- Diagnostic services: Laboratory tests, imaging studies, genetic testing, and cardiac monitoring.
- Therapeutic services: Dialysis, wound care, chiropractic, psychotherapy, physical, occupational, and speech therapies.
- Custodial services: Hospice care, home health services, rehabilitation, nursing services, and medical daycare.

Complementary Therapies

Complementary medicine and therapies are used alongside the standard medical treatment (as opposed to alternative medicine, in which the standard treatment is not used). Some examples include acupuncture, meditation, vitamin therapy, plant-based supplements, special diets, massage therapy, and Ayurvedic medicine.

Complementary medicine can be safe and effective—however, these therapies usually do not have enough research to support their use or safety in specific conditions. For this reason, it is important for patients to discuss these therapies with their healthcare provider before implementation.

Medical Terminology

Abbreviations, Acronyms, and Symbols

°C: Celsius.

°F: Fahrenheit.

a.c.: Before meals (ante cibum).

Abd: Abdomen.

ad lib.: As desired.

AIDS: Acquired immunodeficiency syndrome.

AM, **a.m.**: Before noon.

aq: Water.

ATB, **ABX**: Antibiotic.

BID, **bid**: Two times a day.

BMI: Body mass index.

BP: Blood pressure.

Bx: Biopsy.

C.C.: Chief complaint.

CBC: Complete blood count.

CDC: Centers for Disease Control and Prevention.

CHF: Congestive heart failure.

CMP: Comprehensive metabolic panel.

CMS: Centers for Medicare & Medicaid Services.

CNS: Central nervous system.

COPD: Chronic obstructive pulmonary disease.

CT: Computerized tomography.

CV: Cardiovascular.

D&C: Dilation and curettage.

Derm.: Dermatology.

DM: Diabetes mellitus.

Dx: Diagnosis.

EKG, ECG: Electrocardiogram.

ER, E.R.: Emergency room.

FDA: Food and Drug Administration.

GI: Gastrointestinal.

GU: Genitourinary.

Ht.: Height.

HTN: Hypertension.

Hx: History.

ICU: Intensive care unit.

IM: Intramuscular.

IP: Inpatient.

IV: Intravenous.

Meds.: Medication.

MRI: Magnetic resonance imaging.

N/V: Nausea and vomiting.

NICU: Neonatal intensive care unit.

NPO: Nothing by mouth.

OB/GYN: Obstetrics and gynecology.

OD, **od**: Right eye (oculus dexter).

OP: Outpatient.

OR, **O.R.**: Operating room.

OSHA: Occupational Safety and Health Administration.

p.c.: After meals.

Pap.: Papanicolaou smear.

PM, **p.m.**: After noon.

PNS: Peripheral nervous system.

PO: By mouth.

Post-op: Postoperative.

PPM: Pulsations per minute.

Pre-op: Preoperative.

prn: As needed.

Px, **PE**: Physical exam.

Q#H, **q#h**: Every # hours (q6h = every 6 hours).

QID, **qid**: Four times a day.

ref.: Referral.

Rx, **R**: Prescription.

S/R: Suture removal.

SOB: Shortness of breath.

SQ, **SubQ**: Subcutaneous.

STAT: Immediately.

Supp., **suppos.**: Suppository.

Sx: Symptoms.

Tab.: Tablet.

Temp., **T**: Temperature.

TID, **tid**: Three times a day.

TPR: Temperature, pulse, respiration.

Tx: Treatment.

UA: Urinalysis.

US: Ultrasound.

VS: Vital signs.

Wt., wt.: Weight.

Y.O., **y.o.**: Year old.

The Joint Commission's Official "Do Not Use" List

Do Not Use:

IU (International Unit): It may be mistaken for IV (intravenous) or 10 (ten). Use International Unit.

Lack of leading zero (.*x* mg): The decimal point can be missed. Use 0.*x* mg.

MS: It could mean morphine sulfate or magnesium sulfate. Use morphine sulfate or magnesium sulfate.

MSO4 and **MgSO4**: They could be mistaken for each other. Use morphine sulfate or magnesium sulfate.

Q.D., **QD**, **q.d.**, **qd (daily)**: They may be mistaken for each other. Use daily.

Q.O.D., **QOD. q.o.d.**, **qod (every other day)**: The period after the /Q/ may be mistaken for /I/ and the /O/ for /I/. Use every other day.

Trailing zero (*x*.0 mg): The decimal point can be missed. Use *x* mg.

U, u (unit): It may be mistaken for 0 (zero), 4 (four), or cc. Use unit.

Word Building

Healthcare workers can use word building to recognize and understand various medical terms. Words consist of multiple parts.

Prefix

When present, it is the first part of a word and modifies the root. Examples include

A-: Without.

Anti-: Against.

Auto-: Self.

Bi-: Both.

Dys-: Painful, difficult, bad.

Ec-: Away.

Ecto-: Outside.

Endo-: Within.

Neo-: New.

Poly-: Many.

Retro-: Back, behind.

Root

The main part of the word which holds its most basic meaning.

Suffix

When present, it is the last part of a word and modifies the root.

-ac: Related to.

-form: Resembling.

-iasis: Abnormal condition.

-ism: Condition.

-itis: Inflammation.

-oma: Tumor.

-penia: Deficiency.

-plasia: Development.

-rrhea: Discharge.

-stasis: Stoppage.

-stomy: Creation of an opening.

-tomy: Incision.

Common Lay and Medical Terms

Medical assistants may need to express medical terms simply or understand what a patient may be trying to say. The following is a list of medical terms and their lay equivalents.

Abdomen: Tummy, stomach.

Asthenia: Weakness, lack of strength.

CT scan: X-ray from many angles.

Diarrhea: Loose or watery poo.

Diastolic pressure: The lower number (when referring to the measurement).

Diuretic: Water pill, a medication that makes you pee.

Dyspepsia: Upset stomach, indigestion.

Dyspnea: Shortness of breath, difficulty breathing.

Edema: Puffiness, swelling.

Emesis: Throwing up, vomiting.

Gastroesophageal reflux: Heartburn, burning feeling in the chest.

Hyperglycemia: High sugar, too much sugar, diabetes.

Injection: Shot.

Otalgia: Earache, pain in the ear.

Paresthesia: Tingling, numbness, loss of sensation.

Pruritus: Itching, scratchy.

Somnolence: Sleepiness.

Systolic pressure: The higher or top number (when referring to the measurement).

Upper respiratory infection: Cold, stuffy nose, runny nose.

Varices: Engorged or enlarged veins.

Vertigo: Dizziness, lightheadedness.

Anatomical Terminology

Anatomical terminology includes terms related to the dirction and planes of the body.

Directional terms

Anterior/ventral: Front of the body.

Deep: Farther from the surface of the body.

Distal: Away from the point of attachment or trunk.

Inferior/caudal: Toward the feet, away from the head.

Lateral: Away from the midline.

Medial: Toward the midline.

Posterior/dorsal: Back of the body.

Proximal: Close to the point of attachment or trunk.

Superficial: Closer to the surface of the body.

Superior/cranial: Toward the head, away from the feet.

Body planes

Frontal/coronal: The vertical plane that divides the body into anterior and posterior sections.

Median/mid-sagittal: The vertical plane that travels through the midline.

Sagittal/lateral: The vertical plane that divides the body into right and left sides.

Transverse/axial: The horizontal plane that divides the body into upper and lower sections.

Basic Pharmacology

Pharmacology is the study of substances (drugs) that interact with living organisms. They can affect one or multiple bodily functions and are used for various purposes.

- **Therapeutic** drugs are used to treat a condition. For example, antihypertensive medication is used to treat arterial hypertension.
- **Diagnostic** drugs are used to diagnose a condition. For example, tuberculin (purified protein derivative or PPD) can be used to diagnose tuberculosis.
- **Palliative** drugs are mainly used to treat symptoms. For example, analgesics are used to treat pain.
- **Preventive** drugs are used to prevent a condition. For example, the MMR vaccine prevents measles, mumps, and rubella.
- **Replacement** drugs are used to replace another substance. For example, estrogen is commonly used for hormone replacement therapy in some post-menopausal women.

Medical assistants will work with pharmacologic agents in their day-to-day practice. Therefore, basic knowledge of pharmacology is needed to understand the effects of prescribed medications, administration methods, possible adverse effects, and other functions.

The U.S. Food and Drug Administration (FDA) regulates food, drugs, biologics, medical devices, products that emit radiation, cosmetics, veterinary products, and tobacco.

Drug Classifications, Indications, and Commonly Prescribed Examples

The following (non-exhaustive) list presents a general classification of pharmacologic agents, their clinical uses, and a few examples of commonly prescribed drugs from each group.

Analgesics (painkillers) help to relieve and control pain. They are usually divided into two categories.

Opioids treat severe pain, such as post-surgical pain or cancer.

- Morphine (Avinza).
- Tramadol (Ultram) is classified as an opioid-like analgesic but not a true opioid.
- Oxymorphone (Opana).

Non-opioids treat mild to moderate types of pain.

- Nonsteroidal anti-inflammatory drugs (NSAIDs): Ibuprofen (Advil), naproxen (Aleve), and diclofenac (Cataflam).
- Acetaminophen (Tylenol).

Antacids are used to neutralize stomach acid in patients with heartburn or indigestion.

- Calcium carbonate (Tums).
- Bismuth subsalicylate (Pepto Bismol).

Antiarrhythmics are used to treat arrhythmias (irregular or abnormal heartbeats).

- Amiodarone (Cordarone).
- Diltiazem (Cardizem).

Antibiotics treat bacterial infections. They are formulated to fight a variety of bacteria.

- Broad spectrum: Amoxicillin/clavulanate (Augmentin) or ciprofloxacin (Cipro).
- Gram-positive: Penicillins or cephalexin (Biocef).
- Gram-negative: Aztreonam (Azactam).
- Anaerobic: Metronidazole (Flagyl).

Anticoagulants prevent the formation of blood clots.

- Warfarin (Coumadin).
- Rivaroxaban (Xarelto).

Anticonvulsants (antiepileptics) help to prevent seizures.

- Valproic acid (Depakene).
- Diazepam (Valium).

Antidepressants help to treat depression.

- Tricyclic antidepressants: Amitriptyline (Elavil).
- Monoamine oxidase inhibitors: Selegiline (Eldepryl).
- Selective serotonin reuptake inhibitors (SSRIs): Fluoxetine (Prozac) and Sertraline (Zoloft).

Antiemetics treat nausea and vomiting.

- Metoclopramide (Metozolv ODT).
- Ondansetron (Zofran).

Antifungals treat fungal infections.

- Fluconazole (Diflucan).
- Clotrimazole (Canesten).

Antihistamines are commonly used to treat various types of allergic conditions.

- Cetirizine (Zyrtec)
- Fexofenadine (Allegra).

Some antihistamines, specifically H2 blockers, treat peptic ulcers and gastroesophageal reflux disease. Cimetidine (Tagamet) is an H2 blocker used to treat peptic ulcers and gastroesophageal reflux disease.

Antihypertensives treat hypertension and include multiple types of drugs.

- Enalapril (Vasotec).
- Nifedipine (Adalat).
- Losartan (Cozaar).

Anti-inflammatories decrease inflammation in acute and chronic conditions. They are usually divided into two groups.

- Nonsteroidal: NSAIDs
- Steroidal: Prednisone (Deltasone, Pediapred), methylprednisolone (Depo-Medrol, Solu-Medrol), and hydrocortisone (Hydrocort).

Antineoplastics (chemotherapy) treat various types of cancer.

- Cisplatin (Platinol).
- Methotrexate (Trexall).
- Paclitaxel (Onxol, Abraxane).
- Vincristine (Oncovin).

Antipsychotics treat psychiatric conditions, usually associated with psychosis. Antipsychotics can be divided into two groups.

- First-generation or typical: Haloperidol (Haldol).
- Second-generation or atypical: Risperidone (Risperdal).

Antipyretics are used to treat fever.

- NSAIDs

- Acetaminophen.

Antivirals treat acute and chronic viral infections.

- Acyclovir (Zovirax).
- Zidovudine (Retrovir).
- Remdesivir (Veklury).

Anxiolytics are used to reduce stress and anxiety in patients with panic attacks and anxiety disorders. The most common anxiolytics are benzodiazepines.

- Alprazolam (Xanax).
- Clonazepam (Klonopin).

Barbiturates are sedative drugs used to treat insomnia, seizures, and other conditions. They can be used as anesthesia or to induce coma.

- Phenobarbital (Luminal).
- Methohexital (Brevital).

Beta-blockers act on beta-adrenergic receptors, which help to treat hypertension, tachycardia, arrhythmias, glaucoma, hyperthyroidism, and heart failure.

- Propranolol (Inderal).
- Bisoprolol (Zebeta).
- Carvedilol (Coreg).

Bronchodilators dilate the airways, which promotes breathing. These drugs can treat breathing conditions like asthma and chronic obstructive pulmonary disease.

- Albuterol (Ventolin).
- Ipratropium (Atrovent).

Corticosteroids are synthetic analogs of the steroid hormones produced by the adrenal gland (glucocorticoids and mineralocorticoids). They are anti-inflammatories commonly employed to treat asthma, chronic obstructive pulmonary disease, rheumatoid arthritis, and systemic lupus erythematosus.

- Dexamethasone (Decadron).
- Betamethasone (Diprosone).

Cough suppressants (antitussives) reduce the cough reflex.

- Dextromethorphan (Robitussin).
- Codeine (Cheratussin AC).

Cytotoxins are toxic to cells and, therefore, used to destroy harmful tissue. These agents are commonly used in oncology to treat various types of cancer.

- Cyclophosphamide (Cytoxan).
- Doxorubicin (Adriamycin).

Decongestants reduce nasal congestion (stuffiness) through the constriction of blood vessels. They can be applied locally or taken orally.

- Pseudoephedrine (Sudafed).
- Oxymetazoline (Vicks, Sinex).

Diuretics promote urine excretion (diuresis). They are used to treat various conditions such as hypertension, heart failure, and nephrogenic diabetes insipidus.

- Furosemide (Lasix).
- Bumetanide (Bumex).
- Spironolactone (Aldactone).

Expectorants help clear mucus from the respiratory airways. They may come combined with cough suppressants.

- Guaifenesin (Mucinex).

Hormones are synthetic analogs of naturally occurring hormones used to treat various conditions.

- Insulin (Lantus, Levemir, Apidra, Humalog).
- Thyroid hormones (Synthroid, Euthyrox).
- Corticosteroids.
- Estrogen (Depo-Estradiol).

Hypnotics (sedatives) induce and prolong sleep.

- Benzodiazepines.
- Zolpidem (Ambien).
- Melatonin.
- Barbiturates.
- Nonbenzodiazepines: Zolpidem (Ambien) or eszopiclone (Lunesta).

Hypoglycemics reduce blood glucose levels, most commonly in patients with diabetes. There are multiple drug families that reduce glycemia.

- SGLT2 inhibitors: Dapagliflozin (Farxiga).
- DPP-4 inhibitors: Sitagliptin (Januvia).
- Thiazolidinediones: Pioglitazone (Actos).
- Biguanides: Metformin (Glucophage).
- Sulfonylureas: Glimepiride (Amaryl).

Immunosuppressives decrease the body's normal or pathological immune response (e.g., infections, organ rejection, inflammatory bowel disease, rheumatoid arthritis, and cancer).

- Corticosteroids.
- Tacrolimus (Prograf, Astagraf XL).
- Mycophenolate mofetil (CellCept).

Laxatives are used to treat constipation.

- Magnesium hydroxide (Phillips' Milk of Magnesia).
- Lactulose (Constilac).
- Polyethylene glycol (MiraLAX).
- Mineral oil (Muri-Lube).

Muscle relaxants reduce muscle tone and treat muscle-related pain.

- Carisoprodol (Soma).
- Chlorzoxazone (Lorzone).
- Cyclobenzaprine (Amrix, Flexeril).

Thrombolytics (fibrinolytics) dissolve clots in patients with ischemic strokes, heart attacks, pulmonary embolisms, and other thromboembolic conditions.

- Alteplase (Activase).
- Reteplase (Retavase).
- Streptokinase (Kabikinase, Streptase).

Vitamins and minerals are micronutrients essential for the body to function normally. They need to be acquired via diet or supplementation.

Over-the-Counter Medications

Over-the-counter (OTC) medications (nonprescription medications) can be sold to the general public without a prescription from a healthcare professional. In the United States, OTC drugs are regulated by the Food and Drug Administration (FDA) and must include a *Drug Facts* label to educate the consumer. These drugs are safe to use when the directions on the label (or those dictated by a healthcare professional) are adequately followed.

OTC medications treat and manage many conditions (e.g., a cold, fever, allergic reactions, and pain) without the need for professional help. They include various substances applied locally, such as

- Creams with antibiotics, steroids, and antifungals.
- Medicated shampoo.
- Mouthwash.
- Toothpaste.

Sometimes, a medication enters the market as a prescription drug but becomes available OTC after it earns a proven safety record and FDA approval. Certain drugs may exist in low-dose versions sold over the counter and higher-dose presentations that require a valid prescription by a health professional.

The following list includes some of the most commonly used OTC active ingredients and medications:

- Acetaminophen (analgesic, antipyretic).
- Aspirin (analgesic, antipyretic).
- Bacitracin (topical antibiotic).
- Caffeine (analgesic, diuretic, menstrual analgesic, stimulant).
- Dextromethorphan (cough suppressant).
- Dimenhydrinate (anticholinergic, antiemetic).
- Diphenhydramine (antihistamine, sedative).
- Fexofenadine (antihistamine).
- Guaifenesin (expectorant).
- Hydrocortisone (anti-inflammatory, corticosteroid).
- Ibuprofen (analgesic).
- Lidocaine (local analgesic).
- Mineral oil (laxative, lubricant).
- Omeprazole (antacid).
- Povidone-iodine (topical antimicrobial).

- Pseudoephedrine (decongestant).
- Pyrithione zinc (antimicrobial).

Schedules of Controlled Substances

In 1970, the Federal Comprehensive Drug Abuse Prevention and Control Act (Controlled Substances Act) was created to categorize substances that could be potentially abused. There are five schedules.

Schedule I substances have the highest potential for abuse and do not have any FDA-approved medical indication. Therefore, they are not prescribed. Examples include

- Heroin.
- 3,4-Methylenedioxymethamphetamine (MDMA or ecstasy).
- Lysergic acid diethylamide (LSD).
- Marijuana.
- Mescaline.

Schedule II (C-II) substances have a high abuse potential, but they have clinical applications. Medical professionals must provide written or electronic prescriptions for these substances (oral or fax formats are not allowed). Refills are prohibited. Examples include

- Morphine.
- Cocaine.
- Oxycodone.
- Fentanyl.
- Hydromorphone.
- Adderall (amphetamine salts).

Schedule III (C-III) substances have a moderate to low potential for abuse. Prescriptions may be oral, written, or electronic and include only five refills in six months. Examples include

- Ketamine.
- Anabolic steroids.
- Products that contain less than 90 milligrams of codeine per dosage unit (e.g., Tylenol with codeine).

Schedule IV (C-IV) substances have a low potential for abuse. Prescriptions may be oral, written, or electronic and include only five refills in six months. Examples include

- Tramadol.
- Benzodiazepines (diazepam, clonazepam, midazolam).
- Carisoprodol.
- Phenobarbital.

Schedule V (C-V) substances have the lowest potential for abuse. Prescriptions may be oral, written, or electronic. Examples include

- Products that contain less than 200 milligrams of codeine per 100 milliliters (e.g., Robitussin AC).
- Pregabalin.
- Promethazine.
- Attapulgite.
- Lomotil (diphenoxylate/atropine).

Side Effects vs. Adverse Reactions

The terms *side effect* and *adverse reactions* are often used interchangeably, even among healthcare professionals and organizations (which includes the Centers for Disease Control and Prevention (CDC)). However, this is not entirely correct. Although both describe unintended responses to substances, there is an important distinction.

Side effects can be positive (but unintended) results of medication or negative (but manageable). They are usually more predictable than adverse reactions. For example, drowsiness is a side effect that may occur in patients who use antihistamines to treat allergic reactions. In most cases, patients do not have to stop the medication; they may just need to take it in the evening.

Adverse reactions are inherently negative and unintended. They may occur when the patient is taking the drug correctly. For example, patients who use warfarin may experience gastrointestinal bleeding, and patients who use ophthalmic corticosteroids may develop increased intraocular pressure or glaucoma.

Indications and Contraindications

Indications are valid clinical reasons to use a drug to treat one or more conditions. In the United States, the FDA is responsible for the approval process. The indication can be found on the Prescribing Information label. However, healthcare professionals may prescribe medications for indications not approved by the FDA (off-label indications).

Label indications are often specific to the drug's dosage and presentation. For example, a 1% lidocaine multidose vial can be used subcutaneously as a local anesthetic, and a 2%

lidocaine preservative-free single-dose vial can be used intravenously to treat ventricular arrhythmias. Although it is the same drug (lidocaine), it comes in different presentations (multidose vs. single dose; preservative vs. preservative free) for other indications.

Conversely, contraindications are the opposite of indications. They are valid reasons to avoid the use of a drug. Usually, contraindications are divided into two groups.

- **Relative contraindications** demand caution and a risk-benefit analysis. In these situations, a temporary or potentially manageable factor may need to be resolved before the drug is prescribed. For example, insulin should be used with caution for patients with hypokalemia (low potassium). However, this is not an absolute contraindication because the situation can be corrected before the insulin is administered.

- **Absolute contraindications** may result in a life-threatening event. True absolute contraindications cannot be resolved but are not very common. For example, an intravenous fibrinolytic (like alteplase) cannot be used to treat a patient with an acute ischemic stroke who also has intracranial hemorrhage.

Systems of Measurement and Mathematical Conversions

The metric system (gram, liter, meter) is the world's most commonly used measurement system. However, most people in the U.S. use the imperial system (pound, ounce, mile). Nonetheless, metric measurements are used in technical and scientific fields, which includes the pharmaceutical industry. As a result, not everyone can interpret the numbers in a prescription or medication. In some cases, the medication may be measured using the metric system, and the prescription may contain directions using the imperial system (e.g., various liquid medications taken orally).

Relevant Metric Measurements

- 1 kg = 1,000 g.
- 1 g = 1,000 mg.
- 1 mg = 1,000 mcg.
- 1 L = 1,000 mL.
- 1 mL = 1 cc.

Relevant Abbreviations and Symbols

- Kg or kg: kilogram.
- g: gram.

- mg: milligram.
- mcg: microgram.
- L: liter.
- mL: milliliter.
- m: meter.
- cm: centimeter.
- cc: cubic centimeter.
- lb.: pound
- gtt: drop/drops.
- t or tsp: teaspoon.
- T or tbsp: tablespoon.
- oz: ounce.
- fl oz: fluid ounce.
- c: cup.

Relevant Equivalents and Conversions

- 1 kg = 2.2 lb.
- 1 lb. = 453.6 g.
- 1 mL = 20 gtt.
- 1 tbsp = 3 tsp.
- 1 tsp = 5 mL.
- 1 tbsp = 15 mL.
- 1 oz = 2 tbsp = 29.57 mL.
- 1 c = 8 oz = 16 tbsp = 240 mL.
- 2 c = 16 oz = 473.18 mL.

Conversion tables can convert units or medication orders from one measurement system to another. Nonetheless, mathematical conversions may sometimes be needed to make precise calculations and verify simple conversions. Conversions are calculated by multiplication and division.

For example, a patient must receive the equivalent of 2.7 tsp in milliliters. If 5 mL = 1 tsp, how many milliliters are needed for the complete dose? The problem can be solved in the following manner:

$$1\ tsp : 5\ mL = 2.7\ tsp : x\ mL$$

$$1 \times x = 2.7 \times 5$$

$$x = 13.5\ mL$$

Dosage Calculations

Dosages may vary according to a patient's age, weight, condition, comorbidities, and other drugs they are taking. Additionally, the presentation of the medication (tablets, suspension, intramuscular or intravenous injection) is very important. In most cases, drugs are available in multiple strengths.

To calculate a dose, one must know the following values:

1) Drug strength.
2) Unit strength.
3) Ordered strength.

$$\frac{Drug\ Strength}{Ordered\ strength} = \frac{Unit\ strength}{x\ (Dose)}$$

Example 1: The order reads, "500 mg of amoxicillin taken orally every 12 hours for five days." The available strength is 500 mg capsules.

1) Drug strength = 500 mg.
2) Unit strength = 1 capsule.
3) Ordered strength = 500 mg.

$$\frac{500\ mg}{500\ mg} = \frac{1\ capsule}{x\ capsule}$$

Cross-multiply to calculate x (number of capsules needed)

$$x \times 500\ mg = 500x$$

$$1\ capsule \times 500\ mg = 500$$

Divide each side by the available strength (500 mg)

$$\frac{500x}{500\ mg} = \frac{500}{500\ mg}$$

$$x = 1\ capsule$$

In this case, the patient must take one 500 mg capsule every 12 hours for five days.

Example 2: The order reads, "Administer 800 mg of ampicillin IV." The available vial contains 1 gram / 15 mL.

1) Drug strength = 1,000 mg (1 g = 1,000 mg).
2) Unit strength = 15 mL.

3) Ordered strength = 800 mg.

$$\frac{1{,}000\ mg}{800\ mg} = \frac{15\ mL}{x}$$

$$x \times 1{,}000\ mg = 1{,}000x$$

$$15\ mL \times 800\ mg = 12{,}000$$

$$\frac{1{,}000x}{1{,}000\ mg} = \frac{12{,}000}{1{,}000\ mg}$$

$$x = 12\ mL$$

To administer 800 mg of ampicillin, the dose should be 12 mL.

In some cases, the dosage may be based on body weight. This is especially common when caring for pediatric patients. The dose is usually calculated in kilograms. As a result, weight conversion may be needed to calculate the ordered strength (1 kilogram = 2.2 pounds).

Forms of Medication

Solids and Semisolids

- **Tablet**: A pill made of compressed powder. Delayed-release tablets have a special coating that extends the drug's dissolution rate and effect. Enteric-coated tablets have a special coating that resists the acidic environments, which allows the drug to be absorbed in the intestine.
- **Capsule**: An active ingredient in powder or liquid form enclosed in a shell of gelatin or similar material. Some may come as delayed-release or enteric-coated capsules.
- **Powder**: A drug that is ground until it is pulverized. In some cases, a tablet may be crushed to facilitate administration to certain patients (e.g., an elderly patient who cannot swallow a tablet).
- **Lozenge**: A flat tablet that dissolves inside the mouth.
- **Suppository**: A bolus made of cocoa butter, polyethylene glycol, or similar material combined with an active ingredient. Once inserted into the body via the rectum, vagina, or urethra, it will dissolve and exert its effects.
- **Ointment**: An oily solution infused with an active ingredient.
- **Cream**: A water-based solution infused with a drug.
- **Transdermal patch**: A medicated adhesive patch that delivers a drug through the skin.

Liquids

- **Suspension**: A liquid mixture in which fine drug particles are suspended in a fluid where they are not dissolved. It must be shaken to ensure the particles are evenly distributed throughout the mixture.
- **Syrup**: A mixture of water, sugar, and an active ingredient. It may also contain added flavors.
- **Emulsion**: A mixture of two immiscible liquids (such as oil and water) where one liquid contains a dispersion of the other. It must be shaken before use.
- **Lotion**: An aqueous solution infused with a drug for topical use.
- **Elixir**: A solution made of alcohol (10-20%), sugar, and water.

Injectables

- **Ampule**: A small flask that contains a single dose of medication.
- **Vial**: A small bottle that contains medication. It can be single-dose or multi-dose.
- **Prefilled syringe**: A sterile, disposable, single-dose syringe that contains prepared medication.

Routes of Administration

- **Oral**: The drug is swallowed. This is the most common route.
- **Buccal**: The drug is placed between the gums and cheek and is dissolved.
- **Sublingual**: The drug dissolves under the tongue.
- **Parenteral**: The drug bypasses the gastrointestinal tract and is administered by injection. This includes intravenous, subcutaneous, intramuscular, intrathecal, and intradermal routes.
- **Nasal**: The drug is absorbed through the nasal mucosa.
- **Inhalation**: The drug is absorbed through the airways.
- **Otic**: The drug is applied to the ear.
- **Ophthalmic**: The drug is administered into the eye.
- **Topical**: The drug is applied to a specific area of the skin or mucous membranes.
- **Transdermal**: The drug is absorbed through the skin.
- **Rectal**: The drug is absorbed through the rectum.
- **Vaginal**: The drug is absorbed through the vagina.
- **Urethral**: The drug is administered into the urethra.
- **Intraarterial**: The drug is administered through an artery.
- **Intraosseous**: The drug is administered into a bone. It is mostly employed in emergencies if venous access is too difficult.

Rights of Medication Administration

The safe administration of medication requires familiarity with the rights of medication administration.

- The right drug.
- The right patient.
- The right dosage.
- The right time.
- The right route.
- The right technique.
- The right documentation.

Look-Alike and Sound-Alike Medications

Certain drugs have orthographic and phonetic similarities—look-alike, sound-alike medications (LASA). This may result in medication errors and potential harm to the patient.

Sound-alike problems are often caused by confusion with brand-brand, generic-brand, or generic-generic drug names. Look-alike problems may occur with similar-looking drugs or when multiple drug companies produce the same drug but with a different appearance.

To avoid this, the FDA and the Institute for Safe Medication Practices (ISMP) recommend the use of tall man lettering for certain drug names. The following list includes some FDA-approved generic drug names with tall man letters (Institute for Safe Medication Practices, 2016).

- acetaZOLAMIDE, confused with acetoHEXAMIDE.
- buPROPion, confused with busPIRone.
- chlorproMAZINE, confused with chlorproPAMIDE.
- dimenhyDRINATE, confused with diphenhydrAMINE.
- DOBUTamine, confused with DOPamine.
- prednisoLONE, confused with predniSONE.
- risperiDONE, confused with rOPINIRole.
- sulfADIAZINE, confused with sulfiSOXAZOLE.

Pharmacokinetics

Pharmacokinetics is the study of the interactions between a drug and the body. This includes a substance's absorption, distribution, metabolism, and excretion.

Absorption

After administration, a drug must be absorbed. This process varies according to the administration route and various characteristics of the drug (dissolution rate, concentration, and other biochemical variables). Bioavailability is an essential factor to consider, especially when a drug is taken orally. This is the fraction of the administered drug that reaches systemic circulation. In the case of intravenous administration, 100% of the drug reaches systemic circulation. However, bioavailability varies when drugs are taken orally due to inactivation by digestive enzymes, gastrointestinal absorption rate, and liver metabolism.

Distribution

Drugs spread inside the body according to their biochemical properties. These traits include polarity, binding sites, and size.

Metabolism

Drugs usually metabolize inside the body. In some cases, the substance is administered in an inactive form that becomes activated by metabolic processes. However, metabolism usually inactivates a drug.

Excretion

Finally, drugs are eliminated from the body. The kidneys and the liver excrete most drugs via the urine and bile.

Principles of Storage and Disposal

Adequate storage is necessary to avoid medication errors and other safety issues. Pharmaceutical products are usually stored in the pharmacy but can be kept in other areas (e.g., office, floor stock, night closet). In general, drugs should remain in their original container. However, healthcare professionals should refer to the specific storage directions of each drug. Some drugs may require refrigeration (such as insulin, vaccines, and reconstituted antibiotics).

MAs should dispose of unused, out-of-date, or unlabeled drugs according to local and office guidelines. Drugs are commonly disposed of through the trash following proper guidelines. However, this is prohibited in the case of hazardous waste pharmaceuticals (e.g., warfarin, vaccines with thimerosal, and insulins with m-cresol).

Sources of Drug Information

Drug information can be found in multiple ways. Traditionally, the Physicians' Desk Reference and the United States Pharmacopeia Dispensing Information (USPDI) are the most widely used references. Package inserts and scientific publications also contain relevant information about specific drugs or types of medication. Finally, online sources like Drugs.com and DrugBank Online provide an accessible database with up-to-date information.

Nutrition

Nutrients

Nutrients are substances found in food that the human body needs to live. They are commonly divided into two groups.

Macronutrients include carbohydrates, fats, and amino acids (proteins). They are consumed in large quantities and serve as a source of energy and building blocks for most molecules in the body.

- **Carbohydrates** are monosaccharides (simple sugars) like glucose, disaccharides like sucrose or lactose, oligosaccharides, and polysaccharides like starch. All are important sources of energy. Dietary fiber is a carbohydrate that is not broken down into simple sugars but helps digestion instead.

- **Fats** are either saturated or unsaturated. They have important functions related to energy storage and production and maintenance of the body's core temperature. Fats also help to absorb liposoluble vitamins (A, D, E, and K).

- **Amino acids** are molecules that can be linked together to form proteins. Proteins are necessary for enzymes, hormones, and various structures in the human body, such as the skin and muscles.

Micronutrients include vitamins and minerals. They are consumed in smaller quantities and complement various functions of the human body.

- **Vitamins** are essential molecules that the body needs but cannot produce independently in sufficient quantities. Therefore, it is necessary to obtain them from external sources, such as food. They are divided into water-soluble (B complex and C) and fat-soluble (A, D, E, and K).

- **Electrolytes** are various compounds and dietary minerals that carry an electric charge when dissolved in water. They include potassium, sodium, chloride, calcium, and magnesium.

Dietary Guidelines

The United States Department of Agriculture (USDA) and the Department of Health and Human Services (HHS) develop dietary guidelines for Americans. The most recent guidelines (2020-2025) employ MyPlate to help individuals remember the recommended foods (fruits, grains, vegetables, protein, and dairy).

- Focus on whole fruit.
- Vary vegetables.
- Half of the grains should be whole grains.
- Vary protein routine.
- Move to low-fat or fat-free milk and yogurt or lactose-free fortified options such as soy milk.

The Dietary Guidelines also provide further details on the core elements of a healthy diet.

- Vegetables may be any type.
- Fruits should preferably be whole.
- Grains (at least 50%) should preferably be whole grains.
- Dairy should preferably be low or fat-free.
- Protein may include lean meats, poultry, eggs, seafood, beans, peas, lentils, nuts, seeds, and soy products.
- Oils may include vegetable oils and oils from foods like seafood and nuts.

Food Labels

Food labels are descriptions commonly found on packaging to help consumers understand the nutritional properties of the food. These labels include various types of information.

- **Nutrition Facts Label**: This label is regulated by the FDA and contains information on serving size, calories, nutrients, and their daily value percentage. The nutrient list used to include vitamins A and C, but now includes vitamin D and potassium. When reading this label, it is important to check the number of servings per container because even a small container may include multiple servings and significantly increase the total number of calories or specific nutrients.

- **Front-of-package label**: This label is voluntary, and food manufacturers frequently use it to display the positive nutritional qualities of food. However, this selective display of information may not include negative qualities which could deceive the consumer. For this reason, public health advocates recommend warning labels as front-of-package labels to inform consumers about added sugars, high levels of saturated fats, and other potentially negative qualities of food.

- **Side or back labels**: These labels include a list of ingredients in order of weight (the heaviest ingredient is listed first, and the lightest is listed last). Added sugars may appear with different names, such as honey, evaporated cane juice, or high fructose corn syrup. These labels also contain shelf-life information (sell-by, best-by, use-by dates) and allergy information related to the presence (or potential presence) of milk, fish, tree nuts, peanuts, shellfish, wheat, eggs, and soybeans.

Dietary Needs for Common Conditions

Cardiovascular disease: A healthy diet to help prevent cardiovascular disease or cardiovascular events (e.g., stroke or myocardial infarction) should include vegetables, whole grains, nuts, fish, poultry, and fruits. It should limit the consumption of added sugars, processed foods, refined carbohydrates, and sodium. The Mediterranean, DASH (Dietary Approaches to Stop Hypertension), and plant-based diets are generally recommended for people with cardiovascular disease (or those who want to prevent it) because they combine many beneficial nutrients.

Diabetes: People with diabetes can follow the Dietary Guidelines and eat vegetables (broccoli, leafy greens, non-starchy vegetables like peppers, starchy vegetables like potatoes, corn), grains (especially whole grains), protein (lean meat, eggs, fish, nuts, chicken without the skin, tofu), dairy, and fruits. It is important to avoid foods high in saturated or trans fats (fried foods, processed foods), salt, and foods with added sugar (sweets, juices, soda, sugary energy drinks).

Kidney disease: A diet for people with kidney disease should include low-sodium foods. It should contain mostly fresh foods and limit packaged foods. The consumption of proteins, potassium (bananas, oranges, potatoes, nuts, dairy foods), and phosphorus (dark-colored sodas, bran cereals, nuts, dairy foods) should be monitored and often restricted.

Inflammatory bowel disease: It is important to increase dietary fiber (especially soluble fiber found in beans, oats, and fruits) and, in some cases, avoid gluten. A diet low in FODMAP (Fermentable Oligosaccharides, Disaccharides, Monosaccharides, and Polyols) may be recommended for patients with this condition.

Celiac disease: It is important to avoid the consumption of gluten, which can be found in various foods, such as wheat, barley, rye, and triticale.

Eating Disorders

Binge-eating disorder: A condition characterized by episodes of excessive or uncontrolled eating (binge-eating), which is not followed by purging or other compensatory behaviors. Patients may be of normal weight, overweight, or obese.

Anorexia nervosa: A condition characterized by the severe restriction of food and low body weight. It may be restrictive (severe reduction of food intake) or binge-purge (severe restriction with episodes of binge eating followed by purging via vomiting, laxatives, or diuretics).

Bulimia nervosa: A condition characterized by binge-eating episodes followed by excessive behaviors aimed at preventing weight gain (such as vomiting, excessive exercise, fasting, or use of laxatives or diuretics). In contrast with patients with anorexia nervosa, those with bulimia nervosa may be overweight or have a normal weight.

Avoidant restrictive food intake disorder (ARFID): A condition characterized by excessive selectivity with the amount and type of food consumed and low-calorie intake. ARFID usually starts during early childhood and may impair the child's growth and development. It is not characterized by body image issues or fear of being overweight or obese.

Psychology

Developmental Stages

Erik Erikson postulated the theory of psychosocial development and established eight sequential stages of development.

- **Stage 1: Trust vs. Mistrust**
  Infancy to one year

  Children learn to trust others when caregivers provide reliable care and affection.

- **Stage 2: Autonomy vs. Shame and Doubt**
  One to two years

  Children learn to be autonomous when parents allow them to develop abilities through free will.

- **Stage 3: Initiative vs. Guilt**

Three to five years (preschool)

Children learn to take the initiative when parents provide support and guidance.

- **Stage 4: Competence vs. Inferiority**
  Six years to puberty (elementary school)

  Children develop a sense of competence when they are successful or feelings of inferiority when they are not.

- **Stage 5: Identity vs. Role Confusion**
  Adolescence

  Teens begin to experiment with various roles and work to figure out their identity, or they end up confused about who they are.

- **Stage 6: Intimacy vs. Isolation**
  Young adulthood (20s to early 40s)

  Young adults develop their interpersonal skills and seek intimate interpersonal relationships that may be long-term.

- **Stage 7: Generativity vs. Stagnation**
  Middle adulthood (40s to early 60s)

  Successful adults feel fulfillment through contributions to their work, family, and community.

- **Stage 8: Integrity vs. Despair**
  Late adulthood (65 years and beyond)

  This is a stage of reflection and self-judgment, where older adults contemplate their achievements or perceived failures in life.

Common Mental Health Conditions

Generalized anxiety: A condition characterized by persistent excessive worry that is difficult to control. Symptoms include nervousness, doubt or insecurity, restlessness, irritability, fatigue, muscle tension, sleeping problems, palpitations, and sweating.

Panic attacks: Recurrent and unpredictable attacks of severe anxiety. Symptoms include palpitations, chest pain, feeling of suffocation, dry mouth, derealization, depersonalization, sense of impending doom, or fear of losing control and dying.

Depression: A disorder characterized by a persistent and deep feeling of sadness and lack of pleasure. Symptoms include persistent sadness, anhedonia (loss of interest and pleasure in activities that used to be enjoyable), unwanted weight loss or gain, changes in appetite, sleeping problems, fatigue, feelings of guilt, pain, recurrent thoughts of death, harm, or suicide.

Post-traumatic stress disorder (PTSD): A disorder characterized by delayed responses to a stressful or traumatic situation. Symptoms include vivid flashbacks (reliving the traumatic event), intense fear, guilt, alertness, irritability, sleeping problems, and difficulty concentrating.

Attention deficit hyperactivity disorder (ADHD): A behavioral disorder characterized by disorganized, excessive, and impulsive activity. Symptoms include hyperactivity, difficulty with attention and following instructions, fidgeting or squirming, and excessive talking and interrupting others.

Autism spectrum disorder: A group of disorders characterized by abnormal social interaction, communication, and behavior. Symptoms include failure to make eye contact, delayed or absent spoken language, repetitive behaviors or speech, lack of empathy, rigid routines, and resistance to change.

Environmental and Socioeconomic Stressors

Psychological stressors are various events, activities, or stimuli that cause stress and may result in both psychological and physical issues. Stressors can be classified into two groups.

- **Environmental stressors**: This group of stressors encompasses crowding, traffic jams, noise pollution, light pollution, temperature, and air quality, among others. Individually, these stressors do not usually impact a person's psychological well-being, but they can be insidious and coupled with other stressors, such as personal or socioeconomic stressors.
- **Socioeconomic stressors**: These are stressors that directly affect a person's life. They include income, job, abuse, war, access to housing, health, education, and nutrition. Positive major life events (like marriage or having a baby) may also result in significant stress, especially for people with other socioeconomic stressors.

Psychology of Special Populations

Patients with physical disabilities and chronic medical conditions deal with multiple challenges that may affect their psychological well-being, which include loss, grief, depression, self-esteem, body image issues, stigma, discrimination, and other interpersonal issues.

These patients need support from their family, friends, support groups, and community. Coping methods such as therapy, mindfulness, and cognitive strategies (e.g., positive reframing) can be beneficial.

Developmentally delayed patients may present various deficits in language, intelligence, attention, and other psychological abilities. These patients may also face various interpersonal issues, such as discrimination and stigma. Multiple interventions can help patients with specific delays, such as speech therapy, special education, and behavioral therapy. Individualized education plans can help these patients maximize their education.

Defense Mechanisms

Patients use defense mechanisms to cope with negative feelings. They are often subconscious behaviors that vary in effectiveness. Some may even be harmful. The following are the most common types.

Denial: The patient rejects the issue (e.g., a cancer patient will not accept their diagnosis).

Regression: The patient returns to a happier time in their life. This is more common in children (e.g., a toilet-trained child wets their bed again).

Repression: The patient unconsciously suppresses a traumatic experience (e.g., the victim of a crime does not remember the event).

Rationalization: The patient tries to find an explanation for a result, response, or outcome (e.g., a person insists the test must be faulty because they have no family history of the diagnosis).

Avoidance: The patient ignores an uncomfortable or overwhelming issue (e.g., A person does not seek treatment for their symptoms).

Sublimation: The patient transforms a negative response or feeling into something positive or productive (e.g., a person with depression forms a support group).

Projection: The patient attributes their negative feelings to someone else (e.g., a person with anger management issues is convinced that others lack emotional regulation).

Displacement: The patient transfers their negative emotions onto someone less threatening (e.g., A patient is frustrated with their doctor, but they yell at their nurse).

Stages of Grief

Dr. Elisabeth Kübler-Ross defined the five stages of grief as a response pattern to separation or health threats.

- **Denial and isolation**: The existence of the disease is denied. As a result, the patient does not want to comply with the treatment plan.
- **Anger**: The patient becomes hostile and does not want to talk or be reminded of the disease.
- **Bargaining**: The patient attempts to negotiate or make deals to alter the situation, often with a higher power or in hopes of delaying the inevitable.
- **Depression**: The patient recognizes the disease and feels sadness about the diagnosis and loss of health.
- **Acceptance**: The disease is accepted, and the patient is more likely to use their resources.

Chapter 2: Anatomy and Physiology

Body Structures and Organ Systems

Cell Structure

The cell is the basic unit of life of any organism. Cells have various structural and functional features. Human cells can be divided into three main parts: cell membrane, cytoplasm, and nucleus. Some cells do not have a nucleus (for example, prokaryotes like bacteria and certain human cells like red blood cells).

- **Cell membrane**: A semipermeable bilayer made of phospholipids that regulates the transport of various substances between the intracellular space and the extracellular space.
- **Cytoplasm**: A medium that contains water, nutrients (such as glucose), electrolytes, RNA, and many other organic molecules. This solution is contained within the membrane of the cell, and it contains other structures and organelles, like the nucleus, the mitochondria, and the Golgi apparatus.
- **Nucleus**: The structure that contains the cell's information in the form of DNA as chromosomes. The nucleus has a nuclear membrane that regulates the transport of substances between the nucleus and the cytoplasm.

Other important organelles include:

- Ribosomes: Organelles composed of RNA that help to translate information from the messenger RNA into amino acids during the protein synthesis process.
- Mitochondria: The structure in charge of providing energy in the form of adenosine triphosphate (ATP) through the process of aerobic respiration. Mitochondria have their own membrane.
- Endoplasmic reticulum: A large structural complex composed of tubules that participate in the synthesis of proteins (through ribosomes), metabolism of lipids, and transportation of various substances through the cell.
- Golgi apparatus: A structure that modifies, sorts, and packages newly synthesized proteins and lipids for secretion or use within the cell.
- Centriole: A cylindrical structure of microtubules required during cell division.
- Lysosomes: An organelle that digests molecules, such as nutrients and foreign substances.

Human Tissues

Groups of cells with similar or related functions may work together and form a structure known as a tissue. In the human body, these tissues include (from the exterior to the interior of the body):

- **Epithelial tissue**: A type of tissue that protects and regulates the flow of substances. It is found in the skin and the mucous membranes (the lining of organs or cavities).
- **Connective tissue**: This tissue provides support to other tissues. It includes cartilage, bone, ligaments, fat, etc. It is the most voluminous type of tissue and can be found throughout the body.
- **Muscle tissue**: A type of tissue that allows movement. This tissue can be skeletal muscle (which is connected to the bone and produces voluntary movement), cardiac muscle (which produces heart contractions), and smooth muscle (which is involuntary and can be found within blood vessels or the intestines).
- **Nervous tissue**: This tissue is responsible for the conduction of nerve impulses. It is found in the central nervous system (the brain) and the peripheral nervous system (the nerves).

Homeostasis and the Major Body Systems

Just like individual cells, groups of tissues with similar and related functions can be organized and described as organs, and eventually, body systems. When working correctly, these systems regulate each other and allow the human body to work in a state of balance known as homeostasis.

The major body systems include:

- **Cardiovascular system**: Composed of the heart and its valves, as well as arteries, veins, arterioles, and venules. It is in charge of transporting blood and nutrients to the tissues, and the return of deoxygenated blood and carbon dioxide to the lungs.
- **Gastrointestinal system**: Composed of the mouth, pharynx, esophagus, stomach, small and large intestine, liver, gallbladder, and pancreas. It is required for the digestion and absorption of nutrients and other substances, as well as the excretion of waste. The gastrointestinal process begins with mastication in the mouth and digestion by salivary enzymes and finishes with evacuation in the rectum and anus (the last portions of the large intestine).
- **Respiratory system**: Composed of the lungs, bronchi, trachea, larynx, pharynx, and the nose. The respiratory system is in charge of all the processes

related to inhalation and exhalation, which are required for the exchange of oxygen and carbon dioxide.

- **Musculoskeletal system**: Composed of the muscles, bones, and the structures that connect them (tendons, ligaments, joints, cartilage). It is required for motion and posture. Muscles are also responsible for the production of heat, and bones (specifically, the bone marrow) are responsible for hematopoiesis (production of blood cells).
- **Nervous system**: Composed of the central and peripheral nervous systems. The central nervous system includes the brain and the spinal cord, and the peripheral nervous system includes the nerves and ganglia. The nervous system is in charge of regulating the functions of other body systems, as well as thinking and other cognitive tasks. The adequate functioning of the nervous system as a system regulator is an important part of homeostasis.
- **Endocrine system**: Composed of various glands, such as the pancreas, the thyroid, the pituitary gland, the adrenal cortex, the ovaries, the testes, etc. Each gland and hormone has a particular action, and they usually work together with other body systems.
- **Urinary system**: Composed of the kidneys, the ureters, the urinary bladder, and the urethra. It filters the blood and removes waste or the excess of certain substances via urine production and excretion.
- **Immune system**: Composed of immune cells, lymph, lymph vessels, lymph nodes, thymus, and spleen. It helps to defend the body from foreign substances or organisms.

Pathophysiology and Disease Processes

Common Conditions

Acne: A skin condition that occurs when hair follicles become saturated with sebum and dead cells. It is characterized by local inflammation and pain.

Acute cholecystitis: Acute inflammation of the gallbladder, usually related to biliary stones or sludge obstructing the cystic duct. Clinical findings include fever, pain, nausea, vomiting, and jaundice.

Acute pancreatitis: Acute inflammation of the pancreas caused by the activation of pancreatic enzymes before reaching the duodenum. The characteristic clinical finding is severe pain that usually worsens after eating (mostly with fatty foods).

Allergic rhinitis: Also known as hay fever. An allergic reaction that affects the nose. Clinical findings include sneezing, rhinorrhea, nasal congestion, and itching.

Alzheimer's disease: A common type of dementia that becomes progressively worse with age. It severely affects cognitive abilities, such as memory and thinking.

Angina: Chest pain related to a partially decreased blood flow through the coronary arteries to the heart.

Myocardial infarction: Infarction of the heart tissue due to severely decreased or completely occluded blood flow through the coronary arteries to the heart. Clinical findings include intense oppressive pain that radiates to the left shoulder, shoulder blade, and jaw.

Appendicitis: Acute inflammation of the appendix, usually treated via surgery. Clinical findings include fever, pain in the lower right flank, diarrhea, nausea, vomiting, etc.

Asthma: Chronic lung condition characterized by the inflammation of the airways, usually related to allergic reactions. Clinical findings include wheezing, coughing, dyspnea, etc.

Atrial fibrillation: Irregular and fast heart rhythm that increases the risk of developing clots in the heart, which may result in other medical conditions, such as a stroke. Clinical findings include chest pain, fatigue, dizziness, palpitations, dyspnea, etc.

Bacterial vaginosis: Vaginal discharge (may be white, gray, or watery) with a strong or 'fishy' smell. Patients may also present with itching and a burning sensation upon urination.

Breast cancer: Cancer that affects the breast tissue. It is one of the most common types of cancer and may spread to other tissues (metastasis).

Cellulitis: Bacterial infection of the skin and soft tissues. It occurs in areas of injury (for example, a wound). Clinical findings include fever, pain, inflammation, and redness, and the area may present with warmth and tenderness.

Common cold: A common viral infection characterized by upper respiratory symptoms like cough, sneezing, rhinorrhea, etc.

Conjunctivitis: Also known as pink eye. Inflammation of the conjunctiva of the eye, usually due to viral infection, bacterial infection, and allergies. Clinical findings include redness, irritation, pain, itching sensation, etc.

COVID-19: A viral infection usually associated with mild to moderate flu-like symptoms. It is a highly contagious condition that may result in severe disease and long-term complications.

Crohn's disease: A type of chronic inflammatory bowel disease that results in inflammation of the digestive tract, causing diarrhea, pain, bloating, and other symptoms.

Deep vein thrombosis: Condition related to the presence of a blood clot in a deep vein, usually in the lower limbs. Clinical findings include pain, swelling, and redness of the limb.

Diabetes: Condition characterized by high serum glucose due to the lack of insulin production (type 1 diabetes) or an altered insulin production or sensitivity (type 2 diabetes).

Otitis: Infection of the ear. Otitis externa affects the outer ear canal and otitis media affects the middle ear.

Febrile seizures: A common type of seizure that occurs in children with fever. These seizures are not a sign of epilepsy, and most children will not present seizures later in adulthood.

Food poisoning: A condition caused by consuming contaminated foods (bacteria, viruses, toxins, etc.). Clinical findings include diarrhea, abdominal pain, vomiting, dehydration, and sometimes fever.

Gastroenteritis: Inflammation of the gastrointestinal tract, sometimes called 'stomach flu.' It causes diarrhea, nausea, vomiting, fever, and abdominal pain.

Hepatitis: Inflammation of the liver. It is usually related to hepatitis viruses (hepatitis A, B, C, D, etc.).

Iron deficiency anemia: Anemia characterized by low iron levels, leading to reduced hemoglobin. It is one of the most common types of anemia. Clinical findings include fatigue, dizziness, and pallor, though it is frequently asymptomatic.

Urinary tract infection: Bacterial infection of the urinary tract. Cystitis affects the bladder and is characterized by dysuria and frequent urination. Urethritis affects the urethra with similar symptoms. Pyelonephritis, a kidney infection, is characterized by higher fever, back pain, and sometimes nausea and vomiting.

Pneumonia: Infection of the lung tissue due to bacteria, viruses, or fungi. Clinical findings include fever, pain, cough, dyspnea, etc.

Prostate cancer: This type of cancer affects the prostate gland. It is one of the most common types of cancer in men. Early diagnosis typically leads to a better prognosis.

Vertigo: Sensation of motion, as if the person or the room is spinning. It is usually related to inner ear conditions.

Diagnostic Tests

Laboratory tests:

- **Complete blood count (CBC)**: Blood test for the assessment of blood cells. It is used during the assessment of anemia, infections, conditions that affect clotting, etc.
- **Blood chemistry**: A blood test that investigates various substances in the blood, such as glucose, electrolytes, proteins, bilirubin, etc.
- **Urinalysis**: Analysis of a urine sample, which checks for and measures the presence of cells, chemical substances, pH, etc. It is used during the assessment of urinary tract infections, diabetes, and chronic kidney disease.
- **Stool analysis**: Analysis of various aspects of a stool sample, which includes macroscopic and microscopic examination, chemical analysis, and microbiological studies.
- **Blood gases**: A blood test that measures oxygen, carbon dioxide, bicarbonate, and pH levels in arterial or venous blood.
- **Hormone levels**: Various hormones, such as estrogen, cortisol, thyroid hormones, etc., can be tested whenever required.

Imaging studies:

- **Radiography**: An imaging technique that employs X-rays to visualize various tissues according to the degree of X-ray absorption. Dense tissues like bones absorb the X-rays and are visualized as white. Tissues filled with air like the lungs are seen as black.
- **Computer tomography (CT) scan**: A 3D image of the scanned tissue created with X-rays. It allows a more detailed study of the tissue, in comparison with a simple X-ray.
- **MRI scan**: An imaging technique that employs magnetic fields and radio waves to create a computerized image without X-ray radiation. It is able to provide a more detailed image of soft tissues, including muscles and the brain
- **Positron emission tomography (PET) scan**: Functional imaging technique that employs a tracer, which is a radioactive substance. It helps to visualize blood flow, cancer, and neurological conditions.
- **Ultrasonography**: Imaging method that uses ultrasound to visualize various structures in the body. It is a fast and practical diagnostic method commonly

used to study abdominal organs, muscles, the thyroid gland, the brain, breasts, etc.

Biopsy:

- **Biopsy**: Procedure that involves taking a tissue or cell sample for analysis.
- **Excisional biopsy**: Involves removing the tissue sample by excision, usually during surgery.
- **Punch biopsy**: This type of biopsy involves a special instrument that "punches" a hole in the skin to take a skin biopsy sample.
- **Needle biopsy**: A special needle is used to take a sample from an organ or internal tissue without surgery. It is commonly guided by ultrasound, X-ray, or other imaging techniques.
- **Perioperative biopsy**: A sample is taken and tested during surgery, which allows the surgical team to act immediately if required.
- **Endoscopic biopsy**: A sample is taken during an endoscopic procedure, such as a colonoscopy or gastroscopy.

Other tests:

- **Colonoscopy**: Endoscopic procedure used to diagnose conditions that affect the large intestine. It can be used to take biopsy samples.
- **Gastroscopy**: Endoscopic procedure used to diagnose conditions that affect the gastric tissues. It can be used to take biopsy samples.
- **EKG**: Test that records the electrical activity of the heart. It is used during the assessment of arrhythmias, heart failure, myocardial infarction, altered potassium levels, and other conditions.
- **EEG**: Test that records the electrical activity of the brain. It is used during the assessment of seizures, epilepsy, strokes, and other brain conditions.

Treatments Modalities

Pharmacological therapy: A type of treatment that employs medication to treat or manage a medical condition.

Surgical treatment: The instrumental treatment or management of a medical condition.

Chemotherapy: A type of cancer treatment using special medication that aims to destroy fast-growing cells, such as cancer cells, although chemotherapy can still affect normal and healthy cells.

Radiation therapy: Also known as radiotherapy, it employs X-rays or another types of radiation to treat cancer. It is commonly used in association with other therapies (such as chemotherapy or immunotherapy) during the treatment of various types of cancer.

Immunotherapy: A type of treatment that uses biologics or other agents to modulate the body's immune response to help it destroy cancer cells.

Blood transfusion: Blood components can be administered as a treatment for various conditions. Patients with severe anemia may need transfusion of packed red blood cells, and patients with thrombocytopenia may need a platelet concentrate.

Basic Epidemiologic Concepts

Incidence: The number of new-onset cases of a specific condition during a period of time. It is commonly used to investigate acute conditions.

Prevalence: The number of cases of a specific condition during a period of time. Unlike incidence, it does not exclusively include new-onset cases.

Risk factors: Factors that, when present, increase the risk of developing a specific condition.

Comorbidities: Refers to the simultaneous presence of multiple medical conditions.

Epidemics and Pandemics

Outbreak: The sudden increase in the incidence of a particular infectious disease within a specific facility, institution, or community.

Epidemic: An outbreak that affects a specific group, such as a community or geographical region.

Pandemic: An outbreak that poses a global threat to the health of the general population. Pandemics spread across different countries and continents.

Chapter 3: Clinical Patient Care

Patient Intake and Vitals

Patient Identifiers

Patient identifiers are unique data that belong to a specific patient, and therefore can be used to differentiate one patient from another. This is useful during the delivery of care and to avoid medical errors (such as wrong patient, wrong procedure, or wrong site events).

There are eighteen identifiers recognized by the Health Insurance Portability and Accountability Act (HIPAA):

- Names.
- Street address, zip/county/city codes, and other geographic identifiers below the state level.
- Relevant dates (date of birth, admission).
- Telephone numbers.
- Fax numbers.
- Email addresses.
- Social security number.
- Medical record number.
- Health plan beneficiary number.
- Account numbers.
- Certificate/license numbers.
- Vehicle identifiers.
- Device identifiers and serial numbers.
- Web Universal Resource Locators (URLs).
- Internet Protocol (IP) address number.
- Biometric identifiers.
- Full-face photographic images.
- Any other unique identifying number, characteristic, or code.

Health care workers must understand that not all patient-related information can be used as an identifier. For example, the patient's room number cannot be used as an identifier. Since valid identifiers can be similar (two or more patients with similar names or dates of birth), it is important to always use at least two or more patient identifiers in order to identify a patient.

Elements of a Patient's Medical, Surgical, Family, and Social History

Medical history: A patient's medical history includes all the information related to the patient's health in the past and the present, as well as the patient's allergies and use of medications.

Surgical history: This section involves all surgical procedures that have been performed on the patient. Include the name, site, date, and motive of the surgery, as well as other relevant information.

Family history: This section includes the medical information of immediate family members that may be relevant to the patient's health, such as hereditary conditions and the state of health of family members. If a family member is deceased, include the cause of death in the record.

Social history: A wide variety of information can be included here, such as education level, job, lifestyle, use of drugs, tobacco, and alcohol, diets, sleep habits, etc.

Health Screenings

A screening is a type of health test performed in a preventive manner, usually directed to an asymptomatic population that presents a reasonable risk of developing a medical condition.

The screening of heart disease (such as ischemic heart disease, hypertrophic cardiomyopathy, and valvular diseases) is applied to patients that present risk factors like family history and tobacco consumption. It usually involves the measurement of blood pressure, as well as the assessment of glucose and lipid levels.

The screening of various types of cancer is common as well. Patients at risk of developing lung cancer can be screened annually, frequently through low-dose helical computer tomography scanning. Lung cancer screening is applied to patients with a history of at least thirty pack-years who are between fifty-five and eighty years of age. It also includes patients who stopped smoking in the last fifteen years. The screening should continue until at least fifteen years after smoking cessation.

Other commonly used screening tests are Papanicolaou smears for cervical cancer in women, thyroid-stimulating hormone levels for neonates to check for congenital hypothyroidism, and colonoscopy for patients at risk of colon cancer.

Mental Health Screenings

A mental health screening can be applied to assess a patient's thinking, mood, behavior, and other mental functions. This type of screening is employed to recognize mental disorders early, which helps patients to receive care sooner. It can be applied to patients at risk of developing a mental condition (for example, patients with sleep problems, fatigue, substance abuse, extreme mood swings, feelings of sadness or anhedonia, hearing voices, suicidal ideation, etc.) and can also be used to determine the patient's response to therapy.

Mental Health America provides screening tests for various mental disorders, which include depression, anxiety, attention-deficit/hyperactivity disorder, bipolar disorder, eating disorder, psychosis, addiction, etc. The screenings can be found at the following URL: https://screening.mhanational.org/screening-tools/

Assessment of Wellness

Wellness is an integral state of physical, mental, and social well-being. The assessment of wellness can be carried out through the application of instruments like the Wellness Evaluation of Lifestyle (WEL), Five Factor WEL (5F-Wel), Perceived Wellness Survey (PWS), the Optimal Living Profile (OLP), or the Body-Mind-Spirit Wellness Behavior and Characteristic Inventory (BMS-WBCI), among other assessment tools. OLP, PWS, and BMS-WBCI are relatively short compared to 5F-Wel and WEL.

Factors That Impact Vital Signs

Various factors may naturally affect vital signs, and this is a common occurrence. Both physical and psychological factors come into play, and they usually result in higher measurements.

In the case of physical factors, exercise (or physical activity in general) may increase all vital signs, such as temperature, heart rate, ventilation, and blood pressure. A common example is a patient who is coming late to an appointment and rapidly climbs the stairs to arrive on time. The resulting physical activity will naturally alter the patient's vital signs. It is important to ask the patient to relax and sit down for a few minutes before the measurement of vital signs in order to give them a chance to return to their baseline levels.

There are psychological factors that can affect vital signs. This is common as well, and may also result in higher readings. Psychological factors include anxiety, fear, joy, etc. An example of this is a patient who is anxious about their diagnosis and arrives at the appointment with high blood pressure. This is a good moment to use therapeutic communication to help the patient feel better and feel understood. Once the patient feels more relaxed, you may measure their vital signs.

Blood Pressure

Blood pressure is the pressure that results from blood pushing against the walls of arteries. This results in two measurements: systolic pressure, which is the highest pressure that occurs as the heart contracts, and diastolic pressure, which is the lowest pressure that occurs as the heart relaxes.

Blood pressure is measured in millimeters of mercury (mm Hg) and recorded with the systolic pressure first and diastolic pressure second. Normal blood pressure for healthy adults is generally considered to be around 120/80 mm Hg or lower.

Patients with blood pressure that is persistently above this normal pressure are considered to have prehypertension, stage 1 hypertension, or stage 2 hypertension, according to the measurements.

- A patient is considered to have elevated blood pressure (formerly known as prehypertension) with a systolic pressure of 120-129 mm Hg and diastolic pressure less than 80 mm Hg.
- **Stage 1 hypertension** is characterized by a systolic pressure of 140-159 mm Hg or a diastolic pressure of 90-99 mm Hg.
- **Stage 2 hypertension** is characterized by a systolic pressure higher or equal to 160 mm Hg or a diastolic pressure higher or equal to 100 mm Hg.

Hypotension, or low blood pressure, is generally recognized as a blood pressure below 90/60 mm Hg that is accompanied by other clinical findings, such as dizziness, hemorrhage, dehydration, emotional shock, etc. Low blood pressure without any other clinical signs or symptoms is usually benign and does not require intervention.

Orthostatic hypotension, also known as postural hypotension, is a specific type of hypotension characterized by a sudden drop in blood pressure after changes in position (for example, lying down to sitting up). Symptoms associated with orthostatic hypotension include vertigo, lightheadedness, blurred vision, and syncope. It is relatively common in older patients.

Blood pressure is frequently measured with a sphygmomanometer and a stethoscope, but digital blood pressure monitors are widely available as well. In most cases, blood pressure is measured in the arm, and the cuff should be one inch above the antecubital fossa and cover two-thirds of the surface of the arm.

The palpatory method is commonly employed to measure systolic pressure. Inflate the cuff until the radial pulse disappears, add 20-30 mm Hg of pressure, and slowly release the air to determine the exact moment the pulse is felt again. The pressure reading at the first pulse is the systolic pressure. The diastolic pressure is determined using a stethoscope by placing the diaphragm over the brachial artery. As the pressure is released, the sound of the heartbeat will slowly disappear. The pressure reading at the last heartbeat is the diastolic pressure.

Temperature

The temperature of the body comes from the relation between heat produced (which is largely mediated by metabolism) and heat lost from the body. It can be measured in degrees Fahrenheit (°F) or Celsius (°C). The temperature of an adult varies between 97.6°F to 99°F (or 36.4°C to 37.2°C) across the day (early in the morning to late afternoon, respectively), with an average temperature of 98.6°F (37°C).

The hypothalamus is a major structure that serves as the body's thermoregulation center, usually in accordance with the circadian rhythm, which results in a natural variance of temperature between morning and afternoon temperature readings. Other factors that affect the body's normal temperature are age, gender (which includes the effects of menstrual cycle), physical activity, and consumption of substances (for example, cold or hot beverages, alcohol, etc.).

The measurement of temperature is usually performed in the following parts of the body:

- Oral (average: 98.6°F or 37°C).
- Axillary (average: 97.6°F or 36.4°C).
- Temporal artery (average: 98.6°F or 37°C).
- Tympanic (average: 98.6°F or 37°C).

A reading higher than 100.4°F (38°C) is considered to be febrile. Fever is a common response to infection. Common patterns include continuous fever, intermittent fever (fever with periods of normal temperature), and remittent fever (a continuous fever with significant fluctuations). An extremely high-temperature reading (105.8°F or 41°C) is known as hyperpyrexia. Temperatures above this level are potentially lethal. On the other hand, extremely low temperatures (below 95°F or 35°C) are known as hypothermia, also potentially lethal.

The mathematical conversion formula for Fahrenheit and Celsius is the following:

$$°C = (°F - 32) \times {}^{5}/_{9} \qquad \text{(Fahrenheit to Celsius conversion)}$$

$$°F = \left(°C \times {}^{9}/_{5}\right) + 32 \qquad \text{(Celsius to Fahrenheit conversion)}$$

It is also important to consider that temperature readings vary depending on the measurement site. Specifically, axillary temperatures are typically 1°F or 0.5°C lower than oral readings. Always document the site of temperature measurement (although this might not be necessary for oral readings).

There are various types of thermometers:

- Digital thermometers can be used to measure oral and axillary temperature. They are practical and widely available. Do not use if the patient has recently consumed cold or hot foods or fluids, smoked, or exercised. After application, the thermometer will emit a beep when the reading is available.
- Tympanic thermometers are specifically used for temperature measurements in the tympanic membrane. Do not use if the patient complains of ear pain or has otitis externa.
- Temporal artery scanners are the most reliable noninvasive method for temperature measurement. The application consists of applying the device in the middle of the forehead and pressing the button. After hearing a beep (without releasing the button), continue by placing the device behind the ear lobe. The highest recorded temperature should be documented.

Pulse

The pulse rate is an indirect measurement of the patient's heartbeats. It is created through the pulsations caused by the heart contractions and the flow of blood, which is felt when palpating an artery.

Pulse can be felt and measured in various parts of the body, but the most common and reliable arteries are those pressed against a bone or solid structures. These are the carotid, temporal, femoral, brachial, radial, popliteal, and dorsalis pedis arteries. Heart rate can also be determined through the heartbeat at the apex of the heart, which can be heard with a stethoscope.

Pulse is characterized by its rate, rhythm, and amplitude.

- **Rate** —The number of pulsations measured in one minute. A normal pulse rate is usually sixty to one hundred beats per minute in healthy adults. A higher rate is known as tachycardia, and a slower rate is known as bradycardia.
- **Rhythm** —The regularity of time between pulsations. Normal pulsations have a constant frequency (the time between pulsations is the same). However, abnormal rhythms (known as arrhythmias) can be found in certain cardiovascular diseases, although healthy individuals may experience benign arrhythmias.

- **Amplitude** — Also known as volume, this refers to the strength of the heart contractions and how they are felt during the assessment of the pulse. Amplitude depends on both the force of contraction and the condition of the artery (whether it is hardened or softened).

Respiratory Rate

Respiration is the process of oxygen and carbon dioxide exchange that is achieved through inspiration and expiration. Oxygen is absorbed into the blood during inspiration, and carbon dioxide is expelled during expiration.

It is important to distinguish this process, specifically known as external respiration, from the intracellular process of internal respiration, which occurs in the mitochondria to produce adenosine triphosphate (ATP).

Normal breathing is automatic and silent, and it is characterized by respiratory rate, rhythm, and depth.

- **Rate** —The number of respirations per minute. The normal range in healthy adults is between twelve and twenty respirations per minute. Higher rates are known as tachypnea and lower rates as bradypnea. The absence of respiration is known as apnea.
- **Rhythm** —The regularity of the breathing pattern. In general, breathing is regular, although minor interruptions may occur in the form of sighs.
- **Depth** —The depth of respiration, which modifies the amount of air inhaled and exhaled. An increased depth is known as hyperpnea, and a decreased depth is known as hypopnea.

Other abnormalities may occur in relation to ventilation. Dyspnea is shortness of breath and may present in patients with any respiratory rate. Orthopnea is a type of dyspnea that specifically occurs when patients are lying down, which is common for patients with heart failure and chronic obstructive pulmonary disease (COPD). Wheezing is an abnormal whistling sound heard in patients with partially obstructed airways. It is characteristic of patients with asthma.

The measurement of a patient's respiratory rate is usually performed without the patient noticing. Since respiration is automatic, the respiratory rate may be altered if the patient is actively thinking about breathing. A common technique involves measuring the patient's respiratory rate just after measuring their pulse. Keep your fingers on the patient's wrist, as if you were still measuring their pulse, and start measuring their respiration.

Pulse Oximetry

Pulse oximetry is a simple and noninvasive method to measure oxygen saturation. These devices also display the patient's pulse rate. Oxygen saturation reflects the percentage of oxygenated hemoglobin in relation to total hemoglobin.

A healthy individual should have a reading above 95% saturation. The measurement is usually performed on a finger or earlobe. Oxygen saturation below 90% is compatible with an oxygenation issue, such as a pulmonary infection, asthma, bronchitis, etc. Oxygen therapy and other treatment options may be required to enhance the patient's oxygenation.

Pain Scale

Pain scales are tools to help patients and health care providers describe pain in a relatively standardized manner. The most common way to measure pain is with a numerical scale from zero to ten where zero is the absence of pain and ten is the worst pain of your life. The visual analog scale presents the patient with a horizontal line where the farthest left is no pain at all and the farthest right is the worst pain, and the patient draws a line at the point they feel describes their pain. Many other variations of pain scales exist, and their usage may vary between institutions and age groups.

Menstrual Status and Last Menstrual Period

After their first menstruation (also known as menarche), which usually occurs after puberty and between the ages of nine and seventeen, female patients initiate their menstrual and ovarian cycles. These cycles last approximately a month, and they are characterized by hormonal changes that promote the proliferation of the endometrium and maturation of ovarian follicles for ovulation in preparation for fertilization and pregnancy.

In the absence of fecundation and/or pregnancy, the menstrual phase begins in the form of the discharge of endometrial tissue in a process known as menstruation (also known as periods), which can last up to seven days.

The **last menstrual period (LMP)** is the first day of the patient's last menstrual period. It is most commonly used to determine the beginning of a pregnancy and calculate the estimated date of delivery.

Methods for Body Measures

The measurement of weight and height is an important part of the physical exam. These are simple measurements the health care provider can use during the diagnosis of malnutrition, obesity, and other weight-related problems, as well as for dosing. In small children, the measurement of head circumference is also common.

The measurement of height and weight in children is similar to the process used with adults; however, small children, like infants, require other types of measurements.

Measurement of height in adults:

- Verify the unit of measurement (centimeters or inches).
- Raise the bar so it is above the patient's head and extend the arm.
- Ask the patient to remove their shoes and step on the center of the scale, standing up straight.
- Lower the bar until the extended arm reaches the head of the patient.
- Ask the patient to step off.
- Read the measurement.
- Record the findings in the patient's record.

Measurement of weight in adults:

- Verify the unit of measurement (kilograms or pounds).
- Check the scale and place the weights on the left side.
- Ask the patient to remove their shoes and step on the center of the scale. You can place a disposable towel on the scale to avoid direct contact between the scale and the patient's feet.
- Move the lower weight to the highest number possible which does not cause the balance indicator to drop.
- Move the upper weight carefully until the balance bar is centered at the middle mark.
- Adjust the weights as necessary.
- Use both values to determine the weight of the patient.
- Record the findings in the patient's record.

Measurement of height in small children (recumbent length):

- To maximize the accuracy of this method, two people should participate in the measurement (an assistant helping to hold and position the child and a measurer).
- The child should only be wearing a diaper and a shirt.
- Place a disposable towel on the measuring table.

- The assistant holds the head of the child in the proper position while the measurer aligns the child's head with the midline, with the eyes looking up and perpendicular to the midline.
- Extend the leg of the child and use a pen to mark the heel.
- Lift the child and measure the distance between the head and heel marks with a measuring tape.
- Record the findings in the patient's record.

Measurement of weight in small children:

- The child should be nude or only wearing a clean diaper.
- To maximize the accuracy of this method, two people should participate in the measurement (an assistant helping to hold and position the child and a measurer).
- Place the child on the scale and record the weight to the nearest ounce or 0.01 kg.
- Repeat the measurement at least two times and compare results (look for an agreement within one quarter of a pound or 0.1 kg).
- Record the findings in the patient's record.

Measurement of head circumference:

- Use a measuring tape. Position it just above the eyebrows, above the ears, and surrounding the most prominent part of the occiput.
- Pull the tape so it compresses the hair.
- Take the measurement and record it in the patient's record.

General Patient Care

Room Preparation

A medical assistant may set up the room before the patient arrives. The examination room should be clean and organized, as well as equipped with the necessary instruments and supplies.

The usage of certain instruments or supplies may vary between health care providers. For example, a primary care provider (general patient care) does not need all the equipment an ophthalmologist (specialty patient care) may have in their office.

Some of the most commonly used equipment includes:

- Gloves: The use of sterile and non-sterile gloves is common in general and specialty practice. They can be used during examination, procedures, and disposal. It is important to consider preferences and allergies in relation to glove size and material (for example, nitrile gloves for providers who are allergic to latex).

- Stethoscope: Can be used to listen to sounds from the lungs, the heart, and the abdomen. It is also employed during the measurement of blood pressure. The stethoscope is a basic tool for most health care providers.
- Thermometer: Used to measure the temperature of the patient. It can be used by most health care providers, but it is most frequently used by primary care providers.
- Penlight: A small flashlight that can be used to enhance visualization or check pupil response. It is frequently used by primary care providers, internists, and neurologists.
- Reflex hammer: Used to test neurological reflexes. It is mostly used during neurological examination by neurologists, but is also used during general care.
- Otoscope: Used to examine the ears. Otoscopes can be portable and use batteries, but they can also be wall-mounted. They are mostly used by Ear, Nose, and Throat (ENT) physicians, however, primary care physicians, internists, and pediatricians also use otoscopes.
- Ophthalmoscope: Used to examine the eyes. Similar to the otoscope, it may be portable or wall-mounted. They are commonly used by ophthalmologists, but also by some primary care providers and internists.
- Tongue depressors: Used to examine the throat of patients. It is used by ENT professionals, primary care physicians, internists, and pediatricians.
- Vaginal speculum: This speculum is used to separate the walls of the vagina, which is needed for examination of the vagina and the cervix, as well as for specimen collection during a Papanicolaou test or other tests. It is mostly used by OB-GYN physicians.
- Nasal speculum: Used to examine the nose, They are mostly employed by ENT physicians.
- Lubricant: Can be used to lubricate equipment or gloves for examination (for example, vaginal or rectal examination). It is frequently used by OB-GYN physicians and surgeons.

Bed Preparation and Patient Positioning

The correct use of draping and positioning is important to maintain the patient's privacy and dignity. Aside from cleaning the surfaces of the bed, a blanket may be used to drape the bed. In some cases, the patient should be provided a gown to wear during the examination or procedure.

The positioning process varies from patient to patient, although some practices may repeatedly require a specific set of positions. Below is a list of common positioning techniques and their applications.

Supine position: Also known as horizontal recumbent position. It is the most frequent and basic position. The patient lies flat on their back with the arms resting at each side. It can be used by any type of health care provider for many types of examinations and procedures. The drapes may cover the arms, torso, and legs.

Dorsal-recumbent position: Similar to the supine position, the patient lies on their back, but this position involves flexing the knees and keeping the soles of the feet over the surface of the table. The knees and feet are kept separated. This position can be used to examine the genital and rectal areas, as well as the abdomen and chest. The draping process involves using a diamond-shaped sheet to cover the lower part of the body—one of the tips should point toward the head and the other to the feet.

Lithotomy position: This position is similar to the dorsal-recumbent position but involves the use of stirrups to hold the feet of the patient. It is frequently employed by OB-GYN professionals to examine the vaginal area. Draping is the same as the dorsal-recumbent position.

Prone position: In this position, the patient lies with their face down. This can be useful when examining the back. However, this position may not be recommended for pregnant or obese patients. Draping should cover the lumbar back, buttocks, and legs of the patient.

Erect position: Also known as standing position. The patient can be standing during the evaluation of gait or hernias. Only a gown may be needed.

Sitting position: This position involves sitting on a chair or on the edge of the bed. Draping may include the lower extremities. The sitting position can be used to evaluate reflexes and for other neurological exams, as well as the chest, back, arms, head, and neck.

Knee-chest position: The patient is positioned facing down, with the head and chest touching the surface of the table, the buttocks elevated, and the knees separated and resting on the bed. This position is used for perianal and rectal examination, as well as some proctological procedures. It may be difficult to maintain for older patients. Therefore, it is important to help the patient when moving in and out of this position to avoid falls. Draping involves covering the buttocks.

Proctological position: Also known as jackknife position. The patient lies facing down with their hips flexed at a 90-degree angle, with both their legs and chest/head lowered. As its name implies, it is used for proctological examination.

Sims' position: Also known as lateral position. The patient lies with their left side down. The left arm is resting straight behind the torso and the right arm is flexed close to the face. Both legs are flexed, but the right leg is more flexed to allow the examination of the rectal area. This position is suitable for patients who need a rectal exam but cannot maintain the knee-chest position safely. It is also useful for the administration of suppositories and enemas.

Trendelenburg position: This position involves the patient lying flat on their back with their head lower and their legs raised. It is commonly employed as a therapeutic measure for patients with hypotension. Draping involves the shoulders, chest, and legs.

Modified Trendelenburg position: Similar to the Trendelenburg position, the modified version seeks to position the head lower than the feet by elevating the legs rather than the entire body.

Fowler's position: The patient is sitting on the bed with the head of the bed elevated at a ninety-degree angle, with their legs resting flat on the surface. This position is employed for patients with lower-back problems or those who cannot breathe appropriately in the supine position. The draping may cover the chest, abdomen, and legs of the patient.

Semi-Fowler's position: This is the same as Fowler's position, but the torso of the patient is at a forty-five-degree angle. This modified form is more commonly used. The uses and draping are the same as the standard Fowler's position.

Patient Instructions

A medical assistant must provide clear, complete, and easy-to-understand instructions to patients before and after an exam or procedure. The information should include instructions about what to do before and after, as well as potential complications or adverse events related to the exam or procedure.

For example:

- At least two or three days before a colonoscopy, the patient should eat a plain, low-fiber diet (white rice, bread, plain chicken, broth, eggs, coffee, tea, lemon juice, etc.) and avoid nuts, seeds, raw vegetables, fruits with skin, seeds, brown rice, etc.

- The day before a colonoscopy, the patient should only have a clear-liquid diet (no solids, only water, clear broth, soft drinks, gelatin, tea, or coffee without milk) and laxatives to prepare their bowels for the procedure. The laxatives are specified by the physician and usually begin late in the afternoon or evening. Instruct the patient to remain at home near a toilet, because they will have diarrhea after taking the laxatives.
- After the procedure, it is normal to feel mild abdominal cramping or bloating. A clear diet can be maintained for the rest of the day and semi-solids and solids may be incorporated gradually. The patient must contact their provider immediately if they present severe pain, fever, or rectal bleeding.

Immunization Schedules and Requirements

The CDC is in charge of providing the recommended immunization schedule and its requirements for children and adults. The latest 2024 updated schedule is summarized below.

Childhood immunization schedule (birth to eighteen years) recommended for all children:

Recommended first dose at zero to one month:

- Respiratory syncytial virus (RSV-mAb): one dose from birth to six months according to mother RSV vaccination status.
- Hepatitis B: At zero, one to two, and six to eighteen months with monovalent HepB vaccine.

Recommended start at two months old:

- Rotavirus: RV5: At two, four, and six months for a total of three doses. Patients receiving RV1 only require two doses.
- Diphtheria, tetanus, and acellular pertussis (DTaP): At two, four, and six months for a total of three doses. Includes two booster doses at fifteen to eighteen months and four to six years.
- *Haemophilus influenzae* type b (Hib): At two, four, and six months for a total of three doses and a booster dose at age twelve to fifteen months (ActHIB®, Hiberix®, Pentacel®, or Vaxelis®).
- Pneumococcal conjugate (PCV15, PCV20): At two, four, six, twelve, and fifteen months.
- Inactivated poliovirus: At two, four, and six to eighteen months and four to six years.

Recommended start at six months old:

- COVID-19 (1vCOV-mRNA, 1vCOV-aPS): one or more doses of updated vaccine.
- Influenza (IIV4): Annual vaccination with one or two doses.

Recommended start at twelve months:

- Measles, mumps, rubella (MMR): Second dose at age four to six years.
- Varicella: Second dose at four to six years.
- Hepatitis A: Second dose after six months.

Recommended start at nine years:

- Human papillomavirus vaccination: Recommended start at eleven to twelve years.
- Dengue: A series of three doses (zero, six, and twelve months) is recommended for children in endemic areas with laboratory confirmation of previous dengue infection.

Recommended start at eleven years:

- Tetanus, diphtheria, and pertussis (Tdap): one dose as a booster during adolescence.
- Meningococcal serogroup A,C,W,Y: First dose at age eleven to twelve years and second dose at sixteen years.

Adult immunization schedule (nineteen years and older) recommended for all adults:

- COVID-19: For unvaccinated patients, one dose of the 2023-2024 updated formula of Pfizer-BioNTech or Moderna vaccine, or two doses (zero, and three to eight weeks) of 2023-2024 updated formula of Novavax vaccine.
- Influenza inactivated (IIV4), Influenza recombinant (RIV4), Influenza live attenuated (LAIV4): one dose annually.
- Tetanus, diphtheria, pertussis (Tdap or Td): For patients that did not receive Tdap at or after eleven years, it includes one dose of Tdap and then Td or Tdap every ten years.
- Measles, mumps, rubella (MMR): one dose, unless the patient has evidence of immunity.
- Varicella: A two-dose series (zero, and four to eight weeks) in patients without evidence of immunity.

- Human papillomavirus (HPV): A two- or three-dose series is recommended for all patients up to forty-five years old.
- Hepatitis B: A two-, three-, or four-dose series according to the specific vaccine employed in patients aged nineteen through fifty-nine years.
- Pneumococcal: Vaccination varies based on age and health condition, with recommendations for PCV15 or PCV20 followed by PPSV23.
- Zoster recombinant: A two-dose series (zero, and two to six months) in patients aged fifty years or older.

Allergies

Allergies are hypersensitivity reactions of the immune system to foreign substances (allergens). Allergic reactions are widely variable, from very mild allergies to a life-threatening shock (e.g., anaphylaxis), or from a localized acute reaction (e.g., urticaria) to a chronic disorder (e.g., hay fever or allergic asthma). The hereditary tendency to present allergic conditions that some families present are known as "atopy."

Allergens are usually harmless substances that the immune system does not recognize. In many cases, allergens are relatively easy to avoid, such as those causing specific food allergies. Examples of allergens include:

- Pollen.
- Fungal spores, mold.
- Insect venom from stings and bites.
- Animal products or epithelium (such as fur, wool, or feces from dust mites).
- Foods (such as milk, eggs, fish, crustacean shellfish, tree nuts, peanuts, wheat, soy/soybeans, or sesame).
- Medication (such as penicillins or salicylates).
- Latex.

The clinical findings related to most mild and moderate allergic reactions include:

- **Skin reactions** (for example, a contact allergy): Itching, urticaria (or hives), swelling, and swollen mucous membranes.
- **Gastrointestinal reactions** (for example, a food allergy): Diarrhea, nausea, and vomiting.
- **Respiratory reactions** (for example, the exposure to pollen): Breathing issues, wheezing, runny nose, sneezing, coughing.
- **Ocular reactions** (for example, allergic conjunctivitis): Red, itchy, and watery eyes.

In order to properly diagnose an allergy, a test may be applied:

- **Skin prick test (or scratch test)**: This consists of applying a small drop of various allergens on the skin of the forearm, pricking the skin, and observing the reaction. A reaction is considered positive when the skin presents inflammation, similar to an insect bite.
- **Patch test**: This employs a patch that contains an allergen, which is placed onto the skin for a few days. It is performed when the reaction is expected to occur only after a couple of days.
- **Intradermal allergy test**: A small amount of individual allergens are selected and injected via intradermal injection, and after a few minutes (usually around twenty minutes) the reaction is evaluated.
- **Provocation test**: In this test, a group of probable allergens are applied or tested to see their reactions. For example, if it is believed that an allergic reaction is caused by pollen, a health care provider may expose the patient's nose (via drops or spray) to pollen and evaluate the response under controlled conditions.

The treatment of allergies includes limiting exposure to allergens, administration of medications (antihistamines and steroids), and immunotherapy (allergen-specific immunotherapy, mainly employed with allergies related to pollen or insect venoms).

Anaphylaxis and Anaphylactic Shock

A severe and generalized allergic reaction is known as anaphylaxis. This type of systemic reaction is potentially life-threatening and may occur within seconds or minutes of exposure to an allergen. An episode of anaphylaxis is most commonly uniphasic, but around twenty percent of cases may be biphasic (symptoms may return several hours after resolution).

Anaphylaxis may result in some of the following clinical findings:

- Difficulty breathing.
- Palpitations.
- Wheezing.
- Nausea and vomiting.
- Abdominal pain.
- Urticaria.
- Flushing.
- Swelling of the face, lips, or tongue.
- Hoarseness or stridor.
- Angioedema.

In extreme cases, anaphylaxis may cause cardiovascular collapse or respiratory failure (anaphylactic shock).

The treatment of anaphylaxis is based on early intervention with epinephrine and complementary use of steroids and antihistamines. It is recommended to use intramuscular epinephrine (0.01 mg/kg up to 0.5 mg in adults) as soon as possible after the onset of symptoms. The use of glucocorticoids and intravenous antihistamines (for example, IV diphenhydramine) is complementary and does not replace intramuscular epinephrine. These drugs do not effectively treat acute symptoms, especially life-threatening signs related to acute hypotension and bronchospasm.

Eye Irrigation

Irrigation is used to clean the eye from discharge, foreign bodies, or chemicals, or to relieve inflammation. It is important to maintain a sterile technique throughout the procedure. The irrigation process requires gloves, sterile solution, a bulb syringe, a basin for drainage, sterile gauzes, and a towel.

- Start with adequate handwashing.
- Verify the patient's name matches the record and that they require eye irrigation.
- Verify which eye requires irrigation.
- Verify the required equipment and supplies are available, and double-check that the type of solution is the one requested by the physician.
- Check the appropriate expiration dates.
- Introduce yourself and explain the procedure to the patient.
- Drape the patient's neck and shoulders, and help the patient to position themselves.
- Put the gloves on. If the gloves contain powder, remove the powder by rubbing them together or rinsing them under warm water.
- Place the drainage basin below the affected eye, so the solution falls into it.
- Pour solution into a gauze and use it to clean the eyelid and eyelashes. Begin near the nose and clean laterally (from the inner canthus to the outer canthus). Dispose of the gauze after each wipe.
- Pour the irrigating solution into a basin and use the bulb syringe to irrigate the eye.
- Separate the eyelids with one hand and use the other hand to hold the syringe.
- Place the syringe near the nose and direct the solution to the conjunctiva in the inner canthus so the solution flows to the outer canthus.
- Refill the syringe and repeat until the specified volume of solution has been irrigated.
- Use a sterile gauze to dry the eyelid (from inner canthus to outer canthus).

- Clean the area.
- Remove gloves and wash your hands.
- Document the procedure in the patient's record. Include date, time, type and amount of solution, simple description of the procedure, condition of the eye before procedure, eyes irrigated (left, right, or both), condition of the eye after procedure, relevant observations, and signature.

Eye Instillation of Medication

Eye instillation is employed to administer medication directly to the eye. This may be necessary to treat infections, alleviate inflammation or pain, or dilate the pupils (for example, for treatment or before a procedure or exam like an ophthalmoscopy). The instillation process requires medication (eye drops or ointment), gloves, drape, and sterile gauze.

- Start with adequate handwashing.
- Verify the patient's name matches the record and that they require eye instillation.
- Verify which eye requires instillation.
- Verify the required equipment and supplies are available, double-check that the medication and strength are the ones prescribed by the physician.
- Check the appropriate expiration dates.
- Introduce yourself and explain the procedure to the patient.
- Put the gloves on. If the gloves contain powder, rinse them under warm water.
- Help the patient to sit down or lie down.
- Ask the patient to tilt their head backward and look up.
- Pull the lower eyelid down to form a pocket and administer the required amount of medication into the conjunctival sac. In the case of ointment, squeeze carefully from the inner to the outer canthus.
- Ask the patient to gently close and rotate their eyes.
- If required, dry any excess medication from the inner to the outer canthus.
- Clean the area.
- Remove gloves and wash your hands.
- Document the procedure in the patient's record. Include date, time, medication name and strength, dose, simple description of the procedure, condition of the eye before procedure, eyes treated (left, right, or both), condition of the eye after procedure, relevant observations, and signature.

Ear Irrigation

Irrigation of the ear is used to facilitate the removal of cerumen or a foreign body or to clean the canal with an antiseptic solution. The irrigation process requires gloves, irrigating solution, a bulb syringe (or irrigation device), a basin for drainage and another basin for the solution, sterile gauzes, applicators, and an otoscope.

- Start with adequate handwashing.
- Verify the patient's name matches the record and that they require ear irrigation.
- Verify which ear requires irrigation.
- Verify the required equipment and supplies are available, and double-check that the type of solution is the one requested by the physician.
- Check the appropriate expiration dates.
- Introduce yourself and explain the procedure to the patient.
- Check the ear canal with the otoscope.
- Help the patient to sit with their head tilted toward the affected ear.
- Drape the patient's neck and shoulders, and help the patient to position themselves.
- Put the gloves on.
- Clean the exterior of the ear with gauze.
- Ask the patient to hold the drainage basin below the affected ear, so the solution falls into it.
- Pull the pinna up and back (patients older than three years) or the earlobe down and back (children younger than three years) to straighten the external canal.
- Place the tip of the syringe or irrigation device at the entrance of the external canal, and direct the flow of the irrigation solution gently toward the canal wall.
- Refill the syringe or irrigation device as required.
- Dry the exterior of the ear with gauze. The applicator may be used to dry the superficially visible part of the exterior canal.
- Check the ear canal with the otoscope.
- Let the patient rest their ear over a clean and absorbent towel.
- Clean the area.
- Remove gloves and wash your hands.
- Document the procedure in the patient's record. Include date, time, type and amount of solution, simple description of the procedure, condition of the ear before procedure, ear irrigated (left, right, or both), description of the material expelled from the ear, condition of the ear after procedure, relevant observations, and signature.

Ear Instillation of Medication

Ear instillation consists of administering otic medication into the ear. This includes the use of drops of antibiotics to treat infections, steroids to alleviate inflammation, or solutions to soften cerumen. The instillation process requires gloves and the prescribed medication.

- Start with adequate handwashing.
- Verify the patient's name matches the record and that they require ear instillation.
- Verify which ear requires instillation.
- Verify the required equipment and supplies are available, double-check that the medication and strength are the ones prescribed by the physician.
- Check the appropriate expiration dates.
- Introduce yourself and explain the procedure to the patient.
- Ask the patient to sit and rest their head with the affected side up.
- Take the medication with your dominant hand and use the other hand to pull the pinna up and back (patient older than three years) or the earlobe down and back (patient younger than three years).
- Place the tip near the entrance of the ear canal and instill the required number of drops.
- Ask the patient to remain sitting for three minutes.
- Clean the area.
- Document the procedure in the patient's record. Include the date, time, name, and strength of the medication, dose, simple description of the procedure, ear treated (left, right, or both), relevant observations, and signature.

Basic Management of Medications

Medical assistants can participate in the basic management of medications, which includes storage, verification of labels, and maintenance of medication logs.

The adequate storage of medications consists of protecting medication from contamination and degradation, as well as keeping the drugs away from any unauthorized person. Not all drugs are stored in the same manner. Some require special consideration (especially injectables and liquid solutions):

- **Refrigeration** — Insulin, vaccines, many antibiotics, various eye and ear drops, weight-loss injections (such as semaglutide and tirzepatide), etanercept, adalimumab, dupilumab, growth hormones, etc.

- **Light-sensitivity** — Injectables like vaccines, many antibiotics, esomeprazole, diphenhydramine, indomethacin, various insulins (regular, Lispro, detemir, etc.), ketorolac, methotrexate, nitroglycerin, etc.

It is important to check the medication label for specific storage instructions. Alongside storage instructions, a label contains information about the manufacturer, the trade and generic name of the product, the unit dose, the amount found in the container, the type of medication, and the expiration date. In general, this includes the most useful information needed in relation to the management and administration of medication. Expiration dates are usually printed in the MM/YY format. Therefore, the first number represents the month (from 01 to 12) and the second number represents the year.

Finally, medication logs are simple tools to document the administration of medication and keep track of the inventory. These logs consist of the name of the drug, strength, amount administered, date, time, patient name, prescriber name, and who administered the medication (e.g., in the case of injectables). Medication logs can be kept on paper or electronically.

Administration of Subcutaneous Injections

Subcutaneous injections are used to deliver a medication or substance into the adipose tissue (subcutaneous tissue), which is between the skin and the muscles. Insulin and heparin are among the most common drugs administered subcutaneously.

These injections are usually inserted at a forty-five-degree angle but may be inserted at a ninety-degree angle depending on the length of the needle or the amount of adipose tissue (e.g., ninety degrees of inclination may be needed for obese patients). The adequate technique includes pinching the skin before the insertion to create an accessible skinfold.

Subcutaneous injections can be administered in various parts of the body, such as the upper arm, abdomen, and thighs. In the case of patients who require multiple or frequent injections (such as patients with diabetes), an injection log may be used to rotate injection sites.

Administration of Intramuscular Injections

The intramuscular route is employed when faster absorption is required, when the medication irritates the subcutaneous tissue, or when the administration requires a relatively large volume.

The needle is inserted at a ninety-degree angle, and the most common muscles are the deltoid, the gluteus medius, and the vastus lateralis. The deltoid muscle holds up to 1 mL of medication in adults, and the gluteus medius and vastus lateralis are viable up to 3 mL.

Sutures and Staples

Sutures are surgical stitches that can be used to close wounds and tie a blood vessel (ligature). Various suture materials exist, and they can be classified into absorbable and nonabsorbable sutures.

Absorbable sutures include catgut, polyglactin 910 (Vicryl), polydioxanone (PDS), and poliglecaprone 25 (Monocryl). These sutures absorb or dissolve via enzymatic action after the healing process is completed. As a result, they can be used to suture inner or deep layers of tissue without requiring manual removal.

Nonabsorbable sutures include nylon, silk, polyester, polypropylene (Prolene), and surgical steel. These sutures do not dissolve. Therefore, they must be removed after the healing process is complete. Nonabsorbable sutures are employed in superficial wounds, such as skin wounds.

Staples are another surgical closure tool. Staples are made of stainless steel or titanium and can be used to close skin wounds. However, their application and removal require special equipment.

Suture and Staple Removal

For the removal of sutures, patients will be instructed to return to the office after seven to ten days, and the physician will examine their wounds. If appropriate, the sutures will be removed. The removal process is simple and requires suture removal scissors, gloves, antiseptic solution, gauze, and dressing forceps.

- If the wound presents discharge, a sample for a culture may be needed.
- Count the number of sutures in place.
- The wound is cleaned with an antiseptic solution.
- You may use the forceps to slightly lift the suture and facilitate the passage of the suture removal scissors, which will be used to cut the suture.
- Place the removed suture on a gauze.
- Repeat until all the sutures have been removed.
- Count the number of sutures and verify that they match the initial number.
- If appropriate, cover the incision with Steri-Strips.
- Provide oral and written directions to the patient so they can take care of their wound.

- Document the procedure in the patient's record. This may include the date, time, and condition of the wound before the removal of sutures, a simple description of the procedure, condition of the wound after the removal of sutures, and signature.

The removal of staples follows the same process. However, it requires a surgical staple remover instead of suture removal scissors. The lower jaw of the surgical staple remover should be placed under a staple and squeezed until the device is completely closed. Then, the instrument is moved away and the staple is disposed of inside a sharps container.

Common Types of Wounds and Their Treatments

The most common types of wounds and injuries include:

- Incisions - These are straight and clean cuts, usually made with cutting instruments, such as a knife or a scalpel. They may require closure with sutures or Steri-Strips.
- Lacerations - These are tears characterized by irregular edges. They may require closure with sutures or Steri-Strips.
- Abrasions - These wounds are caused by superficial scrapes of the skin. They can be cleaned and covered with a sterile dressing.
- Contusion - This is a type of non-penetrating injury that damages the skin and deeper tissues without laceration. The rupture of small blood vessels results in a hematoma. It can be treated with cold packs and oral analgesics.
- Sprains and strains - Sprains are the tearing of ligaments, and strains affect the muscles and tendons. The affected joint is painful when moved, and the compromised area usually presents ecchymosis and edema (swelling). Treatment includes elevation of the affected part and application of cold packs in the first minutes and hours. After one to three days, the application of cold packs can be alternated with warm compresses. Immobilization may be required.
- Burns - These injuries are common, and they can be thermal (superficial, partial-thickness, and full-thickness burns), chemical, and electrical.
- Superficial burns - These cause superficial damage with reddening and edema. Sunburns are a typical example. Treatment includes cool water and sterile dressing.
- Partial-thickness burns - These affect the epidermis and dermis. These burns may present blisters alongside pain and red skin. Treatment includes cool water, sterile dressing, and keeping the blisters intact. Do not break the blisters.

- Full-thickness burns - These burns compromise the skin and subcutaneous tissues. In some cases, these burns may reach muscles and bones. This type of burn is an emergency.
- Fractures - These occur when a bone breaks or cracks. Fractures are painful, and motion may be compromised. It is important to immobilize the affected bone (splinting) and apply ice. If the patient presents an open fracture, they must be transferred for emergency care.

It is important to stay up to date with tetanus immunization. If a patient has not had their boosters, its administration will be necessary to protect the patient.

Wound Infection and Wound Stages

A wound infection consists of the microbial invasion of a wound, which ultimately prevents adequate healing. All wounds are at risk of becoming contaminated and infected. However, infection risk may be higher in the following cases:

- Dirty or traumatic wounds.
- Large wounds.
- Presence of necrotic tissue.
- Peripheral neuropathy.
- Peripheral vascular disease.
- Patients with uncontrolled diabetes.
- Chronic use of corticosteroids.
- Malnutrition.
- Hospitalization.

According to the International Wound Infection Institute (2022), wound infection can be classified into five stages: contamination, colonization, local infection, spreading infection, and systemic infection. These stages describe a continuous process.

- Contamination - The wound contains microorganisms, but there is no proliferation or host reaction.
- Colonization - There is limited proliferation without host reaction.
- Local wound infection - In covert cases, there is hypergranulation, bleeding, and delayed healing without overt signs of inflammation. In overt cases, there are signs of inflammation alongside a purulent exudate.
- Spreading infection - The inflammation extends, and there may be dehiscence of the wound and lymphangitis.

- Systemic infection - The infection creates systemic symptoms like malaise, fever, and asthenia. The infection may complicate even further, which can result in sepsis, septic shock, and death.

There are various types of specific wound infections that are commonly found in clinical practice, including surgical site infections, pressure injuries, and diabetic foot ulcers.

Common Types of Surgical Interventions

Appendectomy: The surgical removal of the appendix, which is commonly performed as a treatment for acute appendicitis.

Breast biopsy: A diagnostic test that consists of taking a sample of breast tissue or cells to study the morphology under a microscope. It is commonly performed to rule out malignancy in patients with signs or symptoms of breast cancer or neoplasms.

Cataract surgery: This procedure consists of removing cataracts, which occur when the lens of the eye becomes cloudy, and replacing it with a new and clear artificial lens.

Cholecystectomy: The surgical removal of the gallbladder, which may be required when a person presents gallstones and the gallbladder becomes infected (cholecystitis). It may also be required during the treatment of cancer that affects the gallbladder.

Hemorrhoidectomy: A surgery performed to remove hemorrhoids.

Hysterectomy: This surgery consists of removing the uterus, which may be required when patients present excessively heavy periods or pain, or when a patient has cancer that affects the uterus.

Inguinal hernia repair: A surgical procedure that repairs inguinal hernias, which occur when the small intestine protrudes through a weak point in the abdominal muscles.

Mole excision biopsy: A common procedure that consists of removing a mole to study its cellular composition and morphology. It serves as a diagnostic procedure but can also be therapeutic.

Debridement: This procedure is frequently part of wound care plans. It consists of removing infected and nonviable tissue from wounds, which allows the tissue to heal effectively.

Emergency Action Plans in the Workplace

The medical office should develop an emergency plan to tackle various types of emergency events that may occur in the workplace. This plan is known as an emergency action plan, which is a written document required by the Occupational Safety and Health Administration (OSHA).

The development of the plan takes into account the layout and structural features of the office. One of the most common emergencies to plan for is a fire, but other events exist (such as chemical, radiological, and biological contamination, natural disasters, explosions, civil disorder, etc.) and should be taken into account. The plan includes guidelines for storage, usage, and maintenance of the required equipment or supplies (for example, fire extinguishers).

The emergency action plan should be tested and discussed. It is important that each member of the team knows the plan and is able to perform their duties in case of an emergency.

Urgencies and Emergencies

The terms "urgency" and "emergency" are frequently used interchangeably, even by health care workers. However, although these terms are closely related, they refer to different things.

Urgency is an injury or medical condition that requires immediate examination and/or treatment by a health care provider, usually within twenty-four hours, in an outpatient setting. On the other hand, an emergency is a severe or life-threatening injury or medical condition that requires immediate examination and/or treatment in the emergency department of a hospital.

Common urgencies include:

- Mild or moderate traumatic injuries like sprains, strains, contusions, small cuts, etc.
- Fever.
- Minor fractures.
- Cough.
- Diarrhea.
- Back pain.
- Allergies.

Common emergencies include:

- Myocardial infarction.
- Stroke.
- Shock.
- Choking.
- Seizures.
- Open fracture.
- Traumatic brain injury.

Basic Life Support, Cardiopulmonary Resuscitation, and Automated External Defibrillator

Basic life support (BLS) is a type of care provided by health care professionals to patients with life-threatening cardiorespiratory conditions (such as cardiac arrest or obstructed airway). It incorporates sequential actions that determine responsiveness, breathing, pulse, and use of cardiopulmonary resuscitation (CPR) and automated external defibrillator (AED).

- Evaluate the environment: Is it safe to perform BLS?
- Assess the need for CPR by evaluating CAB: Circulation, Airway, and Breathing.
- Call for help (physician, 911, etc.) or ask someone else to call for help.
- Use AED as soon as it is available.
- Initiate two minutes of CPR with 30:2 (thirty compressions and two breaths) at a rate of one-hundred to one-hundred-twenty compressions per minute using the CAB sequence (Compression, Airway, Breathing).
- Change rescuer every two minutes if possible.
- Repeat until help arrives.

High-quality CPR is characterized by compressions at a depth of at least two inches (five centimeters) and allowing complete recoil of the chest. The airway can be opened by tilting the chin up.

The use of an AED is especially important in patients who have collapsed. In patients with probable asphyxia, high-quality CPR is the priority. Before using the AED, make sure there is no water in the area, remove the patient's clothing, and dry their chest. Announce you are going to use the defibrillator and make sure no one is touching the patient.

Legal Requirements for Transmission of Prescriptions

- The electronic prescription must be transmitted as soon as possible after being signed.

- The electronic prescription can be printed if it was not delivered successfully, as notified directly by the pharmacy or an intermediary. The printed prescription should include the name of the pharmacy, the data, and the time when it was originally sent, as well as a note clarifying that the electronic transmission failed.
- Other copies can be printed, but they must include a label with the following: "Copy only—not valid for dispensing."
- The electronic prescription application must not allow the transmission of an electronic prescription once an original prescription has been printed.
- The contents of the prescription must not be altered during transmission. Any changes will invalidate the electronic prescription.
- An intermediary may not convert an electronic prescription to another form for transmission.

Electronic Prescribing

Electronic prescribing (or e-prescribing) is the electronic generation, transmission, and filling of medical prescriptions with the help of computer-based applications. These applications facilitate the electronic transmission of new or renewed prescriptions. These prescriptions are also easier to read, which reduces the risk of medication errors.

Pharmacies can also request refills directly via the electronic prescription software, which has to be approved or declined by the original prescriber (or someone authorized by them).

Examples of electronic prescribing software include RXNT, Kareo Clinical, Benchmark Systems, CharmHealth, ScriptSure, AthenaOne, and Elation Health, among others.

Specialty Pharmacies

Specialty pharmacies are pharmacies that handle specialty drugs and services, which are usually employed in the management of rare or complex medical conditions. These are drugs that a small portion of the total population needs, and therefore, a typical pharmacy does not keep them in stock.

Patients who may at some point need services from a specialty pharmacy include those with multiple sclerosis, rheumatoid arthritis, hemophilia, cancer, HIV, and Crohn's disease.

Documentation in the Medical Records

The documentation of the patient's chief complaint should include a description of the characteristics of the patient's symptoms, as well as treatments taken and their effectiveness.

The progress notes contain essential information about the clinical evolution of the patient's condition, which should be updated every time the patient is evaluated. This includes information about the progress of signs and symptoms, application and response to treatments or procedures, and consideration of laboratory and imaging results.

The documentation process should not include predictions or plans for future actions or procedures. This promotes accuracy and reduces the presence of mistakes. However, if a mistake is made for any reason, it is important to correct it in a clear manner. First, you should strike through the entry with the mistake (in paper), then write a new entry specifying there was a mistake and proceed with the correction, and finally, date and sign the correction.

Prior Authorizations for Durable Medical Equipment

Durable medical equipment (DME) refers to any medical equipment that a patient may need at home for various reasons, such as their everyday routine (for example, a wheelchair) or medical management (for example, a CPAP machine). A DME is defined as durable, used for medical reasons, mostly useful to people with an injury or medical condition, used at home, and expected to last three years or more.

Some DMEs require prior authorization, and the health care provider must verify the patient's insurance plan to check the equipment's coverage. The Centers for Medicare & Medicaid Services maintain a Master List of their services, which is updated annually.

If prior authorization is required, the healthcare provider must submit and sign a prior authorization request form. They will also have to identify the adequate CPT codes that apply to the prescribed treatment and follow up with the insurance company through calls and emails until there is a resolution for the request.

Computerized Physician Order Entry

A computerized physician order entry (CPOE) is the computer-based process of creating treatment instructions. This avoids the use of paper, telephone, and fax, and helps to improve patient safety in various ways.

Computer programs with CPOE usually allow the automatic check of drugs for interactions and allergies. These applications check when specific medications, laboratory tests, or radiology orders require pre-approval by the insurer, which helps to reduce denied claims.

Telehealth Care

Telehealth care provides health care providers with different ways to deliver care like remote monitoring or chat-based care, as well as extending many benefits of traditional care visits to e-visits, which contributes to the continuum of care (and usually as an on-demand service). For this reason, telehealth should not be seen as a simple replacement for traditional care, but as a complementary approach that can be used alongside traditional care.

Telehealth can be used as a standalone type of care for specific conditions that may not require in-person visits (such as common cold, sore throat, sinus infection, urinary tract infection, various skin conditions, or mental health issues), but it can also be integrated with in-person care to promote patient compliance and patient-provider communication between in-person visits.

However, some patients with a life-threatening condition may contact the medical office and ask for telehealth care. In this situation, a professional medical assistant must be able to recognize the problem and guide the patient so they can receive the care they need. The following tips can be used as a screening method for emergencies:

- Is the patient conscious? Has the patient lost consciousness at any moment? Can the patient speak properly?
- Is the patient bleeding? How much? Where are they bleeding from?
- Does the patient have an injury? What caused it?
- Has this happened to the patient before?
- How is the patient's breathing and pulse?
- What are the other symptoms of the patient?

Use this information to determine if the patient requires emergency medical attention. If they do, call an emergency medical service and stay on the line with the patient. Do not hang up or put the call on hold.

Infection Control and Safety

Organisms and Microorganisms

An organism is any living thing such as animals, fungi, or plants. The term organism usually refers to macroscopic multicellular organisms that are visible to the naked human eye. The term can also be used to denominate any living thing.

A microorganism or microbe refers to any living being that is microscopic and not visible to the naked human eye. It includes both single-cell and multicellular living things such as bacteria, protozoa, fungi, and algae. The inclusion of viruses is debated because they are generally considered not alive. However, they are still studied by the field of microbiology as infectious agents.

Pathogens and Nonpathogens

Not all organisms are pathogens or able to cause illnesses. In fact, most of them (<1%) are nonpathogens for humans. In the human body, a vast amount of microorganisms exist alongside human cells in a symbiotic relationship that is generally beneficial to both parties. This is known as the normal flora of the body. It helps humans in the digestion of various substances, protection against other potentially pathogenic microorganisms, and production of beneficial substances like vitamins.

The use of antibiotic therapy especially during prolonged treatments with broad-spectrum antibiotics may debilitate the normal flora. This increases the risk of opportunistic infections.

Pathogens can be found in all types of microorganisms. Examples of bacteria include:

- *Listeria monocytogenes* - causes listeriosis.
- *Campylobacter jejuni* - causes gastroenteritis.
- *Escherichia coli* - causes gastroenteritis and urinary tract infection.
- *Borrelia burgdorferi* - causes Lyme disease.
- *Bacillus anthracis* - causes anthrax.
- *Vibrio cholerae* - causes cholera.
- *Pseudomonas aeruginosa* - causes pneumonia, urinary tract infection, and sepsis.
- *Salmonella typhi* - causes typhoid fever.
- *Mycobacterium tuberculosis* - causes tuberculosis and leprosy.
- *Staphylococcus aureus* - causes skin infections, necrotizing pneumonia, and endocarditis.
- *Streptococcus pyogenes* - causes skin infections and pharyngitis.

- *Streptococcus pneumoniae* - causes pneumonia.

Examples of viruses include:

- Influenza virus - causes the flu.
- Herpes simplex virus - causes cold sores.
- HIV - causes AIDS.
- Varicella virus - causes chickenpox.
- Hepatitis viruses - cause hepatitis.
- Rubella virus - causes rubella.
- Measles virus - causes measles.
- SARS-CoV-2 virus - causes COVID-19.

Examples of fungi include:

- *Candida albicans* - causes candidiasis.
- *Histoplasma capsulatum* - causes histoplasmosis.
- *Pneumocystis jirovecii* - causes pneumocystis pneumonia.
- *Cryptococcus neoformans* - causes cryptococcosis.
- *Aspergillus fumigatus* - causes aspergillosis.
- *Coccidioides immitis* - causes coccidioidomycosis (Valley fever).

Examples of protozoa include:

- *Giardia duodenalis* - causes giardiasis.
- Plasmodium - causes malaria.
- *Entamoeba histolytica* - causes amoebiasis.
- *Trichomonas vaginalis* - causes trichomoniasis.
- *Toxoplasma gondii* - causes toxoplasmosis.

Chain of Infection

The chain of infection or chain of transmission describes the spread of an infectious condition. It is composed of six elements:

- **Microorganisms**: represented by the pathogen or infectious agent.
- **Source or reservoir**: the environment where the microorganism can multiply.
- **Portal of exit**: the exit portal from the pathogen's reservoir (mucous membranes, skin to surface, skin to skin, blood, feces).

- **Modes of transport**: represented by the way a pathogen moves from the reservoir to the susceptible host (airborne, contact, droplets, bites, sharps, fomites, food).
- **Portal of entry**: the entry portal for the pathogen into the susceptible host (eyes, respiratory tract, mouth, urinary tract, wounds, incisions).
- **Susceptible host**: the person at risk of becoming infected due to other health conditions, age, nutrition, medication use, immunodeficiency.

Conditions for Bacterial Growth

Bacterial growth can be influenced by various factors that are environmental and nutritional. In relation to pH, bacteria can be acidophilic (prefer a pH below 5.5), alkaliphilic (prefer a pH above 8.5), or neutrophilic (prefer a pH from 5 to 8).

An important factor to be considered is temperature. Bacteria can withstand various ranges of temperature. Pathogenic bacteria and bacteria from the human flora live between 25°C and 45°C (mesophiles).

Some microorganisms require oxygen but others do not. Bacteria can be divided into the following:

- **Obligate aerobes** — require oxygen to produce energy.
- **Microaerophiles** — require a small amount of oxygen to grow but high concentrations may be detrimental.
- **Facultative anaerobes** — can use both oxygen and fermentation or anaerobic respiration to produce energy. This is the most common type of bacteria.
- **Obligate anaerobes** — grow in the absence of oxygen and can be damaged by its presence.
- **Aerotolerant anaerobes** — do not use oxygen for energy but can exist and grow in an aerobic environment.

Signs and Symptoms of Infectious Diseases

The clinical findings associated with an infectious disease can be caused by the direct effect of the pathogen's actions. However, the host's immune response against the pathogen also produces a wide variety of responses. Some responses can be more detrimental than the pathologic action of the infectious agent.

Common signs and symptoms associated with an infectious disease include:

- Fever.
- Asthenia.

- Cough.
- Nausea, vomiting.
- Sore throat.
- Inflammation or exudate in wounds.
- Diarrhea.
- Shortness of breath.
- Chills.
- Burning sensation during urination.
- Swollen lymph nodes.
- Headache.
- Pain.
- Neck stiffness.

Universal and Standard Precautions

The universal precautions are a set of recommendations established by the CDC in 1987 to prevent the transmission of HIV, hepatitis B, and other bloodborne pathogens within the healthcare environment. The premise is that it is not possible to know with certainty whether each patient has or does not have these disorders. Therefore, all patients must be treated with this set of universal precautions.

OSHA used the major features of the CDC's universal precautions to develop the Bloodborne Pathogens Standard. This is also known as standard precautions. These precautions apply to the risk of exposure to blood, any body fluids except sweat, non-intact skin, and mucous membranes. They include hand hygiene, use of gloves, masks, face shields, goggles, gowns, adequate patient placement, safe handling of textiles, and safe injection practices.

Needlestick Safety and Prevention

Needlestick accidents are preventable. Agencies have developed guidelines to help workers and employers create a safer work environment. It is recommended to keep a needlestick and sharps injury log to document the type of device used during the accident, location, and other relevant information. Recommendations include:

- Develop a control program compatible with standard precautions.
- Always switch to a new needle device if it is safer and effective.
- Use needle devices with safety features.
- Use sharps containers and consider disposal of needles after use.
- Avoid the use of needles if a safer alternative exists.
- Avoid recapping or bending needles.

Control of Infectious Diseases, Epidemics, and Pandemics

Some infectious diseases can spread rapidly and pose a risk to the health of the general population. This especially affects vulnerable people such as the elderly, pregnant women, and children. To prevent the deleterious effects of outbreaks, epidemics, and pandemics, various research groups and federal agencies study these phenomena and work on the development of response plans.

One of the most important tools for the prevention and response to epidemics and pandemics is the use of vaccines and immunizations. This is important for both the general population and healthcare workers.

Within a healthcare facility, the healthcare team can work together to develop their own preparedness and response plan. This includes following guidelines for the prevention and control of infections through handwashing, use of personal protective equipment, use of sterile instruments, adequate disposal, needle and sharps safety. The needs of the particular facility should also be determined through geographical location and the characteristics of patients served.

Medical and Surgical Asepsis

Medical asepsis – refers to the reduction of the number of microorganisms to minimize their transmission as much as possible. It is also known as the clean technique. It is commonly used in medical settings for non-invasive procedures.

Surgical asepsis – refers to the complete destruction of microorganisms. It is also known as the sterile technique. It is necessary during invasive procedures like surgeries.

Sterilization Techniques and Equipment Maintenance

The sterilization process aims to destroy all microorganisms found on the surface of an item. This helps to reduce the transmission of pathogens and other agents during medical and surgical procedures such as surgeries or phlebotomy. Sterilization techniques include:

- **Steam sterilization** – Steam is the most common sterilization technique. If it is available and appropriate to use with the item that requires sterilization, steam is usually the best choice. It employs an autoclave and relies on the use of steam, pressure, temperature, and time.
- **Flash sterilization** – This is a special type of sterilization technique that involves sterilization of an unwrapped item at 132°C for 3 minutes at 27-28 lbs. of pressure in a gravity displacement sterilizer. It is used for approved medical

devices when strictly necessary. It must not be used as a replacement for traditional and routine sterilization techniques.

- **Low-temperature sterilization** — This includes various methods that, unlike steam sterilization, do not require heat. Examples include ethylene oxide, hydrogen peroxide, and hydrogen peroxide/ozone. If an item cannot be sterilized with high heat or moisture, low-temperature sterilization is commonly employed.
- **Peracetic acid sterilization** — This is a method that employs concentrated peracetic acid. It is commonly used to sterilize endoscopic tubing.

The management process of sterilization includes the following steps:

- **Cycle verification** — All sterilization devices should be tested with chemical and biological indicators to verify the sterilization process occurs effectively. This should be performed when the sterilization machine is installed, relocated, redesigned, receives an important repair, or after sterilization failure. Each sterilization cycle or function is tested separately. The sterilizer must not be used until the process is completed successfully.
- **Decontamination (pre-cleaning)** — All sterilization techniques require decontamination prior to sterilization. This can be achieved by manually pre-cleaning the item to eliminate visible traces of tissues, soil, or fluids.
- **Arrangement** — The items that require sterilization should be arranged in such a way that all surfaces come into contact with the sterilizing agent. This allows complete sterilization and adequate circulation of the agent.
- **Monitoring** — The routine monitoring of sterilization parameters is important to assess the state of the sterilizer and quality of the sterilization process. The indicators may vary between techniques. They include mechanical, chemical, and biological indicators.
- **Recordkeeping** — It is important to keep logs for the sterilizer and the sterilization process. This includes information about sterilizer testing and monitoring.

Sterile Field

To establish a sterile field, a medical assistant will need a Mayo stand or countertop and a sterilized instrument kit wrapped with autoclave paper.

- If required, clean the Mayo stand or countertop. Allow to dry.
- Perform handwashing or hand scrub, if required. Allow to dry.
- Place the sterile kit on the Mayo stand or countertop. Check the indicator tape, if present.
- Position the kit so the uppermost flap opens toward the body.

- Open the uppermost flap and unfold the kit without touching the inside portion or the content.

Handwashing Techniques

Handwashing requires a sink with running water, antimicrobial liquid soap, a disposable nail brush, paper towels, and waste container with a pedal.

- Remove any jewelry.
- Turn on the water. Use a paper towel if necessary and avoid touching the faucet. Use warm or lukewarm water.
- Place hands into the water, apply liquid soap, and lather in a circular motion with fingertips pointing down.
- Rub between the fingers.
- Use a nail brush.
- Place hands into the water again and rinse so the water flows from the wrists to the fingertips.
- If required, repeat handwashing (if hands are evidently contaminated or if this is the first handwash of the day).
- Dry hands with a paper towel but do not touch the dispenser.
- Turn off the water. Use a paper towel (if necessary). Do not touch the faucet.
- Dispose of the paper towel.

An alcohol-based handrub is a washing technique that is simpler and faster than standard handwashing with liquid soap. It requires the following three steps:

- Apply the solution to the palm of a hand.
- Rub hands together and cover all the surfaces of the hands and fingers.
- Keep rubbing hands until the solution is completely absorbed.

Stages of Cleaning

There are six stages of cleaning:

1. The first stage of cleaning is pre-cleaning. This removes visible soil, tissues, and other substances that may be found on the item or surface.
2. The second stage is the main cleaning with cleaning products and warmer water.
3. The third stage is rinsing, usually with hot water.
4. The fourth stage is disinfection. A disinfectant is used on the item or surface for an amount of time according to the specific directions.
5. The fifth stage is the final rinse to remove the disinfectant.
6. The sixth stage is drying.

Types of Cleaning Products

Cleaning products and disinfectants are mainly chemical agents. The most common types include:

- **Alcohol** – This is one of the most common cleaning agents. Alcohol can destroy bacteria, viruses, and fungi. It can be used to disinfect items and the surface of medical equipment.
- **Chlorine** - Hypochlorite is the most frequently used chlorine agent. Hypochlorite is bactericidal, viricidal, and fungicidal. It should be handled carefully because these compounds usually come in high concentrations and must be diluted. It is mostly used on hard surfaces.
- **Iodophors** - These are iodine complexes and have a wide range of action that covers bacteria (includes M. tuberculosis), viruses, fungi, and spores. Povidone-iodine is a commonly used iodophor.
- **Hydrogen peroxide** - This is a commonly used disinfectant that kills bacteria, viruses, fungi, and spores. It can be used to disinfect non-critical equipment and some surfaces.
- **Peracetic acid** - This is an acid employed on devices like hemodialyzers and endoscopes. It has bactericidal, viricidal, fungicidal, and sporicidal properties.
- **Hydrogen peroxide** and **peracetic acid** - This combination is used as a more effective alternative to each single agent. It is commonly used against glutaraldehyde-resistant mycobacteria.
- **Quaternary ammonium compounds** – These are also known as QACs. They can destroy bacteria and fungi but are less effective against mycobacteria, spores, and non-enveloped viruses. They are used on hard surfaces or items that do not touch mucous membranes or damaged skin.
- **Phenolics** - These are disinfectants that kill bacteria, viruses, and fungi. Phenolics can be used on non-porous surfaces.

Safety Data Sheets

A safety data sheet is also known as material or product safety data sheet. It is an occupational safety and health document from the manufacturer of a product that details relevant information related to the product's chemical information and hazards. This includes how to prevent damages and injuries related to the use of the product. Medical assistants must review the safety data sheet of any potentially dangerous chemical product found in the medical office or workplace.

OSHA and other agencies require safety data sheets to contain the following information in the form of a standardized list of sections:

- Identification.
- Hazard(s) identification.
- Composition/information on ingredients.
- First-aid measures.
- Fire-fighting measures.
- Accidental release measures.
- Handling and storage.
- Exposure controls/personal protection.
- Physical and chemical properties.
- Stability and reactivity.
- Toxicologic information.
- Ecologic information.
- Disposal considerations.
- Transport information.
- Regulatory information.
- Other information.

Cautions Related to Chemicals

- Review the product's safety data sheet.
- Use chemical products in accordance with training and duties.
- Do not use a chemical product if you do not know how to handle it.
- Use protective equipment when handling potentially dangerous chemical products.
- Verify that the product inside the container is the correct one as stated by the label.
- Perform handwashing after handling chemical products.
- Do not consume foods or drinks when handling chemical products.
- Do not handle contact lenses or other personal objects when handling chemical products.
- Follow the facility's plan in case of an accident or injury.
- Keep the chemical products stored in a ventilated and dry area.

Disposal Methods

The adequate disposal of medical waste and sharps is essential to protect healthcare workers and the public. Always use sharps containers to dispose of needles and sharps.

Waste must be disposed in red or yellow bags:

- **Reg bags** are used for medical/biohazardous waste. This includes tissues and other organic waste, blood, items with blood (gowns, gauzes, gloves, vials, tubes), body fluids, and sharps containers.
- **Yellow bags** are used for other hazardous waste. This includes items that contain mercury, batteries that contain cadmium, lead, or silver, and IV lines and fluid bags used alongside pharmaceutical products.

Exposure Control Plan

The development of an Exposure Control Plan includes the following elements:

- Develop a written policy for protection from exposure.
- Study facility to determine which workers are exposed to which type of exposure risk.
- Follow universal and standard precautions.
- Implement immunization and vaccination programs.
- Use preventive measures to avoid accidents.
- Structure an exposure action plan such as needle safety guidelines or a chemical exposure plan that includes the adequate use of eyewash stations.
- Report and evaluate exposure events.
- Educate and train healthcare workers.

Point-of-Care Tests and Laboratory Procedures

Point-of-Care Tests

Point-of-care tests are clinical tests that can be performed close to the place where the patient receives care. This may include the patient's bedside, the patient's home, or inside an ambulance. Point-of-care tests represent a practical solution to the need for fast and reliable tests. They bypass the need for a clinical laboratory which may entail longer wait times and logistical requirements. Not all clinical tests are currently available as point-of-care tests. Some tests are still preferably performed in a laboratory setting.

Point-of-care tests include:

- Glucose-monitoring devices (to monitor glucose levels).
- Dipstick urinalysis (to screen for kidney issues and diagnose urinary tract infections).
- Home pregnancy (urine).
- PT/INR (to monitor warfarin therapy).
- Fecal occult blood (to screen for colorectal cancer).

- Oxygen saturation (for assessment of oxygen saturation in the blood).
- Blood gases (for assessment of gas exchange and acid-base disorders).
- Rapid HIV (to screen for HIV).

Some point-of-care tests can be performed by both healthcare workers and laypeople. Point-of-care tests are less complex than their laboratory counterparts and they are generally very reliable. However, the use of wrong techniques or a misinterpreted result may give rise to adverse situations. Therefore, these tests must be used responsibly. It is of utmost importance to adequately educate and provide clear instructions to a patient who will use point-of-care tests at home.

CLIA-Waived Test Regulations

The Clinical Laboratory Improvement Amendments (CLIA) of 1988 are a group of regulations. They apply to facilities in the United States that perform laboratory tests on human specimens through substances such as blood, urine, or stools. These tests are designed for assessment, diagnosis, prevention, or treatment of human health or medical conditions.

The U.S. Food and Drug Administration clears some tests for home use under CLIA regulations. These are known as CLIA-waived tests. They are laboratory tests or procedures that are characterized as very simple with a low risk of error. Therefore, they can be safely performed at home or in ambulatory settings. CLIA-waived tests must represent no unreasonable risk or harm to the patient when the test is performed incorrectly.

Management of Laboratory Requisition

The requisition of a laboratory exam is required when said exam must be performed outside the medical office. A laboratory requisition is a document that contains all the necessary information for the laboratory to adequately perform the desired test on the required specimen of the designated patient.

Laboratory requisitions can be electronic and sent directly from the medical office to the external laboratory center. They can also be written on paper and given to the patient to show at the laboratory. Preprinted paper forms may also exist for specific laboratories. This includes cases in which an insurance company requires the patient to use the services of a specific laboratory.

A complete laboratory requisition includes the following information:

- Identification and contact information of the healthcare provider that orders the exam (full name, address, phone number).

- Identification information of the patient (full name, address, social security number, age, date of birth, gender, insurance information).
- Source of the specimen or specimens.
- Date and time of each specimen collection.
- Specific test or tests to be performed on each sample.
- Provisional diagnosis.
- Any additional information (fasting, dietary requirements, relevant medications).
- Specification if the test must be performed as soon as possible.

Remember to review the patient's results when available and note them in the appropriate healthcare record.

Specimen Collection Techniques and Requirements

The collection of different types of medical specimens is an important skill and responsibility for any medical assistant. The quality of the specimen greatly impacts the potential accuracy of the test results. Each type of specimen may require a different collection technique. Medical assistants must familiarize themselves with each technique.

Some common specimens include blood, urine, feces, and swabs from mucous membranes and wounds. Other specimens such as gastric contents, semen, cerebrospinal fluid, amniotic fluid, peritoneal fluid, and tissues are collected less frequently.

When the specimen must be collected by the patient, the medical assistant should provide clear instructions to enhance the patient's ability to successfully collect the sample on their own.

Collection of Urine Specimens

Urine specimens may be collected through various techniques for different purposes. In most cases, urine samples require a random specimen. This refers to urine that is collected in a clean container at any time of the day. Random specimens can be used for most clinical purposes. Usually, at least 12 mL of urine is necessary. A half-filled container is generally enough. Although urine samples can be refrigerated, they should be processed within 1 hour after collection.

An early or first morning urine specimen is collected just after the patient wakes up. This specimen may be used for assessment of proteins like Bence Jones proteins present in patients with multiple myeloma or to determine pregnancy.

A clean-catch midstream specimen consists of specific steps. The genitals must be cleaned. Then the first stream of urine must be discarded to flush out the distal portion of the urethra. This is followed by a midstream of urine that is collected. This collection technique is commonly used to diagnose urinary tract infections through urine culture. Catheterization can also be used to collect samples for urine culture with a lower chance of contamination.

A 24-hour urine specimen represents a sample collected throughout a total of 24 hours. It can be used to measure clearance rates with creatinine levels to determine glomerular filtration rate.

Collection of Stool Specimens

The collection of stool specimens consists of taking a sample of stool. This is usually done with the help of a container. Some kits come with a plastic potty or similar container to avoid contact with toilet water. Any clean and empty container may work. A plastic spoon or spatula and a specimen container is generally provided. The spoon is used to fill the specimen container which is then closed and sealed in a plastic bag.

The patient should be instructed to preferably include stool samples with diarrhea or liquid, blood, or mucus, and avoid including urine or toilet paper in the specimen.

A stool sample can be refrigerated (2-8°C) but should be taken to the laboratory as soon as possible.

Stool specimens may be required to evaluate medical conditions such as parasitical or bacterial infections as well as gastrointestinal neoplasms like colon cancer or polyps.

Collection of Sputum Specimens

A sample of sputum is also called phlegm or mucus. It is usually collected early in the morning. The patient must be provided with a clean container. Instructions include the following:

- Perform mouth-washing before collection (especially after eating, drinking, or taking medication). Rinsing with water is acceptable.
- Perform handwashing to reduce the chances of specimen contamination. Hands must be dried as well.
- Perform chest clearance exercises (sit down, take a slow, deep breath, and exhale). This should be repeated a few times.
- Only when ready to cough, open the container and cough into it.
- Close the container tightly.

- Take the sputum specimen to the laboratory as soon as possible (within 1-2 hours).

The sample should be sputum which comes from the lung. Remind the patient not to spit into the container. The sterile container must not be opened until ready to use. In the case of tuberculosis assessment, the healthcare provider may request three samples across three consecutive days.

Requirements for Management of Medical Specimens

Medical specimens require various types of care and handling. Appropriate guidelines must be considered for the management of each specimen. This includes temperature requirements, processing requirements, light protection, and sterility.

Under certain circumstances, a specimen may be used as evidence for a legal proceeding. These cases require the medical office to follow the chain of custody. This can be achieved with a chain of custody form or similar document to keep track of the specimen and all workers that come into contact or maintain custody of it. Every member of the team must sign the chain of custody document as they interact with the specimen. If necessary, they may be called to testify in the case.

Quality Assurance

Any analytical procedure can be affected by errors that take place in various steps. Healthcare workers must work together to avoid these errors. This process is known as quality assurance. It can be divided into pre-analytical, analytical, and post-analytical phases.

Preanalytical stage: This stage consists of variables related to the order, collection, storage, transport, and preanalytical processing of a specimen. Errors in this stage may include:

- Orders that are missing, wrong, incomplete, or with deficient patient preparation.
- Collections with incorrect technique, wrong container, lost specimen, or sample contamination.
- Storage with wrong temperature, wrong light conditions, contamination, or lost specimen.
- Transportation with lost, contaminated, or damaged specimen.
- Processing with wrong timing, temperature, or technique.

Analytical stage: This stage consists of variables related to the analysis of the specimen. Errors in this stage may include:

- Calibration issues with lack of quality control, handling error, or wrong technique.
- Reagent issues with lack of quality control, handling error, or wrong technique.
- Machine issues with lack of quality control, handling error, computer or technical error, power failure, or wrong technique.

Postanalytical stage: This stage consists of variables related to report and delivery of results, and disposal of specimen. Errors in this stage may include:

- Disposal error or wrong technique.
- Reporting delay, wrong patient, incorrect result, or documentation error.
- Delivery delay, wrong patient, or incorrect result.
- Interpretation error or wrong diagnosis.

Quality Controls

Quality controls for various tests are performed to compare the patient's results with a set of samples that provide a specific result. A quality control sample can be positive or negative. They should be used daily alongside specimens from patients.

A common test that frequently employs quality control is chemical analysis of a urine specimen. It contains a control strip with synthetic compounds that mimic those found in human urine. The control solution is used to perform quality control of reagent or urine chemical strips.

The reagent strip is immersed in the control solution. The results are compared with the reference ranges stated by the quality control kit. There are positive and negative control strips. The positive control solution will show abnormal results and the negative control solution will show normal results.

This practice provides context to the professional who performs the test. It ensures the result can be trusted. Quality control should be performed every day and when a new reagent package or container is used for testing.

Other examples of quality control include glucose-monitoring devices, pregnancy test kits, and rapid antigen test kits.

Vision Testing

Visual acuity in a clinical setting consists of employment of eye charts like the Snellen or logMAR chart. Refractor devices are specialized vision testing devices. They are frequently used by ophthalmologists and other eyecare professionals.

The Snellen chart uses lines of letters that are each identified with a number and the resulting visual acuity. With one eye covered, the patient tries to read each line from a measured distance until it is no longer possible. The smallest line that can be read correctly represents the patient's visual acuity.

Ishihara charts are used to study color vision or color blindness. This may affect various groups of colors, such as red-green color blindness (deuteranopia and protanopia) and blue-yellow color blindness (tritanopia).

Hearing Testing

Hearing testing is usually performed with the help of an audiometer. The Weber and Rinne tests can be clinically performed with a tuning fork.

An audiometer measures sound intensity in decibels and tone in hertz or cycles per second. The procedure requires the patient to indicate when they hear a tone produced by the device, often by pressing a button or raising their hand. This measures the hearing threshold of the patient.

Respiratory Testing

Respiratory testing usually includes peak flow rate or peak expiratory flow rate measurement, or spirometry.

Peak flow rate is a very simple test that measures the flow rate during a forced expiration after a maximal inhalation. A reusable and small hand-held device is used. It contains a mouthpiece, cylinder, and indicator with red, yellow, and green zones to reflect percentages. A peak flow rate can be used by patients with respiratory conditions to adapt their treatment or identify the need for acute care.

Spirometry is a pulmonary function test that measures general lung function. It requires a spirometer and can be used to determine various respiratory parameters. Spirometry is employed to diagnose various respiratory conditions such as asthma, chronic obstructive pulmonary disease, and pulmonary fibrosis.

Reference Laboratory Values

Urinalysis:

- Color = Yellow (light yellow to amber).
- Odor = Characteristic.
- Turbidity = Clear.
- Specific gravity = 1.010 to 1.025.

- pH = 4.5 to 7.8.
- Blood = Negative.
- Glucose = Negative.
- Leukocyte esterase = Negative.
- Ketones = Negative.
- Bilirubin = Negative.
- Urobilinogen = Negative.
- Nitrite = Negative.
- Protein = Negative.
- Crystals = Negative.
- Casts = Negative.
- Red blood cells = 0 to 4 cells per high-power field.
- White blood cells = 0 to 5 cells per high-power field.
- Squamous epithelial cells = None.

Basic stool analysis:

- Water = 75%.
- pH = 7.0 to 7.5.
- Osmolality = 280 to 325 mOsmol/kg.
- Fat = 2-7 g/d.
- Alpha-1-antitrypsin = <540 mg/L.
- Occult blood = Negative.
- White blood cells = None.

Respiratory testing:

The reference ranges refer to male patients as 40 years old, 75 kg, 175 cm tall, and female patients as 40 years old, 60 kg, 160 cm tall.

- Total lung capacity = 6.9 L (male) / 4.9 L (female).
- Functional residual capacity = 3.3 L (male) / 2.6 L (female).
- Residual volume = 1.9 L (male) / 1.5 L (female).
- Inspiratory capacity = 3.7 L (male) / 2.3 L (female).
- Expiratory reserve volume = 1.4 L (male) / 1.1 L (female).
- Vital capacity = 5.0 L (male) / 3.4 L (female).
- Forced vital capacity (FVC) = 5.0 L (male) / 3.4 L (female).
- Forced expiratory volume in 1 second (FEV1) = 4.0 L (male) / 2.8 L (female).
- FEV1/FVC = 80% (male) / 78% (female).

- Maximal expiratory flow at 50% of expired vital capacity = 5.0 L/s (male) / 4.0 L/s (female).
- Maximal expiratory flow at 50% of expired vital capacity = 5.0 L/s (male) / 4.0 L/s (female).

Phlebotomy

Blood Components

Blood: Whole blood is a body fluid found within the circulatory system. It transports oxygen, nutrients, and other components to the body tissues. Blood also carries waste products for their elimination. It contains various cells (red blood cells, white blood cells, and platelets) and substances (hormones, proteins, lipids, complement and coagulation factors).

Red blood cells: These cells are also known as erythrocytes. They are mature cells with hemoglobin that carry oxygen from the lungs to the rest of the body tissues. They then carry carbon dioxide back to the lungs. These cells are biconcave, disk-shaped, and without a nucleus.

Reticulocytes: These are immature red blood cells that still contain remnants of ribosomal RNA but no longer have a nucleus. Reticulocytes are usually found within the bone marrow. They can also be found in peripheral blood in patients with anemia as the bone marrow releases these slightly immature cells into the blood circulation.

White blood cells: These mature cells protect the body against infection. Unlike red blood cells, they are colorless and have a nucleus. According to the presence of granules in their cytoplasm they can be divided into granulocytes (neutrophils, basophils, and eosinophils) and agranulocytes (lymphocytes and monocytes).

Platelets: Platelets are also known as thrombocytes. They are small clotting cells without a nucleus. Platelets are fragments from megakaryocytes which are bigger cells with a nucleus. Megakaryocytes are found in the bone marrow and rarely present in the blood.

Plasma: Plasma is the liquid portion of the blood and represents approximately 55% of the whole blood volume. It is mostly water (91%) with various substances such as clotting factors, antibodies, albumin, globulins, lipids, carbohydrates, and hormones. To obtain plasma, anticoagulants must be added to the sample to avoid activation of clotting factors.

Serum: Serum is the liquid portion of clotted blood. It is obtained when the clotting factors are naturally activated after the specimen is collected. As a result, serum does not contain clotting factors.

Bloodborne Pathogens

Bloodborne pathogens are microorganisms that can be transmitted through contact with infected blood. These microorganisms can be pathogenic which means they produce disease. The most important are hepatitis B virus, hepatitis C virus, and HIV.

Hepatitis B virus (HBV) is a virus that causes inflammation of the liver. It can be transmitted via blood, contaminated needles or sharps, sexual contact, as well as vertical transmission from infected pregnant mothers to their children. Approximately 10% of patients with acute hepatitis B infection may develop chronic hepatitis B. This may eventually result in liver cirrhosis or liver cancer. This condition is preventable via the hepatitis B vaccine. The vaccine is especially important for healthcare workers.

Hepatitis C virus (HCV) is similar to the hepatitis B virus. It is a virus that causes inflammation of the liver and can be transmitted via blood. However, HCV is predominantly present in recipients of unsafe blood transfusions through lack of blood product screening or those who share needles and syringes when using intravenous drugs. Most patients infected with the hepatitis C virus will develop chronic hepatitis C. While there is no vaccine, chronic hepatitis C can now often be cured with antiviral medications.

Human immunodeficiency virus (HIV) is a virus that destroys lymphocytes and specifically T cells. This weakens the immune system. The damage to the immune system may result in acquired immunodeficiency syndrome (AIDS) especially in patients who do not receive appropriate treatment. HIV can be transmitted via blood, sexual contact, and vertical transmission.

Patient Preparation

The patient's healthcare provider must formally request a phlebotomy before the procedure can begin. This can be achieved with a requisition or laboratory form. The Clinical Laboratory Improvement Amendments (CLIA) establishes the regulations to request laboratory tests. These include the laboratory form requirements. The requisition should contain the following information:

- Identification and contact information of the person who requests an exam (usually the patient's healthcare provider).
- Patient identification information with at least one unique identifier (social security number or healthcare record number), name, and date of birth.

- Specimen information such as time and date of specimen collection. In the case of Papanicolaou smears, include the patient's last menstrual period.
- Specified test to be performed on which specimen or sample.
- Notation of other relevant information related to the sample or test (timing details, patient fasting, use of medications, presence of fever).

To collect blood for laboratory assessment, a medical assistant must assemble the required equipment. Specific items may vary for special collections such as blood cultures or glucose tolerance tests.

Once the patient enters the room, it is important to present yourself and verify that the patient's identity matches the order. Medical records, date of birth, government-issued photo identification are examples of verifications. It is not uncommon for a patient to feel uncomfortable or anxious during this process. Therefore, it is important to be respectful and help the patient relax.

Explain the procedure to the patient and ask for verbal consent. When possible, talk to the patient to help them shift their focus away from the procedure. If the patient is visibly anxious, ask them what would make them feel more comfortable. Other ways to help the patient with their fear or anxiety include lying down in a supine position or counting. Ask the patient about the last successful collection site to help you find the easiest vein to perform the phlebotomy.

Special Considerations for Patient Preparation

In certain cases, patients may need special considerations to adapt to their needs or specific situations. Such cases may include pediatric patients and chain of custody.

Phlebotomy in pediatric patients:

- Phlebotomy in the pediatric population can be particularly difficult. It should be performed by trained healthcare workers. It is normal for children of most ages to feel fearful during the procedure. Healthcare workers may need to employ various techniques to help their patients feel safer and cooperative.
- Medical assistants may try to gain the confidence of the child and parents. It is important to explain the procedure but medical assistants may avoid disclosure of details about potential medical conditions that can be diagnosed with the test.
- The presence of a parent or legal guardian may greatly help a child feel more comfortable. However, it is important to consider the parent's willingness to participate in the procedure. Consider who will make a positive contribution and promote cooperative behavior from the child. If no adult can assist during the

procedure, the facility's policies may be followed if the child requires any type of restraint. This should be a last resort.

- The medical assistant should remain calm and understanding during the blood draw. Each age group may react differently and professionals must understand these differences. Medical assistants should show respect and praise children for their courage to help them overcome the situation.

Chain of custody:

- Chain of custody is the sequential or chronological documentation that follows the sequence of custody, control, transfer, analysis, and disposition of a specific piece of evidence. In the context of phlebotomy, a chain of custody is followed for specimens that will be used as evidence in a legal case. This may include DNA, drug, or alcohol testing.
- To comply with this type of documentation, it is important to keep a record of each worker that handles the sample. This includes information about identification and time of collection, transport, and general custody of the specimen. A specific chain of custody form may be used to help make the process easier to follow.

Factors that Affect Blood Collection and Results

Phlebotomy can be affected by various factors. These may result in unwanted effects such as injury or altered laboratory results.

Hematoma:

- Recognize this common problem associated with phlebotomy.
- Remove the tourniquet before removal of the needle.
- Prioritize straight, superficial, and clearly visible veins.
- Avoid the intersection of veins.
- Apply pressure after removing the needle.

Hemolysis:

- Do not perform venipuncture in an area with a hematoma.
- Verify that the selected site is dry before inserting the needle.
- Gently mix the blood with the anticoagulant additives inside the tube.

Exercise:

- Various laboratory results can be altered after physical exercise.

- These results include higher levels of creatine kinase, lactate dehydrogenase, and platelet count.

Time of day:

- The circadian rhythm may affect levels of certain substances. This includes hormones like cortisol which is higher early in the morning.
- Insulin and glucose levels will be different before and after a meal.

Stress:

- The body responds to stress by releasing various substances.
- This may result in higher levels of cortisol, catecholamines, and white blood cells.

Physiological fluctuations:

- Laboratory results may show normal changes across different ages, genders, and pregnancy.
- Such changes are specified as normal reference ranges provided in reference books or by the laboratory.

Vacuum Tubes

Vacuum tubes or evacuated collection tubes come in various sizes. They contain different additives identified by a colored top. The color coding employed by BD Vacutainer® is as follows:

Plain red — No additives. The tube does not need to be inverted. It is used for serum tests and includes chemistry tests, drug levels, blood bank testing, and serology. Volume: 5 mL.

Red-gray/Gold — Contains clot activators. It requires 5 tube inversions. It is also used for serum tests. Volume: 10 mL.

Green — Contains lithium/sodium/ammonium heparin. It requires 8 tube inversions. It is used for chemistry tests. Volume: 10 mL.

Light green — Contains lithium heparin and gel. This results in plasma separation and allows the determination of plasma levels for chemistry tests. Volume: 2 mL.

Gray — Contains potassium oxalate/sodium fluoride. It requires 8 tube inversions. It is used for glucose testing (sodium fluoride prevents glycolysis). Volume: 10 mL.

Lavender — Contains EDTA. It requires 8 tube inversions and is used for hematology tests that include complete blood count, hemoglobin, and hematocrit. Volume: 7 mL.

Light blue — Contains sodium citrate. It requires 4 tube inversions. It is used in various coagulation tests that include PT, PTT, INR, and D-dimer. Volume: 4.5 mL.

Royal blue — May contain EDTA or no additives. It requires 8 tube inversions if it contains an additive. It is used to study trace elements such as aluminum, mercury, lead, and selenium. Volume: 7 mL.

Yellow — Contains sodium polyanethol sulfonate (SPS). It is used for cultures of blood and other fluids. Volume: 5 mL.

Phlebotomy Site Selection and Preparation

After patient preparation, proceed with selection of the phlebotomy site. Ask the patient to extend their arm and visualize their antecubital fossa. Look for and select a clearly visible and straight vein. The median cubital vein is usually suitable for phlebotomy. It is found between muscles without any arteries or nerves in its vicinity. Avoid vein intersections which result in higher probability of hematoma.

It is important to inspect both arms. If necessary, other sites may be inspected such as the veins found in the back of the hand, foot, or ankle. Check skin anatomy and integrity for the presence of local or regional disorders. These may complicate the procedure or alter the laboratory results:

- **Burns** — Select another site. There is a higher risk of infection in burned skin.
- **Infection** — Infected sites must be avoided. Venipuncture may facilitate the passage of bacteria from the skin to the circulatory system.
- **Scar tissue** — Look for another site. It may be harder to collect blood from scarred skin.
- **Edema** — Look for another site. It may be harder to collect blood from edematous skin.
- **Hematoma** — Look for another site. Samples collected from a hematoma may alter the laboratory results.
- **Petechiae** — The tourniquet may cause the rupture of smaller blood vessels. This may occur when it is held in place for longer than 1 minute.
- **Mastectomy** — Avoid the side of the mastectomy. The impairment of lymphatic flow may result in altered laboratory results.

Once the vein has been selected, place a tourniquet 4 fingers above the site. Clean hands properly and wear gloves. Use 70% isopropyl alcohol to disinfect the area. Chlorhexidine is used instead when collecting blood for a blood culture. Wait approximately 30 seconds for the area to dry.

Blood collection requires a specific order of draws according to the additives inside the tubes. This is outlined by the National Committee for Clinical Laboratory Standards as follows:

1. SPS (yellow stopper).
2. Sodium citrate (light blue stopper).
3. No additive (red stopper).
4. Clot activators (red-gray stopper).
5. Sodium/lithium/ammonium heparin (green stopper).
6. EDTA (lavender stopper).
7. Potassium oxalate/sodium fluoride (gray stopper).

Venipuncture Methods

Venipuncture can be performed through various techniques. These include different blood collection devices and methods such as vacuum tubes, syringes, and safety butterfly needles.

Gather the required equipment and supplies. These include:

- Patient's health record (and other appropriate means to correctly identify the patient).
- Gloves.
- Phlebotomy order.
- Vacuum tubes required for the ordered tests.
- Gauzes.
- Tourniquet.
- Bandages and hypoallergenic tape.
- Alcohol pads (70% isopropyl alcohol).
- Permanent marker for label identification or printed labels.
- Safe disposal method (sharps and biohazard waste containers).
- Required blood collection devices (vacuum tube needle, tubes, syringes, needles).

Vacuum tube method:

- Verify the order.
- Gather equipment and supplies (including vacuum tube needle and needle holder).
- Perform handwashing.

- Put on gloves and required protective equipment.
- Verify the identity of the patient.
- Position the patient (sitting or lying down, arm extended).
- Assemble the equipment and attach the needle.
- Apply the tourniquet (approximately 4 fingers above the antecubital fossa). May ask the patient to clench their hand into a fist.
- Examine the arm and select a venipuncture site.
- Apply alcohol pads (or chlorhexidine in the case of blood cultures) to the skin. Begin at the center and move the pad outward in a circular manner.
- Wait for the alcohol to dry or dry with a sterile gauze.
- Take the assembled vacuum tube (needle, holder, and tube) with your dominant hand and remove the sheath.
- With your nondominant hand, use your thumb to anchor the vein.
- Insert the needle bevel up, aligned with the vein, at a 15-degree angle.
- Wait for the tube to fill.
- Ask the patient to release the fist.
- Remove the tube by pushing the needle holder.
- Invert the tube to mix the blood and additives.
- Insert a new tube and repeat as required.
- Remove the tourniquet, use a gauze to cover the venipuncture site, and remove the needle.
- With the gauze, apply pressure over the venipuncture site.
- Label the tubes with the required information.
- Examine the venipuncture site.
- Apply a bandage or clean gauze held in place with hypoallergenic tape.
- Dispose of contaminated materials and clean the area.
- Complete the required documentation, including the patient's record.

Syringe method:

- Verify the order.
- Gather equipment and supplies (including a syringe with a safety needle and a blood transfer device).
- Perform handwashing.
- Put on gloves and required protective equipment.
- Verify the identity of the patient.
- Position the patient (sitting or lying down, arm extended).
- Assemble the equipment by attaching the needle, pull and depress the plunger to loosen it.

- Apply the tourniquet (approximately 4 fingers above the antecubital fossa). May ask the patient to clench their hand into a fist.
- Examine the arm and select a venipuncture site.
- Apply alcohol pads (or povidone-iodine in the case of blood cultures) to the skin. Begin at the center and move the pad outward in a circular manner.
- Wait for the alcohol to dry or dry with a sterile gauze.
- With your dominant hand, take the syringe and remove the needle sheath.
- With your nondominant hand, use your thumb to anchor the vein.
- Insert the needle bevel up, aligned with the vein, at a 15-degree angle.
- When blood is visible inside the hub of the syringe, use your non-dominant hand to pull the plunger and fill the barrel as required.
- Remove the tourniquet, use a gauze to cover the venipuncture site, and remove the needle.
- With the gauze, apply pressure over the venipuncture site.
- Remove the needle and use a transfer device to transfer blood to the required tubes. Invert the tube to mix the blood and additives as required.
- Label the tubes with the required information.
- Examine the venipuncture site.
- Apply a bandage or clean gauze held in place with hypoallergenic tape.
- Dispose of contaminated materials and clean the area.
- Complete the required documentation, including the patient's record.

Butterfly method:

- Verify the order.
- Gather equipment and supplies (including a safety winged or butterfly needle set and vacuum tube holder).
- Perform handwashing.
- Put on gloves and required protective equipment.
- Verify the identity of the patient.
- Position the patient (sitting or lying down, arm extended).
- Assemble the equipment by attaching the vacuum needle to the vacuum tube holder and place the first tube in the holder.
- Apply the tourniquet above the wrist. Ask the patient to clench their hand into a fist.
- Examine the veins and select a venipuncture site.
- Apply alcohol pads (or povidone-iodine in the case of blood cultures) to the skin. Begin at the center and move the pad outward in a circular manner.
- Wait for the alcohol to dry or dry with a sterile gauze.

- With your dominant hand, insert the needle bevel up, aligned with the vein, at a 15-degree angle. Be careful not to activate the safety device.
- With your nondominant hand, push the tube into the holder until the tube is filled.
- Remove the tourniquet, use a gauze to cover the venipuncture site, and remove the needle.
- With the gauze, apply pressure over the venipuncture site.
- Remove the needle and use a transfer device to transfer blood to the required tubes. Invert the tube to mix the blood and additives as required.
- Label the tubes with the required information.
- Examine the venipuncture site.
- Apply a bandage or clean gauze held in place with hypoallergenic tape.
- Dispose of contaminated materials and clean the area.
- Complete the required documentation, including the patient's record.

Post-Collection Management of Blood Specimen

After collection, the blood sample begins to decay. Therefore, most samples are ideally processed as soon as possible. However, processing may not be possible or ideal at the time of collection. The sample must be stored.

To obtain serum from blood samples without anticoagulant, they should remain in a rack for 15-30 minutes. This depends on the presence of clot activator. The sample should be processed within 1 hour after clot formation. Check the centrifuge's instruction manual to determine the appropriate settings for blood samples.

The centrifuge is also used to separate plasma from the cells. It can be removed via aspiration. Another way to separate plasma is the use of vacuum tubes with lithium heparin.

Storage, Transportation, and Disposal of Blood Samples

The storage of blood samples varies among samples and the type of test. Whole blood samples can be stored for 24 hours at 4-8°C, without freezing. Blood cultures can be stored at room temperature (around 25°C) for less than 24 hours. Blood samples that require analysis of bilirubin must be protected from light sources. The sample can be wrapped with aluminum foil or other materials.

In the case that a specimen requires transportation, it is important to follow the Hazardous Materials Shipping Regulations by the Department of Transportation. Some relevant points to keep in mind to transport specimens are the use of triple packaging, appropriate labeling in the outer package, consideration of temperature requirements for each specimen, packaging certification, and shipment of the specimen with absorbent material within the second container.

In most cases, the remaining blood samples are disposed of via incineration.

Reference Values for Common Bood Tests

Hematology and coagulation:

- Hematocrit (Hct): 42%-50% (in men) / 36%-45% (in women).
- Hemoglobin (Hgb): 14-18 g/dL (in men) / 12-16 g/dL (in women).
- International normalized ratio (INR): 0.9-1.1.
- Mean corpuscular hemoglobin (MCH): 26-34 pg/cell.
- Mean corpuscular hemoglobin concentration (MCHC): 33-37 g/dL.
- Mean corpuscular volume (MCV): 80-100 fL/cell.
- Partial thromboplastin time (PTT): 25-40 seconds.
- Platelet count (Plt): 150,000-350,000 cells/mm^3.
- Prothrombin time (PT): 10-13 seconds.
- Red blood cell count (RBC): 4.5-5.9 million cells/mm^3 (in men) / 4.1-5.1 million cells/mm^3 (in women).
- Reticulocytes: 0.5%-1.5%.
- White blood cell count (WBC): 4.5-11.0 x 10^3 cells/mm^3.

Blood chemistry:

- Alanine aminotransferase (ALT): 10-40 U/L.
- Albumin: 3.5-5 g/dL (in adults) / 3.4-4.2 g/dL (in children).
- Alkaline phosphatase (ALP): 30-120 IU/L (in adults) / 150-420 IU/L (in children).
- Ammonia: 15-45 mcg/dL.
- Amylase: 27-131 U/L.
- Aspartate aminotransferase (AST): 10-30 U/L.
- Bilirubin (direct): 0.1-0.3 mg/dL.
- Bilirubin (total): 0.3-1.2 mg/dL.
- Blood urea nitrogen (BUN): 8-23 mg/dL (in adults).
- Total serum calcium: 8.2-10.2 mg/dL.
- Carbon dioxide (venous) (CO_2): 22-28 mEq/L.
- Chloride (Cl): 96-106 mEq/L.
- C-reactive protein (CRP): 0.08-3.1 mg/L.
- Creatinine kinase (CK): 40-150 U/L.
- Creatinine, serum (SCr): 0.6-1.2 mg/dL (in adults) / 0.2-0.7 mg/dL (in children).

- Creatinine (clearance) (CrCI): 75-125 mL/minute/1.73 m^2.
- Ferritin: 15-200 ng/mL.
- Gamma-glutamyl transpeptidase: 2-30 U/L.
- Serum glucose: 70-110 mg/dL.
- Hemoglobin A1C: 4%-7%.
- Lactate dehydrogenase (LDH): 100-200 U/L.
- Lipase: 31-186 U/L.
- Magnesium: 1.3-2.1 mEq/L.
- Phosphorus: 2.3-4.7 mg/dL (in adults) / 3.7-5.6 mg/dL (in children).
- Potassium: 3.5-5.0 mEq/L.
- Sodium: 136-142 mEq/L.
- Uric acid: 4-8 mg/dL.

Serum lipids:

- Total cholesterol (TC): <200 mg/dL.
- High-density lipoprotein (HDL): ≥40 mg/dL.
- Low-density lipoprotein (LDL): <100 mg/dL.
- Triglycerides (TG): < 150 mg/dL.

Blood gases:

- pH: Arterial 7.35-7.45 / Venous 7.31-7.41.
- Partial pressure of carbon dioxide (PCO_2): Arterial 35-45 mm Hg, Venous 38-52 mm Hg.
- Partial pressure of oxygen (Po_2): Arterial 80-100 mm Hg / Venous 40-50 mm Hg.
- Oxygen saturation (SaO_2): Arterial >90% / Venous 60%-75%.
- Serum bicarbonate (HCO_3): Arterial 22-26 mEq/L / Venous 21-28 mEq/L.

External Databases

Testing.com (formerly LabTestsOnline.org) - https://www.testing.com

Guide to Diagnostic Tests, 7e (Access Medicine) - https://accessmedicine.mhmedical.com/book.aspx?bookID=2032

UCSF Clinical Labs online laboratory manual - https://clinlab.ucsf.edu/ucsf-clinical-laboratories-online-manual

American Society for Microbiology's Protocols - https://asm.org/browse-by-content-type/protocols

EKG and Cardiovascular Testing

Electrocardiography is a diagnostic process that creates a graphical pattern based on the changes in electrical charge generated by cardiac activity. The instrument employed is an electrocardiograph. The record of result is an electrocardiogram. This is commonly known as an ECG or EKG. Electrocardiography is useful for assessment of arrhythmias, cardiovascular conditions like myocardial infarction, and other medical conditions like electrolyte imbalances.

Supplies

Electrocardiograph: instrument employed to produce an EKG.

Electrocardiograph paper: special graph paper that is pressure and heat sensitive. It contains vertical and horizontal lines at 1 mm intervals where the x-axis represents time (1 mm represents 0.04 seconds) and the y-axis represents voltage (10 mm represents 1 mV).

Electrodes: ten electrodes or sensors (one for each arm and leg, and six for the chest). They are used to record the electrical activity of the heart from various angles. Electrodes are usually self-adhesive and disposable.

Lead wires: wires that carry the recorded electrical activity to the electrocardiograph.

Razor: disposable razor may be needed for hair removal if there is excess hair on the chest.

Waveforms, Intervals, Segments

Isoelectric line: the baseline of the EKG which represents the lack of changes in electrical charge.

P wave: small upward wave that represents the depolarization of the atria. It is responsible for the contraction of the atria.

QRS complex: combination of the Q, R, and S waves that represent the depolarization of the ventricles. It is responsible for the contraction of the ventricles.

T wave: upward wave that represents the repolarization of the ventricles. It is responsible for the relaxation of the ventricles.

U wave: small upward wave that can be seen in patients with low serum potassium due to the slow repolarization of Purkinje fibers in the ventricles.

PR interval: interval that begins with the P wave and ends with a point that connects the isoelectric line with the QRS complex. The PR interval represents how long it takes for the electrical impulse to travel from the sinoatrial (SA) node to the atrioventricular (AV) node.

QT interval: interval that begins with the QRS complex and ends with the T wave. It represents the amount of time the ventricles need to depolarize and repolarize.

ST segment: interval that begins with the end of the QRS complex and ends with the starting point of the T wave. It represents the amount of time between the end of ventricular depolarization and repolarization.

Techniques and Methods for EKGs

12-lead EKG: standard method for an EKG. It consists of an electrocardiograph with 10 electrodes to produce a 12-lead EKG. The leads are the standard leads (I, II, III), the augmented leads (aVR, aVL, and aVF), and the precordial leads (V1, V2, V3, V4, V5, and V6). The standard leads are also known as bipolar leads. They are the result of two limb electrodes: lead I represents the electrodes from the right arm and left arm, lead II from the right arm and left leg, and lead III from the left arm and left leg.

Holter monitor: portable EKG recording device that a patient carries for 24 hours or more. It is used to monitor a patient's cardiac activity for prolonged periods of time. It can also be activated periodically such as when the patient presents symptoms. The patient is instructed to keep a journal to record any stressful or symptomatic events. They describe the event and report the time and duration of the occurrence.

Cardiac stress test: specialized test performed to record cardiac activity during a period of cardiovascular stress. The patient participates in an exercise challenge such as running on a treadmill. The cardiologist can use this EKG study to determine if the patient presents an arrhythmia during exercise or other relevant cardiovascular findings.

Event monitor: small cardiac monitor that records the activity of the heart for various intervals, usually up to 30 days. It is used to diagnose conditions that may need more than 24 hours to appear and cannot be accurately determined with a Holter monitor.

Artifacts, Signal Distortions, and Electrical Interference

Patients may present signs and symptoms related to distress, anxiety, and fear during an EKG. As a result, they may present higher blood pressure, tachycardia, dyspnea, and other findings. It is important to use therapeutic communication to help patients feel more comfortable during the procedure to reduce artifacts in the EKG and avoid prolonged procedure.

- **Wandering baseline**: Instead of being a horizontal line, the isoelectric line shifts up or down. It may occur when the patient moves or an electrode is not positioned correctly. Ask the patient to stay still and check the electrodes.
- **Somatic tremor**: This tremor is simply the electrical activity of muscle movement that affects the tracing of the EKG. It looks jagged. Tremors may occur when the patient is anxious, uncomfortable, talking, moving, or when the patient has a condition that causes tremors. Talk with the patient to calm them down and try to make them feel comfortable.
- **Alternating current interference**: These are interferences created by other electrical devices. Ensure the electrocardiograph is connected to a grounded outlet and verify the wires are not crossed. Unplug any unnecessary devices. This interference is seen as spikes in the EKG.
- **Interrupted baseline**: This is the interruption of the isoelectric line. It may occur when the stylus of the electrocardiograph moves up and down erratically. The electrodes may not be placed correctly or the wires may be damaged.
- **Pacemaker spikes**: These are artifacts in the form of spikes. The spikes are vertical and short signals that are normally found in patients with a pacemaker.

Patient Preparation

- The test should be performed in a quiet and well-lit room, far from other electrical devices, X-ray machines, and laboratory equipment.
- The table should be made of wood or an electrically insulated material.
- Place the electrocardiograph in a comfortable position. Usually, it is placed on the left side of the table. All the electrodes must be positioned correctly.
- Explain the procedure to the patient.
- Make sure the patient has not applied any substance to their chest prior to the test.
- Ask the patient to take their clothes off to expose their chest and provide a gown. The lower limbs should be accessible as well.
- Position the patient in the supine position. Arms and legs should rest separate from each other. The semi-Fowler position may be used for patients with dyspnea. In this case, discuss the position with the physician.
- Measure the patient's vital signs.

Placement of Limb and Chest Electrodes

- Use self-adhesive and disposable electrodes. In the case of reusable electrodes, an electrolyte gel or solution may be required before attachment.
- Position the limb electrodes accordingly on the wrists and ankles.
- Position the precordial electrode for V1 on the 4th intercostal space (right parasternal line).
- V2 on the 4th intercostal space (left parasternal line).
- V4 on the 5th intercostal space (left mid-clavicular line).
- V3 midway between V2 and V4.
- V5 on the 5th intercostal space (left anterior axillary line).
- V6 on the 5th intercostal space (left mid-axillary line).
- Attach the lead wires to their respective electrode. They are color-coded and generally follow this standard: right arm = white; left arm = black; right leg = green; left leg = red; V1 = red; V2 = yellow; V3 = green; V4 = blue; V5 = orange; V6 = purple. Note that the color codes for precordial leads can vary by manufacturer, so always refer to the device's manual.

Considerations Related to Patient Characteristics

Amputated limb: In the case of patients with an amputated limb, the electrode can be placed above the site of amputation.

Dextrocardia/situs inversus: In these cases, the limb electrodes are placed in the same manner. The precordial electrodes should be placed on the right side of the chest to mirror the usual position on the left side.

Injuries/incisions: Do not place an electrode on an injury or incision. Place it as close to the site as possible. The modification should be documented.

Children: The placement of electrodes is the same. To adjust for the smaller size of the chest, the fourth precordial lead (V4) can be moved to the right side of the chest to reduce clutter. This lead change is known as V4 right or V4R and should be documented.

Abnormal Rhythms

Sinus arrhythmias: These arrhythmias are characterized by an increased or decreased fire rate of the SA node. This results in tachycardia (>100 beats per minute) and bradycardia (<60 beats per minute), respectively. Sinus tachycardia can be a normal occurrence during exercise or extreme emotions. Sinus bradycardia can be normal in some athletes. In other situations, these findings may be pathologic. Sinus arrhythmias may appear as a relatively normal EKG but with a faster or slower frequency.

Atrial arrhythmias: These are characterized by an abnormal electrical discharge in the atria due to irregular electrical impulse formation in ectopic foci in the atria. Examples include atrial fibrillation and atrial flutter. Atrial flutter can be identified as an extremely fast heartbeat (>200 beats per minute) and a sawtooth pattern (a string of multiple P waves that resembles a sawtooth) followed by a QRS complex.

Ventricular arrhythmias: These can occur due to ectopic foci or altered conduction in the ventricles. The most common examples are ventricular tachycardia and ventricular fibrillation. Ventricular tachycardia is characterized by an increased heart rate with irregular and wide QRS complexes. Ventricular fibrillation is a life-threatening condition in which the ventricles contract erratically. No waves are identifiable.

Metabolic arrhythmias: These include increased or decreased potassium as well as toxicity due to treatment with digitalis.

Calibration and Standardization of the EKG

Electrocardiographs are calibrated according to international guidelines to present a standardized sensitivity that can be interpreted in the same manner anywhere in the world. This international sensitivity standard dictates that 1 mV of electricity translates to a 10 mm vertical movement (y-axis). This is known as 1 STD (one standard) which is the standard mode of an EKG. This can be altered to double standard (1 mV = 20 mm) or one-half standard (1 mV = 5 mm). This can be seen at the start of the tracing (as a short 10 mm trace at 1 STD) or written on the paper.

The standard speed is 25 mm per second. This can be altered as well. A faster speed (usually 50 mm per second) is useful to inspect faster heart rates or waves that are too close together.

Chapter 4: Patient Care Coordination and Education

Preventive Medicine and Screenings

Preventive medicine is the development of preventive health care practices to reduce the prevalence of disease and its consequences (such as disability and death). Preventive medicine has allowed the general population to progress in various areas, such as immunization, maternal and neonatal health, tobacco consumption, vehicle safety, occupational safety, and prevention of cardiovascular disease, cancer, and multiple communicable diseases.

A valuable tool employed in preventive medicine is the screening of medical conditions—this is a diagnostic intervention that aims to identify a specific condition at an early stage. In many cases, screenings take specific risk factors into consideration (for example, patients between fifty to eighty years old with significant history of smoking should be screened for lung cancer). Universal screenings encompass a broader population (for example, all patients older than forty-five years, regardless of whether they are overweight or obese, should be screened for diabetes and prediabetes).

Some of the most common screenings are:

- **Papanicolaou test** — Also known as Pap smears or cervical cytology, this is a cytological sample taken from the cervix in women. The screening is done in women aged twenty-one to sixty-five to help in the detection of cervical cancer.
- **Mammography** — This is performed as a screening test for breast cancer in women after reaching the age of fifty. It should be performed every one or two years.
- **Colonoscopy** — It should be performed for patients after the age of fifty, and earlier in those with a family history of colon polyps or cancer.
- **Prostate-specific antigen (PSA)** — PSA was commonly performed in the screening process of prostate cancer; however, the United States Preventive Services Task Force (USPSTF) now opposes the use of this screening due to overdiagnosis (PSA may be elevated in patients with non-malignant conditions, such as benign prostatic hyperplasia).

Clinical Quality Measures

Clinical quality measures (or CQMs) are tools to determine, quantify, and document the safe, competent, appropriate, and timely delivery of care. Ideally, CQMs are included in the electronic health record. They are used to measure health care performance, identify weaknesses, and find ways to improve.

Types of CQMs include:

- Structure (infrastructure, equipment, staff).
- Process (evidence-based processes or interventions).
- Outcomes.
- Patient-reported outcomes.
- Use/cost/efficiency of resources.
- Composite of various measures.

Strategies for Patient Education

Patient education should include high-quality and accurate information about the patient's condition, medications, procedures, quality of life, and required medical equipment or supplies. In many cases, medical assistants will reinforce and complement the information provided by the physician. This may occur in the office or during virtual visits. Effective patient education requires:

- **The assessment of a patient's needs** — What do patients need to know to understand their condition? Various patient factors, such as age, language, level of education, and cultural background should be considered. Always remember to check the patient's record to understand their context and needs.
- **The determination of teaching priorities** — The information content is important, but an adequate delivery of high-quality information is essential. The educator may determine which information is relevant for the patient now and what is relevant in the long term.
- **The use of teaching materials** — Patient education can be imparted through various means. These include printed or digital materials, informational fliers, approved video material (e.g., from a trusted source on YouTube), apps, etc. Ideally, the materials should be available in the patient's preferred language.
- **The inclusion of family members** — In many cases, the participation of family members in the learning process improves patient compliance. The inclusion of the patient's family may directly help the patient in their learning. This also helps the family comprehend the patient's condition better, which allows them to support the patient in a meaningful and understanding manner.
- **Special considerations for virtual visits** — Although telehealth allows the remote delivery of care via virtual visits, it also introduces new challenges for providers. Always check the patient's record beforehand and prepare a quiet, well-lit place for the visit. Remember to look into the camera (this simulates eye

contact with the patient) and remind the patient that the visit is private. Speak clearly and encourage the patient to ask questions.

Patient Education Related to Nutrition

Patients should learn that nutrition goes beyond losing weight. It helps to lower the risk of various conditions (cancer, cardiovascular disease, diabetes) and promotes better health and quality of life.

There are multiple types of diets (Mediterranean diet, DASH diet, low-fat diet, plant-based diet), and patients may benefit from one over the other due to personal preferences, nutritional needs, cultural or religious background, cost, etc. Diets with limited evidence include the ketogenic diet and gluten-free diet for individuals without celiac disease. In general, the most important components of a healthy diet are:

- Whole grains.
- Fruits.
- Vegetables.
- Fiber.
- Healthy fats (monounsaturated and polyunsaturated fats).
- Proteins.

It is also important to avoid added sugars, processed foods and meats, red meats, alcohol, and unhealthy fats (saturated and trans fats).

People with diet restrictions or specific conditions may need to use supplements. For example, B12 vitamin supplementation may be needed in patients who have a limited consumption of animal products. Similarly, some patients may need to use supplements after a bariatric surgery. Pregnant patients (or those planning to become pregnant) should receive folic acid supplementation daily.

Certain foods and nutrients may interact positively or negatively with specific drugs:

- **Warfarin** – This anticoagulant interacts with multiple foods. Leafy greens can decrease the effectiveness of warfarin, cooked onions increase warfarin activity, charbroiled foods decrease it, and cranberry juice can increase the international normalized ratio (INR).
- **Antidepressants (monoamine oxidase inhibitors)** – These drugs interact with foods that contain tyramine (overripe bananas, matured cheese, salami, yogurt), which may result in a hypertensive crisis.

- **Antibiotics** — Milk consumption may reduce the absorption of certain antibiotics (e.g., ciprofloxacin and tetracycline). Food reduces the absorption of azithromycin.
- **Oral hypoglycemics** — Sulfonylureas like glimepiride should be taken with food (thirty minutes before meals).
- **NSAIDs** — Alcohol consumption increases the risk of gastric bleeding and liver damage.

Resources for Clinical Services and Non-Clinical Services

- **Care Compare** (https://www.medicare.gov/care-compare/) — This is a Medicare tool that helps to compare various Medicare providers (physicians, hospitals, nursing homes, home health services, hospice care, inpatient rehabilitation facilities, long-term care hospitals, dialysis facilities, and medical equipment and suppliers).
- **CDC programs** (https://www.cdc.gov/chronicdisease/center/community-health-worker-resources.html) — This webpage contains resources grouped for community health workers, but they can be useful for other types of providers and related facilities. It includes resources on cardiovascular disease, asthma, cancer, diabetes, and obesity, among others. Content includes guidelines, interventions, fact sheets, and informational material.
- **National Association for Home Care & Hospice (NAHC) Resource Library** (https://nahc.org/nahc-resources/) — This library includes various webinars, links, documents, and fact sheets related to home care and hospice.
- **AHRQ Resources on Patient-Centered Medical Homes** (https://archive.ahrq.gov/ncepcr/tools/pcmh/implement/resources.html) — This webpage includes briefs, white papers, reports, guides, case studies, databases, and other resources related to Patient-Centered Medical Homes.
- **Family Caregiver Alliance (FCA)** (https://www.caregiver.org/connecting-caregivers/services-by-state/) — This resource from the FCA includes information per state on various initiatives and programs directed toward caregivers.
- **Eldercare Locator** (https://eldercare.acl.gov/Public/Index.aspx) — This site is useful for finding services and resources directed toward older adults and their families/caregivers.
- Contact insurers for a **list of in-network providers**.

Barriers to Care

Multiple barriers may obstruct access to care, even for patients with insurance. According to Allen et al. (2018), barriers can be grouped in the following manner:

- **Patient-level barriers**: These are mainly related to the patient's responsibilities that may affect their access to care, such as family, work, and in the case of patients with children, the availability of childcare.
- **Provider-level barriers**: Provider-level barriers: Providers may impose barriers on patients if they do not speak the patient's language, do not understand their culture or religion, or if there is a lack of cultural competence. In some cases, the patient may not trust their provider or may perceive discrimination (due to their gender, race, ethnicity, nationality, ability to pay, or being a beneficiary of a public health care program).
- **Systemic-level barriers**: These include barriers related to coverage (patients do not know their coverage, if they were dropped from their healthcare program, or where to ask), finances (patients worry about the cost of care and medications), and access (patients are not able to attend due to transportation issues or inconvenient office hours, or they do not know where to go).

Roles and Responsibilities of Team Members Involved in Patient-Centered Medical Home and Team-Based Care

The team members in a patient-centered medical home (PCMH) and team-based care (TBC) are:

- **The physician**: in charge of managing patients, especially those with complex conditions. They examine, diagnose, and develop a treatment plan.
- **The nurse**: in charge of administering treatments, taking vital signs, recording medical history, refilling medications, and notifying patients of test results.
- **The physician assistant** and **the nurse practitioner**: in charge of managing patients, examination, diagnosis, and treatment (in relation to their scope of practice).
- **The medical assistant**: in charge of assisting the physician (taking medical history, comprehensive health assessment, vital signs, assistance during procedures) and the nurse (basic handling of medications, logistics), as well as patient education.
- **The pharmacist**: in charge of managing medication and related resources.
- **The social or community health worker**: in charge of coordinating care for high-risk patients (those who require frequent services or have complex and difficult-to-treat conditions).
- **The receptionist**: in charge of patient registration, verification of information, management of calls, emails, appointments, etc.
- **The office manager**: in charge of coordination of the office workflow.

Referral Forms and Processes

A referral is a document provided by a primary care provider when a patient needs to see a specialist due to a specific medical condition. A referral coordinator from the medical office manages the referral process by scheduling the visit with the required specialist, which involves a referral form along with the patient's relevant information.

An efficient referral process requires organization, and the first step is a standardized form, which may be filled out on paper or electronically. Referral forms may include:

- Date of the appointment.
- Name of the primary care provider.
- Current diagnosis.
- Urgency (from immediate to routine).
- Type of specialist required.
- Motive of referral and required service (consultation, diagnosis, follow-up, etc.).

Ideally, the coordination process includes asking the patient about their preferred day of the week or date before scheduling the visit.

The specialist may ask for extra information (in some cases, they may provide their own referral form to include the specific information they need). The exchange of information is important to avoid delays and duplication of imaging or tests.

Once the referral is correctly scheduled, the medical office has to monitor the rest of the process. After the visit, the medical office should receive a letter from the specialist with details about the visit (which includes findings, diagnosis, treatment plan, test results, etc.). In some cases, the patient may miss the appointment or the letter from the specialist may not arrive. At this point, the coordinator should call the patient or the specialist's office to find out what has happened. Usually, the process should be tracked through the electronic health record (when unavailable, the coordinator may create a referral tracking spreadsheet with the referral's information to follow the process). If the patient misses their appointments repeatedly, determine the cause in order to look for a solution.

Prevention of the Transmission of Communicable Diseases

The transmission of communicable diseases (viral hepatitis, salmonella, HIV, tuberculosis, chickenpox, disseminated herpes zoster, etc.) can be prevented through various types of precautions that consider contact, airborne, and droplet transmission. Preventive measures include:

- Adequate use of personal protective equipment (PPE).
- Patients should use a mask.
- Susceptible health care staff should avoid contact with patients known or suspected to have communicable diseases.
- Immunizations, if applicable.
- Place the patient in a single patient room, when available.
- Avoid transport of these patients unless strictly necessary.

Chapter 5: Administrative Assisting

Office Visits

Office visits can serve various purposes. In most cases, patients will go to the medical office to see their health care provider due to new or already-known conditions. However, patients may need to see their provider due to other reasons. As a medical assistant, you may schedule some of the following visits:

- **New patient visit**: This is the first visit between a patient and their new health care provider. It focuses on a thorough assessment of the patient's personal and family medical history. It may also include additional testing. If a patient comes for a specific condition, it may be discussed as well. After three or more years without a visit, a patient may be considered a "new patient."
- **Follow-up visit**: These visits are programmed directly after a standard office visit in order to review the progress of a condition. The health care provider may analyze the patient's diagnostic results to develop a treatment plan or check the patient's response to treatment.
- **Urgent visit**: Patients may need to see their provider as soon as possible without needing to go to urgent care or an emergency room. In these cases, it is important to determine the severity of the situation (triage) and find a place for the patient where they can be seen first.
- **Preventive health exam**: Also known as a physical or annual exam, this is a yearly routine exam to check overall health, schedule screening tests, order immunizations, and identify risk factors.
- **Sports physical**: Also known as preparticipation physical evaluation (PPE), these visits determine if a patient can participate safely in a sport. In many cases, these visits are not covered by insurance.
- **School physical**: This is a routine exam for students that is usually performed by pediatricians or family physicians. It focuses on the early identification of health conditions that may affect the growth and development of the student, a review of the immunization history, and a physical exam.
- **Medicare's Initial Preventive Physical Exam (IPPE) and Annual Wellness Visit (AWV)**: These visits are available for patients enrolled in Medicare Part B. The IPPE is available within the first twelve months of enrollment and focuses on patient and family history. The AWV is available annually after the first twelve months and focuses on developing a personalized prevention plan, routine measurements (height, weight, blood pressure), and an assessment of the patient's health risk. IPPE and AWV are free of charge (note that these visits are different from a physical exam, which is not covered by Medicare).

- **Screening visit**: These visits can be arranged during a previous visit as a personalized screening or prevention plan. They involve the preventive study of a patient with or without risk factors for a specific condition (for example, the performance of a diabetes screen in a fifty-year-old patient).
- **Specialty visit**: This is a visit with a specialist. These visits are usually scheduled with a referral by a primary care provider when the patient needs special care (for example, specific diagnosis, treatment, or procedures that need the help of a specialist).
- **Telehealth visits**: These are appointments that allow patients to receive care via phone or video. Many types of visits can be safely arranged as telehealth visits unless a physical exam is required (for example, the yearly preventive health exam or physical).
- **Pharmaceutical sales representative**: In some cases, providers may meet with sales representatives to discuss and see pharmaceutical products or medical devices.

The scheduling process may vary from patient to patient and between different types of visits. These are some useful tips to have in mind:

- Remember that visits with new patients will usually require more time to discuss medical history, fill out forms, etc.
- Schedule visits early in the morning for patients who require fasting before a procedure.
- Some patients may require frequent visits—schedule visits at the same spot (same day and/or hour) to increase patient compliance with the appointments.
- When referring a patient, verify that the patient's insurance is accepted by the specialist.

The Health Record

A health record is a legal record that documents clinical findings, the progress of treatments, and a patient's medical and family history. At the same time, the health record helps health care providers to communicate with each other by recording relevant information, and it also serves as a research document.

Records can be electronic (electronic health records or EHRs) or paper-based. Each has its benefits and disadvantages. However, EHRs now dominate medical documentation. Paper documentation is harder to share, requires more physical space, may be easier to be misfiled or lost, can only be used by one person at a time, and can be difficult to read. EHRs, on the other hand, are efficient and versatile, can be shared when required, are easy to read and update, etc. In addition, EHR software usually comes alongside other practical features, such as systems to facilitate scheduling and billing.

The health record may include the following sections:

- **Patient demographic information**: This includes patient information like full name, gender, birth date, address, telephone number, e-mail address, occupation, marital status, social security number, and health care insurance information.
- **Medical and family history**: This section describes the patient's health (previous diseases, surgeries, significant injuries, past hospitalizations, etc.) and social history (exercise, nutrition, drug use, alcohol, tobacco, etc.), as well as family history (health information from the immediate family).
- **Chief complaint**: This is an accurate and concise chronology and description of the patient's condition, which includes any treatment the patient has received (and its success or failure).
- **Vital signs and measurements**: These include temperature, respiratory and pulse rate, blood pressure, pulse oximetry, weight, and height.
- **Clinical and paraclinical findings**: These include objective findings from the physical exam, as well as laboratory or imaging reports.
- **Diagnosis**: In this section, the health care provider in charge considers all the information gathered from the patient's medical history, chief complaint, physical findings, laboratory results, imaging studies, etc., to propose a diagnosis, which may be a provisional diagnosis.
- **Treatment**: Based on the diagnosis and the rest of the gathered information, a treatment plan is decided.
- **Progress notes**: As the patient returns for new visits, the patient's progress is recorded in the form of progress notes. Here, various new findings, orders, and events are recorded.
- **Condition at the time of treatment termination**: Upon treatment termination, a final note can be used to detail the patient's condition at the time of discharge from care.
- **Consent forms**: Consent may be signed before certain procedures, especially those that carry some risk, such as surgical procedures or when the patient needs to agree or refuse treatment. For this purpose, a provider must explain the procedure or treatment (as well as the consequences of accepting or refusing such procedure) before the patient (or a legal representative) signs the informed consent.
- **HIPAA forms**: The Health Insurance Portability and Accountability Act (HIPAA) protects patient health information, and disclosure of certain information requires permission. HIPAA forms need to be signed by the patient

or their legal representative for the disclosure or use of health information for research, to share information with a third party, to allow the use of photographs, etc.

The Electronic Health Record

An electronic health record (EHR) is a system that allows health care providers and institutions to optimize their work and save time and money. These computer programs can be tailored to the needs of specific types of medical practice, such as medical and surgical specialties. EHR software usually includes an appointment management system to schedule, remind, and confirm visits, which is especially useful for medical offices. Finally, the software may also allow the management of laboratory tests, imaging, referrals, and medical billing.

However, EHR systems are not perfect—they will not work without electrical energy, which may be affected by natural events or infrastructural issues. Therefore, it is important to create a plan to back up information and work around these issues. The main three strategies are:

- **External storage** — An external storage device is used to back up information from the EHR every day (for example, at the end of the day). The device is ideally an external hard drive or solid-state drive, but it may also be a CD or DVD, USB drive, or memory card. It is a simple solution, but may not be suitable for large amounts of data.
- **Full server backup** — A full backup is performed on a dedicated server, which is located in another location away from the medical facility.
- **Online backup** — This is a full backup performed online. This type of service is usually reliable, but the setup process requires time and preparation.

The Paper-Based Record

Originally, the health record was paper-based. This has changed in the last two decades and the EHR has become the default system. However, the paper-based documentation of medical information is still important, especially when EHR is unavailable for a long period of time.

Common paper records systems are source-oriented and problem-oriented records. Source-oriented takes into account the source of the record (for example, a provider or the laboratory), and it is usually organized in reverse chronological order. Problem-oriented records organize the record in a database that contains the patient's clinical and paraclinical information, which includes the chief complaint and the patient's medical history, a list of problems to be resolved, a treatment plan (to resolve each problem), and progress notes (which follow the progress of each problem).

Chart Review

The chart review is useful for identifying errors in the diagnostic or therapeutic process. It is based on the analysis of retrospective data from the EHR. It is a complex process because there is no golden standard for the identification of these errors. The main questions to answer during a chart review include:

- Did any diagnostic/therapeutic error occur?
- How many errors?
- Did these errors result in harm to the patient? If the answer is no, is there a potential for these errors to result in patient harm?
- When did the error occur or when could it have been prevented?

Some tools can be used to aid in the chart review process, such as the Diagnosis Error Evaluation & Research (DEER) taxonomy tool and the Safer Dx tool.

There are three aspects of a diagnostic error that may occur: missed diagnosis (failure to recognize a condition), delayed diagnosis (diagnosis occurs later than it should have), and incorrect diagnosis (despite the availability of adequate evidence, there is an incorrect diagnosis).

Electronic Referrals

Electronic referral systems, also known as e-referral, are electronic platforms that allow the direct transfer of patient information between health care providers.

An electronic referral system can enhance productivity, reduce costs, and facilitate the safe sharing of patient information. However, implementation of e-referral systems may be difficult. Many countries have successfully implemented such systems for referrals within their facility (for example, within a hospital), but regional implementation and integration is more difficult (each facility, clinic, and medical office may have a different management software).

Health Insurance Fundamentals

Health insurance, also known as medical insurance, represents protection against financial loss due to unplanned medical events. Coverage may be partial or total. Therefore, the patient will pay, usually a monthly premium, and the insurance will cover part or the whole cost of certain medical expenses (hospitalization, medicines, visits, etc.) depending on coverage.

A health insurance plan or policy is a coverage package that describes the items and services that will be covered, how much the insurance will pay for each one, and how long the coverage will last (it usually lasts a year, which is known as policy year, but some plans may have a shorter duration).

In general, health care coverage can be public (less common, provided via government programs like Medicaid) or private (more common, usually provided by the patient's employer). In certain cases, patients have limited plans that only cover a specific type of condition (for example, cancer plans).

Health insurance plans may have a network of health care professionals and facilities (in-network providers), and the plan encourages their customers to see this pool of providers. The health care plan may still work with other providers (out-of-network providers) at a higher price for the consumer. In some cases, the plan only covers in-network providers, and the patient has to pay the full price of items and services provided by out-of-network providers.

The federal government of the United States provides coverage through Medicare, Medicaid, TRICARE, and CHAMPVA.

Medicare

Medicare provides the Original plan, which provides insurance to patients who are over sixty-five years old or to younger patients with disabilities or End-Stage Renal Disease (ESRD).

- Medicare Part A helps to cover inpatient care in hospitals and skilled nursing facilities, and may also help to cover hospice and home health care in some cases.
- Medicare Part B helps to cover outpatient care, home health care, services from physicians, durable medical equipment (such as walkers, beds, wheelchairs), and certain preventive services (screenings, immunization, IPPE, and AWVs).
- Medicare Part C, also known as Medicare Advantage plans, are plans provided by private companies with the approval of Medicare (Part A and Part B coverage).
- Medicare Part D provides prescription drug coverage in outpatient settings. It is provided by private insurance companies approved by Medicare.

Medicaid

Medicaid plans are plans jointly managed by federal and state governments that provide health benefits for indigent or low-income patients. The federal government defines the standard for the programs, but Medicaid is mostly administered at the state level. As a result, Medicaid has different names in each state: Medi-Cal (California), Oregon Health Plan (Oregon), TennCare (Tennessee), etc.

TRICARE and CHAMPVA

TRICARE provides benefits to military personnel, retired personnel, veterans, and the families of uniformed and retired personnel. The Civilian Health and Medical Program of the Veterans Administration (CHAMPVA) benefits the families of veterans with total and permanent disabilities related to their service.

Health Insurance Terminology

Premium: Coverage cost for the health insurance plan or policy.

Coinsurance: Fixed percentage of costs of a covered service or item paid by the patient/consumer after paying a deductible.

Cost sharing: Share of costs for covered services or items paid out of pocket by the patient/consumer.

Deductible: Amount paid by the patient/consumer for a covered service or item before the insurer pays the rest of the expenses.

Copayment or copay: A fixed amount paid by the consumer for a covered service or item after the payment of the deductible.

Insurance benefits: The payments for services or items submitted by the insurer under a predefined plan or policy.

Health maintenance organization (HMO): This type of plan mostly covers in-network providers, but may accept out-of-network providers in certain situations, such as emergencies or after a prior authorization has been approved.

Exclusive provider organization (EPO): This type of plan generally only works with in-network providers with the exception of an emergency.

Point of service (POS): This type of plan encourages using in-network providers by providing discounted prices. A referral is required to see a specialist.

Preferred provider organization (PPO): This type of plan encourages using in-network providers by providing discounted prices. Patients/consumers can use out-of-network providers without referral and additional cost.

Insurance claim: Request for payment to the insurance company after an incident (hospitalization, accidental injury, etc.).

Paper claim: This is the CMS-1500 claim form, which is the most commonly used and obligatory for all Medicare patients.

UCR: Usual, customary, and reasonable (UCR) fee. This compares the fee charged by the doctor with the fee charged by most doctors in a community and the appropriate price for such service.

Medical billing cycle: This is the process that allows the payment of the health care provider for their services.

Third-party payer: A plan that carries the risk of paying for the services of the patient (i.e., the insurance company, Medicaid, Medicare).

Carrier: Insurer, insurance company, third-party payer.

Acceptance of assignment: The agreement by the provider of the amount established by the insurer.

Allowed charge: The maximum charge that will be covered by the insurer.

Disallowed charge: The difference between the amount billed by the provider and the amount paid by the insurer (the resulting amount is written off and not paid by the patient/consumer).

Limiting charge: For providers that do not accept assignments, this is the highest charge for a specific service.

Subscriber: The insured person in an insurance contract.

Beneficiary: The person who receives the benefits from the insurance plan.

Waiting period: The time during which the insured person is not eligible to receive the benefits from the plan.

Explanation of benefits: A document that describes the determination of the amount of the benefit.

Exclusions: Expenses not covered by the plan.

Utilization: Usage pattern for the service.

Health information management: The hospital department that manages the medical records.

Patient encounter form: Document with details from a visit, used for billing.

Advanced Beneficiary Notice: Also known as ABN, this a notice issued by health care providers to Medicare beneficiaries when a medical service or item may not be covered or paid for by Medicare. If the patient wants to receive the medical service or item, the health care provider may ask the patient to pay upfront and bill Medicare If Medicare accepts the claim, the patient receives a refund. If Medicare denies the claim, the patient may appeal the decision.

Government Regulations

The Promoting Interoperability Programs, previously known as Meaningful Use, are incentive programs established by the Centers for Medicare and Medicaid Services (CMS) in 2011 that encourage eligible providers to adopt, implement, upgrade, and demonstrate meaningful use of certified electronic health record technology (CEHRT). Eligible providers include eligible professionals, eligible hospitals, and critical access hospitals—upon meeting the program criteria, they may receive incentive payments. In 2018, the CMS expanded the purpose of the plan beyond meaningful use to include interoperability and information exchange.

The Medicare Access and CHIP Reauthorization Act (MACRA) is a law that regulates payments to physicians by Medicare. MACRA adopts the value-based payment program, the Quality Payment Program (QPP). QPP allows physicians to pick the Merit-based Incentive Payment System (MIPS) track or the Advanced Alternative Payment Model (AAPM) track.

CMS Billing and Documentation Requirements

The CMS is in charge of developing guidelines for billing and documentation, which aim to promote accountability, transparency, and accuracy in the billing process—this includes adherence to coding, compliance regulations (Health Insurance Portability and Accountability Act and the False Claims Act), and documentation standards.

A transparent and efficient billing process requires knowledge of diagnostic and procedural coding, such as the Current Procedural Terminology (CPT), which allows accurate communication between health care providers, patients, and payers. Adequate coding is not only necessary for communicating the billed services, but is also necessary to facilitate reimbursements and avoid fraud.

The main role of documentation regulation is to ensure that the billed services are medically appropriate. Therefore, documentation must accurately reflect the patient's health information. The Evaluation and Management (E/M) guidelines describe the documentation requirements for visits.

The use of online banking through deposits and electronic transfers has increased significantly in recent times, which allows the fast processing and error reduction of incoming payments from payers (patients, insurers, and third-party payers).

Prior Authorizations

Prior Authorization (PA) is a request that is necessary before a health care provider can provide a medical service, such as surgery, laboratory test, imaging study, prescription, or other types of medical services. PA is required when the insurance plan does not cover a medical service or item without first evaluating their medical necessity or cost-effectiveness. These authorizations can be declined by the insurer, and the health care provider may appeal the decision or modify the therapeutic option for one approved by the insurance company.

In some cases, PAs are confused with referrals. It is important to note that referrals are issued by primary care providers so their patients can see a specialist. The insurance plan may require a referral with an in-network specialist, but this is not a PA.

Diagnostic and Procedural Codes

There are two basic medical coding systems—diagnostic and procedural, and they are used during the billing process to standardize and simplify the evaluation of medical necessity and identification of each medical service or item. Each diagnostic or procedural code references a specific diagnosis or procedure.

The International Classification of Diseases (ICD) is a commonly used classification system in the United States. The United States uses the ICD-10-CM (for diagnostic codes) and ICD-10-PCS (for procedure codes in inpatient settings).

The Current Procedural Terminology (CPT), which is published by the American Medical Association, is used for procedure codes for physicians or outpatient settings. These codes are five-digit numbers, which are divided into six sections.

The Health Care Financing Administration Common Procedure Coding System (HCPCS) is the system employed to report medical services for Medicare patients and includes three levels: level I codes (repeats CPT codes), level II codes (eighteen sections with new codes, not listed in CPT), and level III codes (local codes used only by insurance companies in their specific region).

Aging Reports, Collections Due, Adjustments, and Write-Offs

Aging reports are used to monitor how long claims and balances have been outstanding. In most cases, the reports are organized into different ranges (zero to thirty days, thirty-one to sixty days, sixty-one to ninety days, and so on), and the amount for each range is presented in dollars and percentages. This information helps to evaluate the liquidity of the office and which insurance companies are paying.

Collections due is the amount of money that payers (insurance companies, patients, third-party payers) owe to the medical office or facility.

Adjustments are the amount subtracted from the total charges when the health care provider or the facility, for any reason, has decided not to charge.

A write-off is the amount that the health care provider or facility deducts from a charge. In this case, the payment is considered to be uncollectible due to payer bankruptcy, insolvency, or other motives. The practice "writes off" the debt. It is important to follow the regulatory guidelines to avoid fraud.

Auditing Methods, Processes, and Sign-Offs

Auditing is the systematic review and verification of financial data to evaluate its accuracy. The auditing process can be internal (performed by an in-house group) or external (outsourced to a medical billing company).

In general, auditing will cover various processes. The team will collect all the relevant data (billing documents, medical records, relevant regulations, etc.), although this may vary according to the needs of each auditing process (for example, an audit may be focused on regulatory compliance or coding accuracy). Then, the relevant data is analyzed, and the final report includes findings, observations, and recommendations to implement.

Sign-offs are used for approval at various stages of the auditing process. The team may sign off on the auditing plan, process, and implementation of recommendations.

Data Entry and Data Fields

Data entry is an integral part of recording, coding, and billing processes. The management of patient and insurance data demands accuracy and the adequate use of standardized terminology (diagnostic and procedural codes), as well as agility during the data entry process to avoid unnecessarily slowing down the delivery of medical care. Data management in medical offices and other health care settings also implies the use of private and confidential patient information. Therefore, MAs must be compliant with HIPAA regulations when handling private information.

Some of the most important data fields in various health care settings include:

- Health care provider information (name, address, phone number, and professional information).
- Patient demographic information (name, gender, date of birth, address, insurance information).
- Medical history.
- Family history.
- Chief complaint.
- Vital signs and clinical findings.
- Paraclinical findings.
- Diagnosis.
- Treatments.
- Patient consent.
- Billing and coding data (insurance information, diagnostic and procedural codes, received payments, outstanding payments).
- Appointment information (date, contact information, appointment management information).

Equipment in Health Care Facilities

Hospitals, medical offices, and other health care facilities require facility (vacuum systems, elevators, air compressors, etc.) and medical (ventilators, IV infusion equipment, electrosurgery units, etc.) equipment for the adequate delivery of care, and these facilities have to keep accurate inspection or maintenance logs.

The CMS (2013) recommends to keep an equipment inventory with the following information:

- Unique identification number.
- Manufacturer.
- Model number.
- Serial number.
- Description of the equipment.
- Location (when the location is generally fixed).
- Department that owns the equipment.
- Identification of the service provider.
- Acceptance date.
- Any additional information that may be useful for the management of the equipment.

The required inspection schedule may vary between devices due to their function, usage, and safety profile. For example, stethoscopes or wheelchairs do not need frequent inspections, especially when compared with sterilization equipment.

The main regulatory bodies in relation to equipment inspection and maintenance of equipment in health care facilities are the U.S. Food and Drug Administration (FDA) and the Occupational Safety and Health Administration (OSHA), and the CMS (2013) provides thorough guidance in "Hospital Equipment Maintenance Requirements."

Telehealth and Virtual Visit Technologies

Telehealth, also known as telemedicine, is an emerging way of providing various health care services and health-related information without needing an in-person appointment. Although telehealth started with remote consultations via telephone or radio, this practice has become prevalent now in the digital era, especially after the COVID-19 pandemic in 2020. Virtual visits, remote patient monitoring, remote surgery, telepharmacy, patient portals, and other health care services can be provided through telehealth.

The adequate delivery of telehealth services requires a robust telecommunication infrastructure that supports fast and secure internet connections. As a result, telehealth technologies may include:

- **Video communication software** (Zoom, Google Meets, Microsoft Teams, and other platforms) — These programs usually allow users to communicate via video, audio, and text. Most of them are also available for various devices and operating systems.
- **Mobile health care apps** — These apps provide various services. Apps like Teladoc, MDlive, and Amwell provide medical consultation for patients. Apps like Lecturio and Osmosis Med provide education to health care students. Apps like Epocrates, UpToDate, and Drugs.com provide clinical and drug information for health care providers.
- **Remote monitoring** — This can be achieved via wearable devices like smartwatches, but it also includes remote monitoring from pulse oximeters, blood pressure monitors, EKG monitors, glucose monitors, etc. These devices can send information directly to the patient's health care provider in inpatient or outpatient settings, which can be used during diagnosis and treatment.

Barriers to Access for Virtual Visits

- Some patients or health care providers may not have the knowledge required to manage telehealth software and apps.

- It is not possible to perform a thorough physical exam during a virtual visit. Examination can only employ visual examination and remote monitoring, when available.
- The patient and the health care provider may not speak the same language.
- Technical issues like incompatibility, software bugs, and poor internet connection.

Chapter 6: Communication and Customer Service

Cultural, Religious, Psychosocial, and Economic Considerations That Impact Provision of Care

Holistic considerations in health care delivery include cultural, religious, psychosocial, and economic factors. These considerations are necessary in many instances to maximize care in inpatient and outpatient settings

Cultural factors shape the way patients view health, drugs, diseases, and the healing process. An important cultural consideration, for example, is the concept of "face" in Asian cultures, which references the need to preserve dignity and prestige throughout the diagnosis and treatment process. Latin American patients, on the other hand, tend to favor the use of home remedies alongside traditional medicine and rely on familial support.

Religious beliefs can significantly affect the preferred therapies of patients. Jehovah's Witnesses are against blood transfusions, and some individuals in certain Christian evangelical groups may reject the use of vaccines (Swan, 2020). Certain religious groups may also have dietary restrictions or may require accommodations for prayer as an inpatient.

Mental health can have an impact on the effectiveness of medical treatments for physical conditions. Anxiety and depression, both relatively common during disease, may impair patient compliance and result in less favorable outcomes. Similarly, economic concerns due to health care costs and insurance coverage may affect the psychosocial landscape of the patients.

Gender Identity and Use of Pronouns

Gender is the group of characteristics associated with being male or female. These are associated with psychosocial, cultural, and behavioral factors. Gender identity is the inner sense of gender, which may align with being male, female, both, or neither. Similarly, gender may or may not align with the person's sex assigned at birth. As a result, it is important to know how to use pronouns, not only as a courtesy to patients but as a way to connect with them and provide the best care possible.

Pronouns are words used to replace a noun. Examples of pronouns are "I," "me," us," "he," "she," "him," "her," "they," "them," "theirs," "myself," "herself," etc. Pronouns denote someone's gender, which may or may not align with the person's gender identity. In most cases, if the pronouns used do not align with a person's gender, the person will correct you. To avoid such situations, MAs can ask their patients about their preferred pronouns or use gender-neutral pronouns like the singular form of "they" (they, them, theirs).

Patient Factors That Affect Communication

- **Biological barriers**: A patient's condition or disability may affect their capacity to engage meaningfully in a conversation, which limits their understanding and involvement in their own care when not taken into account. Examples include patients with dementia, stroke, or hearing loss. Biological barriers also include age and development. Pediatric patients may have a harder time understanding and expressing their symptoms and concerns.
- **Language barriers**: In some cases, patients and health care providers do not speak the same language. However, language barriers may go beyond that: patients may not have health literacy and may misinterpret certain words. It is important to speak clearly and avoid excessive use of medical terms.
- **Physical and infrastructure barriers**: The advent of telehealth has reduced the issue of geographical distance for various medical services. However, poor technological infrastructure may introduce new problems for patients during virtual visits, such as poor internet connection or lack of proper equipment.
- **Psychosocial factors**: Depression, fear, anxiety, and other psychological factors may affect the way patients understand and convey information to their health care provider.

Nonverbal Cues for In-Person and Telehealth Communication

Nonverbal communication refers to communication that does not have linguistic content, which includes eye contact, facial expressions, posture, hand gestures, and voice characteristics (pitch, rate, volume). These cues are relevant for both in-person and virtual visits, but MAs may need to consider certain factors to apply them effectively in each setting.

Nonverbal cues during in-person visits can be used to comfort a patient, transmit empathy, and enhance the patient's sense of safety, as well as create rapport with them.

Most strategies used during in-person visits can also be used during virtual visits, but camera positioning, camera angle, and lighting play an important role in the process. There is no physical proximity with the patient, but nonverbal cues like nodding and eye contact can be used to let the patient feel heard. Remember that looking at the camera emulates eye contact during video communication.

The Communication Cycle

The communication cycle represents the interactions between patient and health care provider with the purpose of exchanging information. Both participants are responsible for receiving and transmitting information. An important consideration is noise, which may affect how the information is transmitted or interpreted. Noise can be loud or distracting sounds, but it can also include pain, anxiety, fear, etc.

Therapeutic Communication

Therapeutic communication is a group of communication techniques with the objective of improving interactions with patients. It involves the use of nonverbal cues, being a good listener, taking cultural and religious context into consideration, and controlling your emotions.

Interviewing and Questioning Techniques

- Introduce yourself.
- Practice active listening.
- Use nonverbal cues appropriately.
- Do not use leading questions. These questions may prompt specific responses from the patient, which greatly affects the information provided by the patient.
- Take cultural and religious context into consideration.
- Use open-ended questions. It is important that patients elaborate their responses, but closed questions limit the patient's response to "yes" or "no," which results in a loss of context.
- Closed questions can be used when you need to ask about specific information. Closed questions can be followed by an open question.
- Do not hesitate to return to the patient to clarify or ask for more information when necessary.

Scope of Permitted Questions and Boundaries

MAs have to take patient privacy during the interviewing process, as well as keep the patient's trust and dignity intact. The scope of permitted questions includes the gathering of relevant information for the patient's health record: past procedures, medication history, allergies, past hospitalizations, family history, current symptoms, and other clinically relevant information. All questioning should be respectful.

An important factor to take into consideration during history taking is context, which helps to set the boundaries to avoid inappropriate questions. In health care, uncomfortable questions are not uncommon. It is the job of professionals to use their expertise to avoid embarrassing their patients. Avoid asking personal or unnecessary questions that are not directly related to the care of the patient. If an MA has to ask a potentially uncomfortable question, closed questions can be used so the patient does not feel the need to unnecessarily elaborate their answer.

For example, in a situation in which it is necessary to know if the patient has engaged in a specific sexual behavior recently, an open question like "What kind of sexual acts do you do with your partner?" is unnecessary, invasive, and personal. An appropriate question could be "Have you had oral sex in the last couple of weeks?" Also, do not forget to provide context to the patient, explain to them why you are asking such questions, and let them know you are not judging them.

Active Listening Techniques

The main task of an active listener is to understand what the patient is trying to say. Active listening does not only involve hearing what the patient is saying. Active listening is bidirectional, and the active listener asks questions and encourages the patient the elaborate. This is in contrast with a passive listener, who only listens.

Active listening allows the patient to feel heard, encourages the clarification of information, and takes the patient's feelings into consideration. The main tools used by active listeners are:

- **Clarification**: Attempt to clarify the patient's message with phrases and questions like "Can you explain this in more detail?" or "Can you give me an example of that?"
- **Restatement**: Paraphrase what the patient is saying. For example, "Then, what you are trying to say is that..." or "So the problem is..."
- **Reflection**: Acknowledge the patient's feelings by reflecting on them. For example, "You seem to be frustrated by..."

Feedback and Coaching

MAs can use feedback and coaching as communication tools to the benefit of patients in various ways. Feedback is mainly retrospective and can be used to reflect on past actions or events. For example, it can be used to highlight positive behaviors and encourage the patient. Feedback can also be constructive, which helps the patient to identify a problem and improve.

Coaching, on the other hand, is developmental and aims toward the future. It can be used to enhance the patient's development through active listening and guidance. This is useful to help the patient understand their medical condition and treatment options, which increases patient compliance and capacity for self-care. It also allows the patient to participate meaningfully in their care.

Telephone Etiquette

MAs may handle various types of calls as part of their work activities. Calls from patients (for scheduling new and recurring patients, or answering questions from patients) are common, but MAs will also interact with laboratories, insurance companies, other medical offices, and salespeople. Regardless of who is calling, everyone should be treated with attention and respect.

When handling calls, remember to greet the person calling and introduce yourself. The scheduling process requires you to ask for certain information. For new patients, do not forget to ask about insurance details and the name of the referring physician when applicable. For recurring patients, ask for the patient's name, reason for visiting, and if any insurance information has changed.

In all cases, MAs must avoid disclosing protected health information. For example, if a caller asks about the condition of a specific patient (by name), no information should be disclosed without proper authorization.

Email Etiquette

- Emails are useful for non-urgent communication.
- Emails should have a concise subject line that accurately describes the contents of the email.
- Start an email with a salutation, such as "Dear..." and finish with a closing, such as "Best regards," alongside your name and contact information.
- Double-check the contents of the email for errors.
- Upon receiving an email, it is important to confirm the receipt of the message and provide a response as soon as possible.

Business Letter Format

A basic business letter is composed of the following:

- Letterhead, which includes the sender's address.
- Date (Month XX, 20XX; e.g., February 24, 2024).
- Inside address (recipient's address).
- Salutation.
- Subject.
- Body.

- Closing.
- Signature block.
- Identification line.
- Notations.

Professional-looking fonts like Times New Roman and Arial (size 12) are frequently used. The block format is the most common, and it consists of using single spaces between lines and double spaces between paragraphs with all text left justified.

Patient Satisfaction Surveys

Patient satisfaction surveys are used to assess the quality of care provided in a health care facility. These surveys can be varied, and they can be created by the facility or commissioned to a third party.

Most hospitals use the Hospital Consumer Assessment of Healthcare Providers and Systems Survey (HCAHPS), which was created by the CMS alongside the AHRQ to facilitate the evaluation and comparison of care quality between hospitals. The HCAHPS is a standardized survey with twenty-seven questions.

Conflict Management

Conflicts occur all the time in human relationships, and they also occur in health care settings. Patients may become frustrated, fearful, or anxious. In some cases, their medical condition may result in or facilitate agitation and aggressive responses (for example, delirium in elderly patients with electrolyte imbalances). Therefore, health care professionals should be equipped with tools to de-escalate these situations.

De-escalation consists of recognizing the aggressive patient and defusing the aggressive situation. The aggressive patient may be verbally abusive or yelling, refuse to eat or drink, engage in self-harm, breathe heavily, have a threatening appearance (clenched fists, stares, poor hygiene), or be actively violent against objects or people (throwing objects, punching walls, hitting people).

The Dix and Page model is a de-escalation model based on three components: assessment, communication, and tactics (ACT). Assessment refers to the recognition of an aggressive behavior. Communication refers to verbal and nonverbal communication strategies used during de-escalation (therapeutic communication, active listening, avoiding physical contact, avoiding medical terminology, being sincere). Finally, tactics refer to context-specific situations and they are used to invalidate the patient's need for aggression.

Some strategies to de-escalate aggressive behavior may include:

- Early recognition of aggression.
- Active listening.
- Non-threatening body language.
- Gain the trust of the patient by answering to their problem and acknowledging their feelings.
- Provide solutions.
- Practice de-escalation with all the staff.

Escalation of Problematic Situations

Whenever a professional identifies that the severity of a situation is greater than expected or a conflict cannot be resolved with the current approach, it may be necessary to escalate.

The AHRQ developed the CUS ("Concern-Uncomfortable-Stop") method to encourage health care professionals to speak up and escalate when necessary by stating they are concerned and why. If unresolved, the health care professional states, "I am uncomfortable." If the concern remains, the health care professional declares that there is a safety issue in place. At this point, if the issue persists unresolved, the health care professional may escalate the concern to a defined contact in the office or department.

Incident/Event/Unusual Occurrence Reports

Any unwanted or unexpected event, incidental or accidental, that may potentially result in harm to the staff, patients, or visitors must be documented and reported to a superior and/or someone in charge of risk management in the facility. The tool utilized for reporting these issues is an Unusual Occurrence Report (also known as an Incident Report or Event Report).

The exact reporting protocol may vary from one facility to the other, but it usually includes the following information:

- Who was directly affected, where, and when?
- Witnesses.
- Objective summary of the event.
- Description of the area (floor, walls, illumination).
- Who was notified of the event?

Do not include subjective information in the report. Do not assign blame or provide personal opinions.

Cause and Effect Analysis

Cause and effect analysis, also known as root cause analysis, is a system that helps to identify the causes of a problem, such as adverse events.

Diagrams are frequently used during this analysis. For example, the fishbone diagram, which resembles a fishbone with a head and spine. This consists of writing the problem on the right side (head) and a central line to the left (spine) with diagonal lines (bones). Each diagonal line contains a group (equipment, patient, provider, environment, etc.) and possible causes. Each cause is analyzed and discussed among professionals, which helps to identify the most important causes and find a solution.

Professional Presence

A professional presence is necessary to establish a positive relationship with patients and colleagues—it inspires and transmits respect, integrity, responsibility, and confidence.

An MA should work on their presence as a health care professional, and should consider the various key components of professional presence:

- **Appearance** — Patients prefer when health care providers dress formally or wear scrubs. Hygiene and grooming are also very important.
- **Mindfulness** — Health care settings can be very tense, and as a result, emotional intelligence plays a major role. MAs should be able to stay focused in stressful situations. It is important to display empathy and compassion without emotionally involving yourself with the patient.
- **Ethics** — MAs must follow their Code of Ethics (for example, the NHA Code of Ethics), which includes honesty, protecting and respecting the dignity and privacy of patients, and acting in the interest of the general public.
- **Communication** — Remember to be an active listener and use nonverbal cues in your daily work.

Chapter 7: Medical Law and Ethics

Laws and Regulations

Health Insurance Portability and Accountability Act (HIPAA) – This is a privacy rule that addresses the disclosure and use of protected health information.

Affordable Care Act (ACA) or **Patient Protection and Affordable Care Act (PPACA)** – This includes comprehensive health insurance and health care reforms. It facilitates access to health insurance for more people within the federal poverty level. It is commonly called "Obamacare."

Controlled Substances Act (CSA) – This regulates various processes (the manufacturing, distribution, use, etc.) associated with certain regulated substances organized via the Scheduling System (schedules I, II, III, IV, and V).

Health Information Technology for Economic and Clinical Health (HITECH) Act – This is a law that aims to promote the use of technology and EHRs to favor efficiency, privacy, and safety in the health care system.

Public Readiness and Emergency Preparedness (PREP) Act – This is a law that authorizes the Secretary of HHS to provide liability protection through a PREP Act declaration to individuals or groups in relation to the administration of medical countermeasures.

HHS Acquisition Regulation (HHSAR) – This implements the Federal Acquisition Regulation in the HHS.

21st Century Cures Act – This is a rule that provides resources to the National Institutes of Health to promote research in biomedical sciences.

Social Security Act – This is a law that provides general welfare by establishing a federal system of benefits for people who are retired, jobless, or have a disability.

Patient Self Determination Act (PDSA) – This requires health care workers, facilities, and organizations to inform patients of their rights, which includes their right to participate in the decision-making process related to their own medical care.

Consent in Health Care

Consent is the permission, granted by the patient, to allow any action by a health care worker, such as touching, receiving treatment, or disclosing information. Consent is not permanent, and a patient may withdraw their consent whenever they want. Consent is not required for treatment during an emergency situation in which the delay of said treatment threatens the well-being and/or life of the patient.

There are three basic types of consent: informed, implied, and expressed:

- **Informed consent** — Consent is formally granted (e.g., a written and signed informed consent) by a mentally competent person after receiving adequate information about the treatment or procedure, which includes a description of the procedure, as well as its risks and benefits.
- **Implied consent** — Consent is granted without an explicit communication of consent—the patient accepts a treatment or procedure through their actions (or inaction). For example, consent is implied for an unconscious patient who requires emergency treatment.
- **Expressed consent** — Consent is granted by the patient through explicit communication.

Advanced Directives

An advanced directive, also known as a living will or advance decision, is a legal document that specifies in advance a person's wishes and preferences in relation to their health in case they are no longer capable of deciding for themselves in the future due to an illness. Furthermore, one or more people may serve as spokespersons on behalf of the patient in such circumstances.

Advanced directives may include preferences related to various medical interventions that may be needed in emergency situations, such as cardiopulmonary resuscitation (CPR) or endotracheal intubation. Examples include Do-Not-Resuscitate (DNR), Do-Not-Intubate (DNI), Allow Natural Death (AND), and orders related to organ or tissue donation.

Legal Guardianship and Power of Attorney

Although the concept of a legal guardian and power of attorney are similar at first glance, there are important differences to consider.

Legal guardianship is a person (guardian) appointed by a court that is in charge of managing health care and finance decisions for someone who is unable to make said decisions.

Power of attorney is a legal document in which a person grants another person the power to act on their behalf. However, a power of attorney is nullified once a person becomes incapacitated for any reason (except for a durable power of attorney).

Legal guardianship requires a hearing before being effective but power of attorney does not. Legal guardianship is appointed by a court and can be contested, while power of attorney is requested by the person that desires to appoint an agent.

Legal Requirements Related to Maintenance, Storage, and Disposal of Records

Maintenance of records may vary between states, but they will usually require a minimum time during which it is legally required to maintain records. However, insurance providers or plans may also require a specific retention period. If this period is different from the state-mandated period, use the longer period. There is no definite maximum time to maintain patient records.

Health information must be safely stored and protected from natural damage, theft, and accidental disclosure. The management of a large volume of records may require a record storage company with experience in confidentiality and health information.

The disposal or destruction of records (according to the HIPAA Medical Records Destruction Rules) requires an assessment to consider potential privacy risks associated with the destruction process. Destruction of paper records must render the information permanently indecipherable (e.g., shredding). In some instances, deleted information in digital storage devices can be restored. Therefore, the device carrying this information should be destroyed via pulverization, melting, incineration, etc.

If unsure in relation to the maintenance, storage, and destruction of records, it is recommended to seek professional advice on compliance.

Conditions for Sharing or Releasing Information

The release of patient information is a process regulated by the HIPAA Privacy Rule. According to HIPAA, information can be shared with family members and friends if the patient gives express permission (for example, by inviting their friend or family member into the room so they can hear the treatment plan) or if the provider determines through professional judgment that sharing the information is in the best interest of the patient (for example, an emergency physician communicating the condition of an unconscious patient to their family member).

The formal request for the release of any type of patient information (the Release of Information form) from the health care facility/provider to a third party (Medicare, private insurance companies, friends and family members, etc.) requires the approval of the patient (generally in a written document, but electronic signatures can be accepted, too).

The legal guardian or parents of a minor are generally allowed access to the information of the minor, except for situations in which the minor is able to consent, care is authorized by a court, or whenever the minor and provider agree that the minor can have a confidential relationship.

A lawsuit may require the release of patient information (for example, in the case of a liability suit initiated by the patient against the provider). If the request form for information release during the lawsuit's discovery process is signed by the patient, the provider may proceed and comply with the request.

Medical Malpractice

Medical malpractice stems from negligence or substandard care due to a lack of knowledge or experience of a health care professional during a professional act that results in harm to the patient. To avoid malpractice claims, it is important to follow professional guidelines and learn to communicate effectively with patients. Malpractice can be categorized as:

- **Misfeasance**: Inappropriate execution of a legal act (e.g., the inadequate use of a non-sterile instrument during a sterile procedure).
- **Malfeasance**: Performance of an illegal act (e.g., a medical assistant prescribing medication).
- **Nonfeasance**: Failure to perform a required act (e.g., failure to call a physician during an emergency).

Mandatory Reporting

The reporting of mistreatment and abuse is a legal duty for workers (such as health care providers) who are frequently in contact with vulnerable populations. The exact populations protected may vary from state to state, but generally include children, people with disabilities, and the elderly.

In the particular case of health care professionals, reporting laws also include certain infectious diseases. The National Notifiable Conditions is published annually by the CDC.

Test 1

(1) Which of the following is regarded as an administrative duty of a medical assistant?

(A) Assist during examinations.

(B) Manage appointments and office supplies.

(C) Provide wound care.

(D) Perform cardiopulmonary resuscitation.

(2) Which of the following roles is not regarded as a clinical duty of a medical assistant?

(A) Dispose of waste.

(B) Prepare examination and treatment areas.

(C) Perform medical transcription.

(D) Assist during examinations.

(3) What is the main role of a licensed practical nurse (LPN)?

(A) Provide basic nursing care.

(B) Perform surgical procedures.

(C) Administer anesthesia.

(D) Manage patient records.

(4) Which of the following is a common treatment option for back acne?

(A) Topical retinoids.

(B) Antifungal creams.

(C) Moisturizing lotion.

(D) Sunscreen.

(5) What is the difference between a certification and a license in the healthcare field?

(A) A certification is only required in certain states.

(B) A certification is a third-party verification, while a federal, state, or local government agency grants a license.

(C) A license allows professionals to practice in any state.

(D) A license is a third-party verification, while a federal, state, or local government agency grants a certification.

(6) Which type of patient care necessitates admission of the patient into a healthcare facility?

(A) Hospice care.

(B) Outpatient care.

(C) Inpatient care.

(D) Home healthcare.

(7) Which type of care involves healthcare providers with advanced and specialized training in areas like cardiology, neurology, and dermatology?

(A) Primary care.

(B) Specialty care.

(C) Ancillary care.

(D) Complementary care.

(8) What is the main difference between complementary and alternative medicine?

(A) Complementary medicine is used alongside standard medical treatment, while alternative medicine is not.

(B) Complementary medicine is only used for chronic conditions.

(C) Alternative medicine is always supported by extensive research.

(D) Complementary medicine is not safe or effective.

(9) Why is it important for patients to discuss complementary therapies with their healthcare provider before implementation?

(A) To ensure they are covered by insurance.

(B) To receive a prescription for the therapy.

(C) To ensure there is enough research to support their use and that they are safe for specific conditions.

(D) To avoid any additional costs.

(10) Which of the following is an example of therapeutic services?

(A) Laboratory tests.

(B) Genetic testing.

(C) Dialysis.

(D) Cardiac monitoring.

(11) Which of the following constitutes the last part of a word and modifies the root?

(A) Prefix.

(B) Root.

(C) Suffix.

(D) Both prefix and suffix.

(12) What does the prefix ecto- indicate?

(A) New.

(B) Painful.

(C) Both.

(D) Outside.

(13) Which of the following describes the condition of *otalgia*?

(A) Shortness of breath.

(B) Pain in the ear.

(C) Itching.

(D) Puffiness.

(14) Which of the following describes the condition of *dyspnea*?

(A) Shortness of breath.

(B) Upset stomach.

(C) Lack of strength.

(D) Numbness.

(15) Which of the following would describe the condition of *hyperglycemia*?

(A) High blood sugar.

(B) Low blood sugar.

(C) Puffiness.

(D) Heartburn.

(16) Which term describes a position that is closer to the surface of the body?

(A) Superficial.

(B) Deep.

(C) Lateral.

(D) Proximal.

(17) If a structure is described as *distal*, where is it located in relation to the point of attachment or trunk?

(A) Close to the point of attachment or trunk.

(B) Away from the point of attachment or trunk.

(C) Toward the midline of the body.

(D) Farther away from the surface of the body.

(18) Which directional terms describe movement toward the head and away from the feet?

(A) Superior/cranial.

(B) Inferior/caudal.

(C) Anterior/ventral.

(D) Posterior/dorsal.

(19) Which terms refer to the back of the body?

(A) Superior/cranial.

(B) Inferior/caudal.

(C) Anterior/ventral.

(D) Posterior/dorsal.

(20) Which term describes a location that is closer to the point of attachment or trunk?

(A) Proximal.

(B) Distal.

(C) Superficial.

(D) Deep.

(21) Which plane divides the body into anterior and posterior regions?

(A) Sagittal/lateral plane.

(B) Frontal/coronal plane.

(C) Transverse/axial plane.

(D) Oblique/diagonal plane.

(22) Which plane divides the body into upper and lower regions?

(A) Sagittal/lateral plane.

(B) Frontal/coronal plane.

(C) Transverse/axial plane.

(D) Oblique/diagonal plane.

(23) Which plane divides the body into right and left sides?

(A) Sagittal/lateral plane.

(B) Frontal/coronal plane.

(C) Transverse/axial plane.

(D) Oblique/diagonal plane.

(24) A patient who recognizes the disease and feels sadness experiences which stage of grief?

(A) Denial and isolation.

(B) Anger.

(C) Bargaining.

(D) Depression.

(25) All of the following describe the main parts of a human cell except:

(A) Cell membrane.

(B) Cytoplasm.

(C) Nucleus.

(D) Ribosomes.

(26) Which organelle translates information from messenger RNA into amino acids during protein synthesis?

(A) Ribosomes.

(B) Mitochondria.

(C) Golgi apparatus.

(D) Lysosomes.

(27) All the following are functions of the endoplasmic reticulum except:

(A) Protein synthesis.

(B) Lipid metabolism.

(C) Transportation of substances.

(D) Photosynthesis.

(28) Which type of muscle tissue is voluntary and connected to the bone?

(A) Skeletal muscle.

(B) Cardiac muscle.

(C) Smooth muscle.

(D) Neural muscle.

(29) Which tissue is mainly responsible for the body's movement?

(A) Epithelial tissue.

(B) Connective tissue.

(C) Muscle tissue.

(D) Nervous tissue.

(30) Which system is responsible for transporting blood and nutrients to the tissues?

(A) Cardiovascular system.

(B) Gastrointestinal system.

(C) Respiratory system.

(D) Musculoskeletal system.

(31) Which system is responsible for motion, posture, and heat production?

(A) Cardiovascular system.

(B) Gastrointestinal system.

(C) Musculoskeletal system.

(D) Nervous system.

(32) Which two major components does the central nervous system include?

(A) Brain and spinal cord.

(B) Nerves and ganglia.

(C) Kidneys and ureters.

(D) Immune cells and lymph nodes.

(33) Which system helps defend the body from foreign substances or organisms?

(A) Urinary system.

(B) Endocrine system.

(C) Immune system.

(D) Respiratory system.

(34) Which condition is characterized by inflammation and pain in the hair follicles?

(A) Alzheimer's disease.

(B) Acute cholecystitis.

(C) Allergic rhinitis.

(D) Acne.

(35) Which condition severely affects cognitive abilities and memory?

(A) Acne.

(B) Alzheimer's disease.

(C) Myocardial infarction.

(D) Appendicitis.

(36) A patient's medical history usually includes all of the following information except:

(A) A patient's past and present health concerns.

(B) Education and job history.

(C) Allergies.

(D) Medication usage.

(37) What does the family history section of a patient's record include?

(A) The medical information of immediate family members.

(B) The patient's allergies and medication usage.

(C) The patient's social habits and lifestyle choices.

(D) The patient's previous surgical procedures.

(38) All of the following information is usually included in the social history section of a patient except:

(A) Education level.

(B) Sleep habits and diet.

(C) The patient's previous surgical procedures.

(D) Job.

(39) The main purpose of health screenings is to:

(A) Decrease the rate of surgical procedures.

(B) Treat existing medical conditions.

(C) Monitor the progress of chronic diseases.

(D) Detect medical conditions in asymptomatic individuals.

(40) What test is commonly used to screen for cervical cancer?

(A) Blood pressure measurement.

(B) Papanicolaou smear.

(C) Thyroid-stimulating hormone level assessment.

(D) Pelvic MRI.

(41) Which screening test is conducted for patients at risk of colon cancer?

(A) Blood pressure measurement.

(B) Papanicolaou smear.

(C) Colonoscopy.

(D) Abdominal MRI.

(42) Which of the following is not a function of a mental health screening?

(A) Assess a patient's thinking, mood, and behavior.

(B) Determine the patient's response to therapy.

(C) Recognize mental disorders early.

(D) Diagnose medical illnesses early.

(43) What does wellness assessment monitor?

(A) Physical well-being only.

(B) Mental well-being only.

(C) Social well-being only.

(D) Physical, mental, and social well-being.

(44) What factors can naturally affect vital signs?

(A) Physical factors only.

(B) Psychological factors only.

(C) Physical and psychological factors.

(D) Physical and psychological factors do not affect vital signs.

(45) Which of the following vital sign derangements is not expected after physical exercise?

(A) Increased BP.

(B) Decreased temperature.

(C) Increased HR.

(D) Increased breathing rate.

(46) How is a patient's blood pressure recorded?

(A) Systolic pressure, followed by diastolic pressure.

(B) Diastolic pressure, followed by systolic pressure.

(C) Pulse rate, followed by respiratory rate.

(D) Systolic pressure, followed by pulse rate.

(47) Which blood pressure range indicates prehypertension?

(A) Systolic pressure: 120-139 mm Hg, diastolic pressure: 80-89 mm Hg.

(B) Systolic pressure: 140-159 mm Hg, diastolic pressure: 90-99 mm Hg.

(C) Systolic pressure: ≥160 mm Hg, diastolic pressure ≥100 mm Hg.

(D) Systolic pressure: ≥180 mm Hg, diastolic pressure: ≥120 mm Hg.

(48) What blood pressure measurements indicate stage 2 hypertension?

(A) Systolic pressure: ≥160 mm Hg, diastolic pressure ≥100 mm Hg.

(B) Systolic pressure: 140-159 mm Hg, diastolic pressure: 90-99 mm Hg.

(C) Systolic pressure: 120-139 mm Hg, diastolic pressure: 80-89 mm Hg.

(D) Systolic pressure: ≥180 mm Hg, diastolic pressure ≥120 mm Hg.

(49) What blood pressure measurement is generally considered hypotension or low blood pressure?

(A) Systolic pressure: <90 mm Hg, diastolic pressure: <60 mm Hg.

(B) Systolic pressure: >90 mm Hg, diastolic pressure: >60 mm Hg.

(C) Systolic pressure: <120 mm Hg, diastolic pressure: <80 mm Hg.

(D) Systolic pressure: >120 mm Hg, diastolic pressure: >80 mm Hg.

(50) Which tool is commonly used to measure a patient's temperature?

(A) Gloves.

(B) Stethoscope.

(C) Thermometer.

(D) Penlight.

(51) Reflex hammers are used to:

(A) Measure blood pressure.

(B) Enhance visualization.

(C) Check pupil response.

(D) Test neurological reflexes.

(52) Which healthcare providers commonly use a reflex hammer in their practice?

(A) Surgeons.

(B) Ophthalmologists.

(C) Neurologists.

(D) Radiologists.

(53) Ophthalmoscopes are used to:

(A) Examine the ears.

(B) Examine the eyes.

(C) Examine the throat.

(D) Examine the vagina.

(54) Which healthcare providers often use a vaginal speculum in their practice?

(A) Ear, nose, and throat (ENT) physicians.

(B) Primary care physicians.

(C) OB-GYN physicians.

(D) Surgeons.

(55) Who usually uses a nasal speculum for examinations?

(A) Ear, nose, and throat (ENT) physicians.

(B) Primary care physicians.

(C) Internists.

(D) OB-GYN physicians.

(56) Which position involves the patient lying flat on their back with arms resting at each side?

(A) Supine position.

(B) Dorsal-recumbent position.

(C) Lithotomy position.

(D) Prone position.

(57) What is the main purpose of the dorsal-recumbent position?

(A) To examine the genital and rectal areas.

(B) To examine the back.

(C) To examine the vaginal area.

(D) To examine the chest.

(58) Which position involves the use of stirrups to hold the patient's feet?

(A) Supine position.

(B) Dorsal-recumbent position.

(C) Lithotomy position.

(D) Prone position.

(59) The prone position is commonly used to:

(A) Examine the genital and rectal areas.

(B) Examine the back.

(C) Examine the vaginal area.

(D) Examine the chest.

(60) Which position is used to evaluate gait or hernias?

(A) Erect position.

(B) Sitting position.

(C) Knee-chest position.

(D) Proctological position.

(61) All of the following areas can be evaluated in the sitting position except:

(A) Reflexes and other neurological exams.

(B) Chest, back, arms, head, and neck.

(C) Lower extremities.

(D) Perianal area.

(62) What is the main purpose of the knee-chest position?

(A) Perianal and rectal examination.

(B) Lower extremities examination.

(C) Gait evaluation.

(D) Reflex assessment.

(63) The primary purpose of the Trendelenburg position is to:

(A) Examine the chest and abdomen.

(B) Evaluate gait and hernias.

(C) Provide a therapeutic measure for patients with hypotension.

(D) Assess lower-back problems.

(64) When is Fowler's position commonly used?

(A) Chest and abdomen examination.

(B) Gait and hernia evaluation.

(C) For patients with hypotension.

(D) For patients with lower-back problems or breathing difficulties in the supine position.

(65) What should a patient eat at least two or three days before a colonoscopy?

(A) A plain, low-fiber diet.

(B) Nuts, seeds, and raw vegetables.

(C) Fruits with skin and brown rice.

(D) Coffee and tea with milk.

(66) What type of diet should a patient follow the day before a colonoscopy?

(A) High-fiber diet.

(B) Clear-liquid diet.

(C) Solid food diet.

(D) Protein-rich diet.

(67) What symptoms are normal to experience after a colonoscopy?

(A) Mild abdominal cramping or bloating.

(B) Severe abdominal pain.

(C) Fever.

(D) Rectal bleeding.

(68) How many doses of the rotavirus vaccine are recommended for patients receiving RV5?

(A) One dose.

(B) Two doses.

(C) Three doses.

(D) Four doses.

(69) When should the first dose of the measles, mumps, and rubella (MMR) vaccine be administered?

(A) Two months.

(B) Six months.

(C) Twelve months.

(D) Sixteen years.

(70) When should the first dose of the meningococcal serogroup A, C, W, and Y vaccine be administered?

(A) Two months.

(B) Six months.

(C) Eleven to twelve years.

(D) Sixteen years.

(71) What is the correct option for COVID-19 vaccination for unvaccinated adults?

(A) One dose of Pfizer-BioNTech or Moderna vaccine.

(B) One dose of Novavax vaccine.

(C) Three doses of Pfizer-BioNTech or Moderna vaccine.

(D) Four doses of Novavax vaccine.

(72) When should the zoster recombinant vaccine be administered to adults?

(A) At eighteen years of age.

(B) At thirty years of age.

(C) At fifty years of age or older.

(D) At sixty-five years of age or older.

(73) What is the term used to describe the hereditary tendency to present with allergic conditions?

(A) Hypersensitivity reactions.

(B) Anaphylaxis.

(C) Atopy.

(D) Urticaria.

(74) What is the normal flora of the body?

(A) Microorganisms that cause illnesses.

(B) Nonpathogens for humans.

(C) Microorganisms that exist in a symbiotic relationship with human cells.

(D) Pathogens that protect against other microorganisms.

(75) How does antibiotic therapy affect the body's normal flora?

(A) It strengthens the normal flora's ability to protect against pathogens.

(B) It eliminates all microorganisms in the body.

(C) It debilitates the normal flora, which increases the risk of opportunistic infections.

(D) It does not affect the normal flora.

(76) Which of the following entities are not considered living things?

(A) Bacteria.

(B) Fungi.

(C) Viruses.

(D) Protozoa.

(77) Which bacteria causes skin infections, necrotizing pneumonia, and endocarditis?

(A) Listeria monocytogenes.

(B) Campylobacter jejuni.

(C) Escherichia coli.

(D) Staphylococcus aureus.

(78) Which of the following bacteria causes Lyme disease?

(A) Listeria monocytogenes.

(B) Campylobacter jejuni.

(C) Escherichia coli.

(D) Borrelia burgdorferi.

(79) Which bacteria causes typhoid fever?

(A) Listeria monocytogenes.

(B) Campylobacter jejuni.

(C) Escherichia coli.

(D) Salmonella typhi.

(80) Which type of bacteria requires oxygen to produce energy?

(A) Obligate anaerobes.

(B) Microaerophiles.

(C) Facultative anaerobes.

(D) Obligate aerobes.

(81) Which type of bacteria requires a small amount of oxygen to grow, but high concentrations may be detrimental?

(A) Microaerophiles.

(B) Facultative anaerobes.

(C) Obligate anaerobes.

(D) Aerotolerant anaerobes.

(82) Which type of bacteria can use both oxygen and anaerobic respiration to produce energy?

(A) Obligate aerobes.

(B) Microaerophiles.

(C) Facultative anaerobes.

(D) Obligate anaerobes.

(83) Which type of bacteria grows in the absence of oxygen and can be damaged by its presence?

(A) Obligate aerobes.

(B) Facultative anaerobes.

(C) Obligate anaerobes.

(D) Aerotolerant anaerobes.

(84) Which type of bacteria can exist and grow in an aerobic environment but does not use oxygen for energy?

(A) Microaerophiles.

(B) Facultative anaerobes.

(C) Obligate anaerobes.

(D) Aerotolerant anaerobes.

(85) Which of the following tests can be performed close to the patient's location?

(A) Point-of-care tests.

(B) Laboratory tests.

(C) Clinical tests.

(D) Home tests.

(86) Which point-of-care test is used to assess the coagulation profile of a patient?
(A) Glucose-monitoring devices.
(B) Dipstick urinalysis.
(C) Home pregnancy tests.
(D) PT/INR tests.

(87) All of the following are purposes of a dipstick urinalysis except:
(A) Screen for kidney issues.
(B) Monitor warfarin therapy.
(C) Diagnose urinary tract infections.
(D) Screen for diabetic ketoacidosis.

(88) All of the following are point-of-care tests except:
(A) Glucose-monitoring.
(B) Oxygen saturation.
(C) CT scan.
(D) Rapid HIV test.

(89) Which point-of-care test can screen for colorectal cancer?
(A) Glucose-monitoring devices.
(B) Dipstick urinalysis.
(C) Rapid HIV.
(D) Fecal occult blood.

(90) Who can perform point-of-care tests?
(A) Healthcare workers.
(B) Laypeople.
(C) Both healthcare workers and laypeople.
(D) Laboratory professionals.

(91) What is a laboratory requisition?

(A) A document with information for a laboratory test.

(B) A written prescription for medication.

(C) A paper with the results of a laboratory test.

(D) A document used for patient identification at the laboratory.

(92) What information is not required on a complete laboratory requisition?

(A) Healthcare provider's identification.

(B) Patient's financial information.

(C) Source of the specimen.

(D) Patient's identification.

(93) What is a random urine specimen?

(A) Urine collected early in the morning after waking up.

(B) Urine collected at any time of the day in a clean container.

(C) Urine collected over twenty-four hours.

(D) Urine collected after cleaning the distal portion of the urethra.

(94) All of the following might be an indication for an early morning urine specimen except:

(A) Assessment of proteins like Bence Jones proteins.

(B) Pregnancy assessment.

(C) To quantify the twenty-four-hour protein clearance.

(D) For TB diagnosis.

(95) What is a clean-catch midstream specimen?

(A) Urine collected after cleaning the genitals and discarding the first stream.

(B) Urine collected over twenty-four hours.

(C) Urine collected with a catheter.

(D) Urine collected in a clean container at any time of the day.

(96) Which type of investigation requires light protection when not immediately processed?

(A) Bilirubin analysis.

(B) Urine analysis.

(C) Stool analysis.

(D) Sputum analysis.

(97) How should a stool sample be stored before taking it to the laboratory?

(A) Frozen (-20°C).

(B) Room temperature.

(C) Refrigerated (2-8°C).

(D) Heated (40°C).

(98) All of the following are components of whole blood except:

(A) Red blood cells.

(B) White blood cells.

(C) CSF.

(D) Plasma.

(99) What is the main function of red blood cells?

(A) To transport oxygen.

(B) To fight infections.

(C) To stop bleeding.

(D) To give the blood its red hue.

(100) What are reticulocytes?

(A) Mature red blood cells.

(B) Immature white blood cells.

(C) Immature platelets.

(D) Immature red blood cells.

(101) What is the main function of platelets?

(A) To transport oxygen.

(B) To fight infections.

(C) To stop bleeding.

(D) To give the blood its red hue.

(102) How can plasma be extracted from whole blood?

(A) Add naturally activated clotting factors and then centrifuge.

(B) Separate from clotted blood.

(C) Add anticoagulants and then centrifuge.

(D) With fractional distillation.

(103) Which division of white blood cells lacks granules in their cytoplasm?

(A) Neutrophils.

(B) Basophils.

(C) Eosinophils.

(D) Lymphocytes.

(104) Which of the following statements regarding serum is correct?

(A) It is the solid portion of clotted blood.

(B) A centrifuge is needed to obtain it.

(C) It does not have clotting factors.

(D) Anticoagulants must be added to whole blood to obtain it.

(105) All of the following are the components of plasma except:

(A) Water.

(B) Antibodies.

(C) Red blood cells.

(D) Albumin.

(106) In which of the following conditions are reticulocytes observed in peripheral blood?

(A) Asthma.

(B) Anemia.

(C) COPD.

(D) They are only observed in healthy individuals.

(107) All of the following statements regarding red blood cells are true except:

(A) They are biconcave.

(B) They are disk-shaped.

(C) Their deficiency results in anemia.

(D) They have a nucleus.

(108) What part of whole blood is estimated to be plasma in a healthy adult?

(A) 10%.

(B) 30%.

(C) 55%.

(D) 85%.

(109) How is hepatitis B virus (HBV) mainly transmitted?

(A) Through respiratory droplets.

(B) Via contaminated food and water.

(C) During sexual contact.

(D) From needle stick injuries.

(110) All of the following are the modes of hepatitis B virus (HBV) transmission except:

(A) Respiratory droplets.

(B) Contaminated needles or sharps.

(C) Sexual contact.

(D) Vertical transmission from infected mothers.

(111) What percentage of patients with acute hepatitis B may develop chronic hepatitis B?

(A) 5%.

(B) 10%.

(C) 25%.

(D) 50%.

(112) All of the following are potential long-term consequences of chronic hepatitis B infection except:

(A) Liver cirrhosis.

(B) Liver cancer.

(C) Lung cancer.

(D) Portal hypertension.

(113) Which of the following statements accurately differentiates hepatitis B (HBV) from hepatitis C (HCV)?

(A) The risk of chronic HCV infection is higher than chronic HBV infection.

(B) HBV is transmitted mainly through unsafe blood transfusions, while HCV is mainly transmitted through sexual contact.

(C) HBV causes liver cirrhosis and liver cancer, while HCV does not.

(D) Chronic HBV infection is curable with available treatments, while HCV has no cure.

(114) What information can help a medical assistant determine the best vein for a phlebotomy procedure?

(A) Patient’s age and gender.

(B) Patient’s last successful collection site.

(C) Patient’s blood type.

(D) Patient’s current medications.

(115) A medical assistant should do all of the following to help a patient feel more comfortable during a phlebotomy procedure except:

(A) Ask the patient to lie down in a supine position.

(B) Engage in conversation to distract the patient.

(C) Administer sedatives to help the patient relax.

(D) Ask the patient about their fear or anxiety and address their concerns.

(116) All of the following information should be included on the requisition for a phlebotomy procedure except:

(A) The requesting healthcare provider's identification and contact information.

(B) The patient's social security number or health record number.

(C) The date and time of specimen collection.

(D) The patient's insurance information.

(117) All of the following instruments and products are required for a phlebotomy procedure except:

(A) Safe disposal container.

(B) Lidocaine.

(C) Tourniquet.

(D) Alcohol pads.

(118) A restraint can be used in all of the following conditions during pediatric phlebotomy procedures except:

(A) When the child is fearful or anxious.

(B) When no adult is available to assist with the procedure.

(C) When the child exhibits aggressive behavior.

(D) When the child refuses to cooperate.

(119) Which of the following statements regarding the strategies to prevent a hematoma during a phlebotomy procedure is not correct?

(A) Remove the needle before removing the tourniquet.

(B) Avoid the intersection of veins.

(C) Apply pressure after removing the needle.

(D) Prioritize straight, superficial, and clearly visible veins.

(120) Which of the following test results is expected to fluctuate with the circadian rhythm?

(A) Platelet count.

(B) WBC count.

(C) RBC count.

(D) Serum cortisol level.

(121) All of the following are purposes of electrocardiography (ECG) except:

(A) Assess arrhythmias.

(B) Diagnose electrolyte imbalances.

(C) Diagnose colorectal cancer.

(D) Evaluate cardiovascular conditions like myocardial infarction.

(122) What is represented on the y-axis of electrocardiograph?

(A) Voltage.

(B) Current.

(C) Time.

(D) Electrode number.

(123) How is time represented on the electrocardiograph?

(A) 1 mm represents 0.04 seconds.

(B) 1 mm represents 0.1 seconds.

(C) 1 mm represents 0. 4 seconds.

(D) 1 mm represents 4 seconds.

(124) How many electrodes are usually used in electrocardiography?

(A) Two electrodes.

(B) Four electrodes.

(C) Six electrodes.

(D) Ten electrodes.

(125) When might a disposable razor be needed during EKG testing?

(A) It is always required to remove any hair present.

(B) It is not required.

(C) It is contraindicated as it can alter the electrical activity of the hair.

(D) It is sometimes required if the chest has excess hair.

(126) Which waveform represents the depolarization of the atria?

(A) P wave.

(B) QRS complex.

(C) T wave.

(D) U wave.

(127) What does the QRS complex represent on an EKG?

(A) Depolarization of the ventricles.

(B) Repolarization of the atria.

(C) Relaxation of the ventricles.

(D) Baseline of the EKG.

(128) Which waveform represents the repolarization of the ventricles?

(A) P wave.

(B) QRS complex.

(C) T wave.

(D) U wave.

(129) Which waveform might be observed in patients with low serum potassium?

(A) P wave.

(B) QRS complex.

(C) T wave.

(D) U wave.

(130) What does the PR interval represent on an EKG?

(A) Time for atrial depolarization.

(B) Time for ventricular depolarization.

(C) Time for ventricular repolarization.

(D) Time the electrical impulse travels from the SA node to the AV node.

(131) What segment represents the time between the end of ventricular depolarization and the beginning of ventricular repolarization?

(A) P wave.

(B) QRS complex.

(C) ST segment.

(D) PR interval.

(132) In which of the following conditions can sinus bradycardia be considered normal?

(A) Patients with heart failure.

(B) Young individuals.

(C) Women.

(D) Athletes.

(133) Sinus tachycardia is defined as:

(A) HR >50 beats per minute.

(B) HR >75 beats per minute.

(C) HR >100 beats per minute.

(D) HR >125 beats per minute.

(134) What is the recommended age range for undergoing colonoscopy screening?

(A) Below the age of forty.

(B) Between forty and fifty years old.

(C) After the age of fifty.

(D) After the age of sixty.

(135) What is the main purpose of medical screenings?

(A) To diagnose specific diseases at an early stage.

(B) To provide treatment for well-advanced conditions.

(C) To reduce the transmission of disease.

(D) To provide immunization.

(136) Who should undergo a Papanicolaou test?

(A) Sexually active men between the ages of fifty and sixty-five.

(B) Women below the age of sixty-five.

(C) Women above the age of sixty-five.

(D) Sexually inactive women.

(137) When should mammography be performed for breast cancer screening?

(A) After the age of forty.

(B) After the age of fifty.

(C) After the age of sixty.

(D) Every five years.

(138) Why does the United States Preventive Services Task Force (USPSTF) oppose the use of prostate-specific antigen (PSA) screenings?

(A) They do not effectively detect prostate cancer.

(B) They are only recommended for men over seventy.

(C) They may result in overdiagnosis and extra medical costs for unnecessary treatment.

(D) They are a costly screening method.

(139) Who examines, diagnoses, and develops treatment plans for patients in a patient-centered medical home?

(A) Physician.

(B) Nurse.

(C) Physician assistant.

(D) Medical assistant.

(140) Which team member is responsible for coordinating care for high-risk patients?

(A) Physician.

(B) Nurse.

(C) Social or community health worker.

(D) Medical assistant.

(141) What is the primary concern when a patient presents with torsion of a limb?

(A) Pain management.

(B) Preventing infection.

(C) Restoring blood flow.

(D) Applying ice to reduce swelling.

(142) What is the initial step a medical assistant should take when a patient presents with a suspected bone fracture?

(A) Apply a warm compress to the affected area.

(B) Immobilize the affected area.

(C) Encourage the patient to move the affected area gently.

(D) Administer over-the-counter pain medication.

(143) Which team member manages medication and related resources?

(A) Nurse.

(B) Physician assistant.

(C) Pharmacist.

(D) Social or community health worker.

(144) A legal record that documents clinical findings, the progress of treatments, and a patient's medical and family history is known as a:

(A) Chief complaint.

(B) Health record.

(C) Progressive note.

(D) Consent form.

(145) All of the following are advantages of electronic health records except:

(A) Easy to read.

(B) Easy to update.

(C) Can only be used by one person at a time.

(D) Efficient.

(146) All of the following are disadvantages of paper-based health records except:

(A) Easy to lose.

(B) Can be used by multiple persons at a time.

(C) Requires more physical space.

(D) Difficult to read.

(147) Which section of the health record includes information about the patient's main concern for visiting the health center?

(A) Medical and family history.

(B) Chief complaint.

(C) Vital signs and measurements.

(D) Progress notes.

(148) Which section of the health record documents the patient's evolution of disease during their visits?

(A) Medical and family history.

(B) Chief complaint.

(C) Progress notes.

(D) Condition at the time of treatment termination.

(149) Which section of the health record may require the patient's or their legal representative's written permission?

(A) Chief complaint.

(B) Consent forms.

(C) Progress notes.

(D) Medical and family history.

(150) All of the following sections of the health record help establish a diagnosis except:

(A) Medical and family history.

(B) Chief complaint.

(C) Clinical findings.

(D) Consent form.

(151) Which section of the health record usually includes the healthcare professional's objective discoveries from the physical exam?

(A) Clinical findings.

(B) Medical and family history.

(C) Chief complaint.

(D) Vital signs and measurements.

(152) Which type of office visit focuses on a thorough assessment of a patient's personal and family medical history?

(A) New patient visit.

(B) Follow-up visit.

(C) Urgent visit.

(D) Preventive health exam.

(153) Which type of office visit is scheduled to review the progress of a condition?

(A) New patient visit.

(B) Follow-up visit.

(C) Urgent visit.

(D) Preventive health exam.

(154) Which type of office visit is a yearly routine exam to check overall health and schedule screening tests?

(A) New patient visit.

(B) Follow-up visit.

(C) Urgent visit.

(D) Preventive health exam.

(155) Which type of office visit is prioritized for patients who need to see their provider as soon as possible?

(A) New patient visit.

(B) Follow-up visit.

(C) Urgent visit.

(D) Preventive health exam.

(156) Appointments that allow patients to receive care via phone or video are known as:

(A) Telehealth visit.

(B) Specialty visit.

(C) VIP visit.

(D) Screening visit.

(157) Which type of visit involves the preventive study of a patient with or without risk factors for a specific condition?

(A) Telehealth visit.

(B) Specialty visit.

(C) VIP visit.

(D) Screening visit.

(158) Which type of visit is usually scheduled with a referral by a primary care provider when the patient needs special care?

(A) Telehealth visit.

(B) Specialty visit.

(C) VIP visit.

(D) Screening visit.

(159) All of the following statements regarding medical office visits are true except:

(A) Follow-up visits usually require more time than new patient visits.

(B) It must be verified that the specialist accepts the patient's insurance before they are referred.

(C) Visits should be scheduled at the same location (day or hour) to increase patient compliance.

(D) A school physical exam includes the review of immunization history.

(160) Which of the following forms must be signed by the patient or their legal representative to allow healthcare professionals to disclose health information or use it for research?

(A) Consent forms.

(B) Wellness forms.

(C) HIPAA forms.

(D) Legalization forms.

(161) Which Asian cultural factor is important to highlight during the diagnosis and treatment process?

(A) Concept of *face*.

(B) Reliance on home remedies.

(C) Preference for traditional medicine.

(D) Familial support.

(162) What medical treatment are Jehovah's Witnesses against due to their religious beliefs?

(A) Blood transfusions.

(B) Vaccinations.

(C) Surgery.

(D) Chemotherapy.

(163) How can mental health conditions such as anxiety and depression impact patient compliance with medical treatments?

(A) They improve compliance.

(B) They have no effect.

(C) They impair compliance.

(D) They enhance outcomes.

(164) Which religious groups are known to reject the use of vaccines in healthcare?

(A) Jehovah's Witnesses.

(B) Christian evangelical groups.

(C) Buddhists.

(D) Hindus.

(165) How can economic concerns about healthcare costs and insurance coverage impact patients?

(A) Improve mental health.

(B) Have no impact.

(C) Improve patient outcomes.

(D) Affect psychosocial well-being.

(166) Which barrier can limit understanding and involvement in patients with dementia, stroke, or hearing loss?

(A) Biological.

(B) Language.

(C) Physical and infrastructure.

(D) Psychosocial.

(167) What barrier may arise when patients and healthcare providers do not speak the same language?

(A) Biological.

(B) Language.

(C) Physical and infrastructure.

(D) Psychosocial.

(168) How can poor technological infrastructure impact patient communication during virtual visits?

(A) Improve communication.

(B) Have no impact.

(C) Introduce problems.

(D) Enhance understanding.

(169) All of the following are psychological factors that may affect how patients communicate with their healthcare providers except:

(A) Depression.

(B) Fear.

(C) Anxiety.

(D) Hearing loss.

(170) What is gender identity?

(A) A group of characteristics associated with being male or female.

(B) The inner sense of gender, which may align with being male, female, both, or neither.

(C) The assigned sex at birth.

(D) The psychosocial factors associated with gender.

(171) What should medical assistants do if they are unsure about a patient's pronouns?

(A) Assume based on appearance.

(B) Avoid using pronouns altogether.

(C) Ask the patient about their preferred pronouns.

(D) Use generic pronouns like *he* or *she*.

(172) All of the following are ways medical assistants can use to avoid misgendering patients except:

(A) Use gender-neutral pronouns.

(B) Assume based on appearance.

(C) Use the singular form of *they*.

(D) Ask patients about their preferred pronouns.

(173) Which of the following statements regarding preferred pronouns in healthcare settings is not correct?

(A) It shows courtesy to patients.

(B) Pronouns should be avoided altogether.

(C) It helps provide the best care possible.

(D) It helps connect with patients.

(174) Which act provides resources to promote research in biomedical sciences?

(A) Health Information Technology for Economic and Clinical Health (HITECH) Act.

(B) Public Readiness and Emergency Preparedness (PREP) Act.

(C) HHS Acquisition Regulation (HHSAR).

(D) 21st Century Cures Act.

(175) Which law establishes a federal system of benefits for people who are retired, jobless, or have a disability?

(A) Health Information Technology for Economic and Clinical Health (HITECH) Act.

(B) Public Readiness and Emergency Preparedness (PREP) Act.

(C) Social Security Act.

(D) Patient Self Determination Act (PDSA).

(176) Which law promotes the use of technology and electronic health records (EHRs) in the healthcare system?

(A) Health Information Technology for Economic and Clinical Health (HITECH) Act.

(B) Public Readiness and Emergency Preparedness (PREP) Act.

(C) HHS Acquisition Regulation (HHSAR).

(D) Social Security Act.

(177) Which law provides liability protection in relation to the administration of medical countermeasures?

(A) Health Information Technology for Economic and Clinical Health (HITECH) Act.

(B) Public Readiness and Emergency Preparedness (PREP) Act.

(C) 21st Century Cures Act.

(D) Social Security Act.

(178) Which regulation implements the Federal Acquisition Regulation in the HHS?

(A) Health Information Technology for Economic and Clinical Health (HITECH) Act.

(B) Public Readiness and Emergency Preparedness (PREP) Act.

(C) HHS Acquisition Regulation (HHSAR).

(D) 21st Century Cures Act.

(179) Which law addresses the disclosure and use of protected health information?

(A) Health Insurance Portability and Accountability Act (HIPAA).

(B) Affordable Care Act (ACA).

(C) Controlled Substances Act (CSA).

(B) Public Readiness and Emergency Preparedness (PREP) Act.

(180) Who is able to grant consent in the context of healthcare?

(A) Medical doctor.

(B) Patient.

(C) Family members.

(D) Medical assistant.

Test 1 Answers and Explanations

(1) (B) Manage appointments and office supplies.

As part of their administrative duties, medical assistants

- Manage appointments, patient records, and correspondence.
- Inventory and order office supplies.
- Perform medical transcription.
- Arrange hospital admissions.
- Complete billing and bookkeeping tasks.

(2) (C) Perform medical transcription.

Medical assistants (MAs) are flexible members of the healthcare team who aid physicians. They are trained in various clinical and administrative roles and often work in outpatient settings (clinics and medical offices).

As part of their clinical duties, MAs

- Interview patients and document relevant information (medical history).
- Prepare examination and treatment areas.
- Assist during examinations and basic laboratory and other diagnostic testing.
- Perform first aid, wound care, and cardiopulmonary resuscitation.
- Provide patient education.
- Dispose of waste.

(3) (A) Provide basic nursing care.

Licensed practical nurses (LPNs) are licensed nurses who work under the direction of registered nurses, nurse practitioners, or physicians. They provide basic nursing care. The following are duties often performed by LPNs.

- Take patient vital signs.
- Provide basic medical care (e.g., change dressings, apply bandages).
- Assist patient with basic care (e.g., dressing, bathing).
- Communicate with physicians and RNs about patient needs.
- Explain treatments, procedures, and medications to patients.
- Clean and organize equipment.

(4) (A) Topical retinoids.

Topical retinoids are a common treatment option for back acne because they help to unclog pores and reduce inflammation. These medications are derived from vitamin A and promote cell turnover, which helps prevent the formation of new acne lesions.

(5) (B) A certification is a third-party verification, while a federal, state, or local government agency grants a license.

A certification is a third-party verification a professional may receive after proving their ability to perform a specific job or skill. However, a license is a verification granted by a federal, state, or local government agency that allows a professional to practice a regulated occupation or profession in a specific location.

(6) (C) Inpatient care.

Inpatient care requires a patient to be admitted into a healthcare facility, such as a hospital. Issues that warrant this type of care include serious injuries or illnesses and complex surgical procedures. Outpatient care does not require admission into a healthcare facility. Consultations, follow-ups, and many medical concerns are handled in an outpatient setting. Hospice care focuses on end-of-life care and can take place in various settings. Home healthcare is provided in a patient's home.

(7) (B) Specialty care.

Specialty care includes all healthcare providers with advanced and specialized training in different areas of medicine, like cardiology, pneumology, neurology, gastroenterology, and dermatology. Specialty care is for patients with complex conditions that primary care providers cannot treat.

(8) (A) Complementary medicine is used alongside standard medical treatment, while alternative medicine is not.

Complementary medicine and therapies are combined with standard medical treatment. Some examples include acupuncture, meditation, vitamin therapy, plant-based or other special diets, massage therapy, and Ayurvedic medicine. However, alternative medicine is not used in conjunction with standard treatment.

(9) (C) To ensure there is enough research to support their use and that they are safe for specific conditions.

Complementary medicine can be safe and effective. However, there is often a lack of research to support the use of these therapies or their safety in specific conditions. For this reason, patients must discuss them with their healthcare provider before implementation.

(10) (C) Dialysis.

Therapeutic services include dialysis, wound care, physical therapy, chiropractic service, occupational therapy, language therapy, and psychotherapy. Laboratory tests, imaging studies, genetic testing, and cardiac monitoring are examples of diagnostic services.

(11) (C) Suffix.

A suffix is an affix that appears at the end of a word and modifies the root. Examples include

-ac: Related to.
-form: Resembling.
-iasis: Condition.
-ism: Condition.

-itis: Inflammation.
-oma: Tumor.
-penia: Deficiency.
-plasia: Development.
-rrhea: Discharge.
-stasis: Stoppage.
-stomy: Surgical aperture.
-tomy: Incision.

(12) (D) Outside.

A prefix is an affix that appears at the beginning of a word and modifies the root. Examples include

A-: Without.
Anti-: Against.
Auto-: Self.
Bi-: Both.
Dys-: Painful, difficult, bad.
Ec-: Away.
Ecto-: Outside.
Endo-: Within.
Neo-: New.
Poly-: Many.
Retro-: Back, behind.

(13) (B) Pain in the ear.

Otalgia refers to pain in one or both ears. This can be caused by many ailments such as wax accumulation, trauma, ear infections, and transferred pain from other regions like the throat or jaw. Sharp or dull discomfort, itching, or the sensation of ear fullness are possible symptoms. Depending on the underlying cause, treatment options include ear drops, medicine, and, in extreme circumstances, surgery.

(14) (A) Shortness of breath.

Dyspnea is the medical term for difficulty or discomfort in breathing. The symptoms include breathing difficulties, shallow or fast breathing, or a suffocating sensation. It can be caused by numerous illnesses, including heart failure, pneumonia, asthma, and chronic obstructive pulmonary disease (COPD). It can significantly impact an individual's quality of life and range in severity from minor to life-threatening.

(15) (A) High blood sugar.

Hyperglycemia is defined by high blood glucose (sugar) levels. It usually happens when the body can not control blood sugar levels, which is frequently brought on by inadequate insulin synthesis or insulin resistance. Signs and symptoms include increased thirst, frequent urination, weariness, and impaired eyesight. If it is not diagnosed and managed correctly, it may result in significant side effects and complications like diabetic ketoacidosis.

(16) (A) Superficial.

In medical terminology, the term *superficial* describes a region or position closer to the body's surface. It characterizes places or structures that are not very deep. It denotes the outermost layer or the outermost portion of a tissue or organ. This term differentiates structures deeper within the body from those closer to the surface during medical tests, treatments, and anatomical descriptions.

(17) (B) Away from the point of attachment or trunk.

Distal is a term used to describe a region or position farther away from the body's trunk or a structure's point of attachment. It is used to clarify the location of anatomical structures, like limbs or arteries, by describing their relative positions.

(18) (A) Superior/cranial.

Superior or cranial are terms used to describe a direction or region that is nearer the head than the feet. They delineate the relative locations in the body. In medical settings, these terms precisely identify the placement and orientation of various anatomical parts, such as bones, organs, or blood vessels.

(19) (D) Posterior/dorsal.

Dorsal or posterior are terms that refer to a direction or position near the back of the body. They delineate the relative location of an anatomical structure compared to another structure. These terms are essential for accurate anatomical descriptions and orientation.

(20) (A) Proximal.

Proximal is a term that refers to a place or location that is closer to the body's trunk or a structure's point of attachment. It is used to describe the relative location of regions or structures. This term provides clarity and detail.

(21) (B) Frontal/coronal plane.

The frontal/coronal plane lies vertically and separates the body into anterior (front) and posterior (back) sections. It is perpendicular to the sagittal plane. The body is frequently evaluated from various angles and orientations in medical imaging, surgical planning, and anatomical descriptions. Knowledge of anatomical planes is necessary to understand the relative locations of the body's structures and regions.

(22) (C) Transverse/axial plane.

The transverse/axial plane lies horizontally and separates the body into upper and lower portions. It is perpendicular to the frontal and sagittal planes. Healthcare professionals use the transverse/axial plane to help visualize and describe the relative position of anatomical components. Medical imaging procedures like CT and MRI scans use anatomical planes to gather comprehensive data about structures at certain levels of the body.

(23) (A) Sagittal/lateral plane.

The sagittal/lateral plane lies vertically and separates the body into left and right sides. It is perpendicular to the frontal plane and extends from front to back. Healthcare professionals use the sagittal plane to help visualize and describe the relative position of anatomical components. In particular, the median/mid-sagittal plane crosses the body's midline. This plane is frequently utilized to evaluate structures and anomalies from a lateral perspective in medical imaging, such as MRIs and X-rays.

(24) (D) Depression.

Dr. Elisabeth Kübler-Ross defined the five stages of grief as a response pattern to separation or health threats. They are described as follows.

- **Denial and isolation**: Patients deny the existence of the disease. As a result, they do not want to comply with the treatment plan.
- **Anger**: Patients become hostile and do not want to discuss or be reminded of the disease.
- **Bargaining**: Patients want to negotiate about various aspects of the disease and try to buy time or privileges.
- **Depression**: Patients recognize the disease and feel sadness about the diagnosis and loss of health.
- **Acceptance**: Patients accept the disease and are more likely to use most resources.

(25) (D) Ribosomes.

Cells are the basic building blocks of all organisms. They have various structural and functional features. Human cells can be divided into three main parts:

- **Cell membrane**: A semipermeable phospholipids bilayer that regulates the transport of various substances between the intracellular and extracellular spaces.
- **Cytoplasm**: A solution found within the cell membrane that contains structures and organelles, like the nucleus, mitochondria, and Golgi apparatus. It comprises water, nutrients (such as glucose), electrolytes, RNA, and other organic molecules.
- **Nucleus**: A structure that contains DNA, which stores the cell's information in the form of chromosomes. It has a nuclear membrane that regulates the transport of substances between the nucleus and the cytoplasm. Some cells do not have a nucleus, such as prokaryotes like bacteria, or a few human cells like red blood cells.

(26) (A) Ribosomes.

Ribosomes are essential for the production of proteins. They translate the information in messenger RNA (mRNA) into amino acids, which are the building blocks of proteins. Ribosomes use the instructions supplied by mRNA to bind amino acids together in a specific order to produce proteins. These proteins perform several tasks for the cell, such as molecular signaling, enzymatic activity, and structural support. Ribosomes are necessary for cells and organisms to develop and operate correctly.

(27) (D) Photosynthesis.

The endoplasmic reticulum is a large structural complex composed of tubules that synthesize proteins (through ribosomes), metabolize lipids, and transport various substances through the cell.

(28) (A) Skeletal muscle.

Skeletal muscles are made of striated muscle fibers that are affixed to bones. They receive signals from the nervous system that allow the body to move consciously. The body uses voluntary muscles (e.g., skeletal muscles) to run, walk, and lift items. They give the skeletal system strength, mobility, and stability. Additionally, skeletal muscles help produce heat and maintain posture.

(29) (C) Muscle tissue.

Muscle is a type of tissue that allows movement. This tissue includes

- **Skeletal**: Muscle that is connected to the bone and produces voluntary movement.
- **Cardiac**: Muscle that produces heart contractions.
- **Smooth**: Muscle that is involuntary and can be found within blood vessels and intestines.

(30) (A) Cardiovascular system.

The cardiovascular system is composed of the heart and its valves, as well as arteries, veins, arterioles, and venules. It transports blood and nutrients to the tissues and returns deoxygenated blood and carbon dioxide to the lungs.

(31) (C) Musculoskeletal system.

The musculoskeletal system is composed of the muscles and bones, as well as the structures that keep them together (tendons, joints, cartilage). It is required for motion and posture. Muscles also produce heat, and bones (precisely, bone marrow) are responsible for hematopoiesis (production of blood cells).

(32) (A) Brain and spinal cord.

The nervous system is composed of the central and peripheral nervous systems. The central nervous system includes the brain and the spinal cord, and the peripheral nervous system consists of the nerves and ganglia. The nervous system regulates the functions of other body systems, as well as thinking and other cognitive tasks. The nervous system must adequately regulate these systems to achieve homeostasis.

(33) (C) Immune system.

The immune system is composed of immune cells, lymph, lymph vessels, lymph nodes, thymus, and spleen. It mainly helps to defend the body from foreign substances or organisms.

(34) (D) Acne.

Acne is a common skin ailment characterized by the accumulation of dead skin cells and sebum in hair follicles. This causes inflammation, which makes pimples, blackheads, and whiteheads appear. It is especially problematic in adolescence and can be uncomfortable or painful. It can even damage self-esteem. Oral drugs, topical creams, and lifestyle modifications are available as treatments.

(35) (B) Alzheimer's disease.

Alzheimer's disease is a neurological illness that worsens over time and mainly impacts cognitive and memory abilities. It is the most prevalent type of dementia. As the condition worsens, it can cause mood swings, memory loss, confusion, language difficulties, and finally, a loss of independence. Alzheimer's disease does not currently have a cure, but there are several interventions and treatments that can help control symptoms and enhance quality of life.

(36) (B) Education and job history.

A patient's medical history includes a variety of information, such as the patient's past and present health concerns, allergies, and use of medications.

(37) (A) The medical information of immediate family members.

The family history section includes the medical information of immediate family members relevant to the patient's medical care, such as hereditary conditions and each member's state of health. If a family member is deceased, the cause of death should be included in the record.

(38) (C) The patient's previous surgical procedures.

In the social history section, a wide variety of information will be incorporated, such as the patient's education level, job, lifestyle, diet, sleep habits, and use of drugs, tobacco, and alcohol.

(39) (D) Detect medical conditions in asymptomatic individuals.

Screenings are preventative health tests usually performed on asymptomatic individuals with a reasonable risk of developing a medical condition. Heart disease screenings detect ischemic heart disease, hypertrophic cardiopathy, and valvular diseases. They are performed on patients with risk factors like family history and tobacco consumption. They often measure blood pressure and assess glucose and lipid levels.

(40) (B) Papanicolaou smear.

A Papanicolaou smear (pap smear) screens for abnormal cells in the cervix that may be an early sign of cervical cancer. A medical professional collects a tiny sample of cervical cells and examines them under a microscope. Women are advised to get Pap screenings as part of standard gynecological treatment to help detect and prevent cervical cancer. This test has considerably lowered cervical cancer death rates.

(41) (C) Colonoscopy.

A colonoscopy is a screening procedure used on patients at risk for colon cancer. A flexible tube is inserted into the colon to check the lining and rectum for any anomalies, such as polyps or cancer. Healthcare professionals can then remove precancerous polyps, which lowers the chance of colon cancer development. This screening test is an essential tool in the early identification and prevention of colon cancer.

(42) (D) Diagnose medical illnesses early.

Mental health screenings assess a patient's thinking, mood, behavior, and cognitive functions. They are employed to recognize mental disorders early, which helps patients receive care sooner. They can help monitor symptoms that indicate a risk of developing mental conditions, such as sleep problems, fatigue, substance abuse, extreme mood swings, feelings of sadness or anhedonia, hearing voices, or suicidal ideation. They can also be used to determine the patient's response to therapy.

(43) (D) Physical, mental, and social well-being.

Wellness is an integral state of physical, mental, and social well-being. Wellness assessment instruments include:

- Wellness Evaluation of Lifestyle (WEL).
- Five-factor WEL (5F-Wel).
- Perceived Wellness Survey (PWS).
- Optimal Living Profile (OLP).
- Body-Mind-Spirit Wellness Behavior and Characteristic Inventory (BMS-WBCI).

The OLP, PWS, and BMS-WBCI are relatively short compared to 5F-Wel and WEL.

(44) (C) Physical and psychological factors.

Vital signs are the measurement of the body's basic functions. They are naturally affected by both physical and psychological factors. Changes in vital signs can indicate an underlying health condition.

(45) (B) Decreased temperature.

Physical activity may increase all vital signs, such as temperature, heart rate, ventilation, and blood pressure. A common example is a patient who arrives late to an appointment and rapidly climbs the stairs. The sudden physical activity naturally alters the patient's vital signs. The patient should be instructed to relax and sit for a few minutes before the healthcare professional measures their vital signs. This ensures they have a chance to return to their baseline levels.

There are also psychological factors that can result in higher readings. These include anxiety, fear, and joy. An example of this is a patient who is anxious about their diagnosis and arrives at the appointment with high blood pressure. This is an opportune moment to use therapeutic communication to reassure the patient and help them feel understood. Once the patient relaxes, the healthcare worker may measure their vital signs.

(46) (A) Systolic pressure, followed by diastolic pressure.

Blood pressure is measured in millimeters of mercury (mm Hg) and recorded with the systolic pressure first and diastolic pressure second. Normal blood pressure in healthy adults should be below 120/80 mm Hg.

(47) (A) Systolic pressure: 120-139 mm Hg, diastolic pressure: 80-89 mm Hg.

Patients with blood pressure that is persistently above normal are considered to have prehypertension, stage 1 hypertension, or stage 2 hypertension.

Prehypertension

- Systolic pressure: 120-139 mm Hg.
- Diastolic pressure: 80-89 mm Hg.

Stage 1 hypertension

- Systolic pressure: 140-159 mm Hg.
- Diastolic pressure: 90-99 mm Hg.

Stage 2 hypertension

- Systolic pressure: ≥160 mm Hg
- Diastolic pressure: ≥100 mm Hg.

(48) (A) Systolic pressure: ≥160 mm Hg, diastolic pressure: ≥100 mm Hg.

Patients with blood pressure that is persistently above normal are considered to have prehypertension, stage 1 hypertension, or stage 2 hypertension.

Prehypertension

- Systolic pressure: 120-139 mm Hg.
- Diastolic pressure: 80-89 mm Hg.

Stage 1 hypertension

- Systolic pressure: 140-159 mm Hg.
- Diastolic pressure: 90-99 mm Hg.

Stage 2 hypertension

- Systolic pressure: ≥160 mm Hg
- Diastolic pressure: ≥100 mm Hg.

(49) (A) Systolic pressure: <90 mm Hg, diastolic pressure: <60 mm Hg.

Hypotension or low blood pressure is generally recognized as a blood pressure below 90/60 mm Hg that is accompanied by other clinical findings, such as dizziness, hemorrhage, dehydration, and emotional shock. Low blood pressure without any other symptoms is usually benign and does not require intervention.

(50) (C) Thermometer.

Temperature is one of the vital signs measured by a healthcare worker. A thermometer is used to measure a patient's temperature. It is most frequently used by primary care providers but can be used by anyone.

(51) (D) Test neurological reflexes.

Reflex hammers are used to test neurological reflexes. Neurologists use them during neurological examinations, but other healthcare professionals utilize them during physicals.

(52) (C) Neurologists.

Neurologists frequently use reflex hammers. However, they are also used by other medical professionals in general care settings. The main purpose of the hammer is to assess neurological reflexes, which might yield important diagnostic information.

(53) (B) Examine the eyes.

Ophthalmoscopes are used to examine the eyes. Similar to the otoscope, it may be portable or wall-mounted. They are commonly used by ophthalmologists but also by some primary care providers and internists.

(54) (C) OB-GYN physicians.

Vaginal speculums separate the walls of the vagina to examine it and the cervix, as well as specimen collection during a Papanicolaou test or other tests. OB-GYN physicians often use them.

(55) (A) Ear, nose, and throat (ENT) physicians.

ENT doctors often utilize a nasal speculum to examine the nasal passageways. The nasal speculum is a vital instrument to diagnose and treat disorders pertaining to the ears, nose, and throat. ENTs use them to spot any anomalies or problems that might be there.

(56) (A) Supine position.

The supine position is also known as the horizontal recumbent position. The patient lies flat on their back with the arms resting at each side. Drapes may be used to cover the arms, torso, and legs. It is the most frequently used position by healthcare providers to examine patients and perform procedures.

(57) (A) To examine the genital and rectal areas.

In the dorsal-recumbent position, the patient lies on their back with flexed knees and the soles of the feet pressed to the surface of the table. The knees and feet are kept separated. This position can be used to examine the genital and rectal areas, as well as the abdomen and chest. The draping process uses a diamond-shaped sheet to cover the lower part of the body—one of the tips should point toward the head and the other to the feet.

(58) (C) Lithotomy position.

The lithotomy position is very similar to the dorsal-recumbent position but involves the use of stirrups to hold the patient's feet. OB-GYN professionals frequently employ it to examine the vaginal area. Draping is the same as the dorsal-recumbent position.

(59) (B) Examine the back.

In the prone position, the patient lies with their face down, which is useful to examine the back. However, this position may not be recommended for pregnant or obese patients. Draping should cover the patient's lumbar back, buttocks, and legs.

(60) (A) Erect position.

The erect position is sometimes referred to as the standing position. It is the posture utilized to assess hernias or gait. The patient stands straight during the examination in this position. This allows medical professionals to evaluate walking style and look for irregularities or hernia-related symptoms. A gown provides appropriate coverage for this evaluation and guarantees the patient's privacy and comfort.

(61) (D) Perianal area.

The sitting position involves sitting on a chair or the edge of the bed. Draping may include the lower extremities. The sitting position can be used to evaluate reflexes and other neurological exams, as well as the chest, back, arms, head, and neck.

(62) (A) Perianal and rectal examination.

In the knee-chest position, the patient is positioned facing down, with the head and chest touching the table's surface, the buttocks elevated, and the knees separated and resting on the bed. This position is used for perianal and rectal examination, as well as some proctological procedures. It may be difficult for older patients to maintain. Healthcare workers must help patients to move in and out of this position to avoid falls. Draping should cover the buttocks.

(63) (C) Provide a therapeutic measure for patients with hypotension.

The Trendelenburg position involves the patient lying flat on their back with their head lower and their legs raised. It is commonly employed as a therapeutic measure for patients with hypotension. Draping should cover the shoulders, chest, and legs.

(64) (D) For patients with lower-back problems or breathing difficulties in the supine position.

In Fowler's position, the patient sits straight on the bed, with their legs resting flat on the surface at a ninety-degree angle. This position is employed with patients with lower-back problems or those who cannot breathe appropriately in the supine position. The draping may cover the patient's chest, abdomen, and legs.

(65) (A) A plain, low-fiber diet.

At least two or three days before a colonoscopy, the patient should eat a plain, low-fiber diet (white rice, bread, plain chicken, broth, eggs, coffee, tea, and lemon juice). They should avoid nuts, seeds, raw vegetables, fruits with skin, and brown rice.

(66) (B) Clear-liquid diet.

The day before a colonoscopy, the patient should only have a clear liquid diet (water, clear broth, soft drinks, gelatin, tea, or coffee without milk) and laxatives to prepare their bowels for the procedure. The physician specifies the laxatives and usually recommends that they be taken late in the afternoon or evening. Since they cause diarrhea, patients should be instructed to remain at home near a toilet.

(67) (A) Mild abdominal cramping or bloating.

After a colonoscopy, it is normal to feel mild abdominal cramping or bloating. Patients can maintain a clear liquid diet for the rest of the day and incorporate semi-solids and solids gradually. Patients should contact their provider immediately if they experience severe pain, fever, or rectal bleeding.

(68) (C) Three doses.

RV5 is a specific type of the Rotavirus vaccination. Patients should receive three doses at the ages of two, four, and six months. It is important to adhere to the suggested schedule and finish the entire course of immunization so that children can achieve optimal success.

(69) (C) Twelve months.

The recommended age to receive the first dose of the measles, mumps, and rubella (MMR) vaccination is twelve months. This first dosage provides the primary immunity against measles, mumps, and rubella. As part of the recommended regimen, a booster dose of the MMR vaccine is usually given between the ages of four and six. The MMR vaccine is essential for children to be protected against these viral infections and avoid any consequences.

(70) (C) Eleven to twelve years.

The meningococcal serogroup A, C, W, and Y vaccine should be given for the first time at eleven or twelve years old. This vaccine protects people in their early teens against these meningococcal serogroups, which are known to cause serious infections. A booster dose is usually advised to ensure ongoing protection at sixteen years old.

(71) (A) One dose of Pfizer-BioNTech or Moderna vaccine.

For unvaccinated patients, one dose of the 2023-2024 updated formula of the Pfizer-BioNTech or Moderna vaccine or two doses (0, 3-8 weeks) of the 2023-2024 updated formula of the Novavax vaccine.

(72) (C) At fifty years of age or older.

Adults fifty years of age and above should receive the recombinant zoster vaccination. It helps prevent the varicella-zoster virus, which causes shingles. The vaccination is delivered in two doses, the second of which is given two to six months following the first. Adults can lower their chance of shingles and its complications by adhering to the suggested timetable.

(73) (C) Atopy.

Allergies are hypersensitivity reactions of the immune system to foreign substances (allergens). Allergic reactions have various presentations, such as very mild allergies, life-threatening shock (i.e., anaphylaxis), localized acute reactions (i.e., urticaria), and chronic disorders (e.g., hay fever or allergic asthma). Some families present a hereditary tendency for allergic conditions, which is known as *atopy*.

(74) (C) Microorganisms that exist in a symbiotic relationship with human cells.

Not all organisms are pathogens (able to cause illnesses). In fact, most of them (<1%) are nonpathogens for humans. In the human body, a vast amount of microorganisms exist alongside human cells in a symbiotic relationship that is generally beneficial to both parties. This is known as the normal flora of the body, and it helps humans digest various substances, protect against other (potentially pathogenic) microorganisms, and produce beneficial substances like vitamins.

(75) (C) It debilitates the normal flora, which increases the risk of opportunistic infections.

Antibiotic therapy (especially prolonged treatments with broad-spectrum antibiotics) may debilitate the normal flora, which increases the risk of opportunistic infections.

(76) (C) Viruses.

An organism is any living thing (animals, fungi, plants), although the term usually describes macroscopic (visible with the naked human eye) multicellular organisms. However, a microorganism (or microbe) refers to any living being that is microscopic (not visible to the naked human eye), and it includes both single-cell and multicellular living things (bacteria, protozoa, fungi, algae). The inclusion of viruses is debated because they are not generally considered alive. However, they are still studied in microbiology as infectious agents.

(77) (D) Staphylococcus aureus.

The bacterium Staphylococcus aureus is the source of endocarditis, necrotizing pneumonia, and skin infections. This gram-positive bacterium is frequently discovered on mucous membranes and the skin. It can cause mild skin ailments, e.g., cellulitis and boils. It can also result in more serious and invasive infections, e.g., endocarditis (infection of the inner lining of the heart chambers and valves) and necrotizing pneumonia (infection that damages lung tissue).

(78) (D) Borrelia burgdorferi.

Lyme disease is caused by the bacteria Borrelia burgdorferi. It is a spirochete bacterium that is spread to people via the bite of a black-legged tick, which carries the infection. It has numerous symptoms, such as fever, exhaustion, headaches, muscle and joint aches, and a distinctive skin rash known as erythema migrans. Lyme disease can cause more serious side effects that impact the heart, joints, and neurological system if it is not treated.

(79) (D) Salmonella typhi.

The Salmonella typhi bacteria causes typhoid fever. This bacterium is gram-negative and spreads through polluted food and water. A high fever, headache, stomach pain, and gastrointestinal symptoms like constipation or diarrhea typify a systemic of this illness. If untreated, serious consequences that impact several organs may arise. Hygiene, immunization, and good sanitation help stop the spread of Salmonella typhi and lower the risk of typhoid fever.

(80) (D) Obligate aerobes.

Obligate aerobes are oxygen-dependent organisms, and they are unable to survive in a setting without oxygen.

(81) (A) Microaerophiles.

Microaerophiles are types of bacteria that can grow with very little oxygen present. They prefer low-oxygen surroundings since high oxygen concentrations can be detrimental to them.

(82) (C) Facultative anaerobes.

Facultative anaerobes are diverse bacteria that can adjust to varying oxygen levels. They can transition between anaerobic respiration (fermentation) when oxygen is not present and aerobic respiration when it is.

(83) (C) Obligate anaerobes.

Obligate anaerobes can only proliferate when oxygen is absent. Their biological components may be harmed by oxygen.

(84) (D) Aerotolerant anaerobes.

Aerotolerant anaerobes are bacteria that can withstand the presence of oxygen but do not require it for energy. Despite needing anaerobic respiration (fermentation) to produce energy, they can grow and survive in aerobic settings.

(85) (A) Point-of-care tests.

Point-of-care tests are clinical tests that can be performed near where a patient receives care (e.g., at the patient's bedside, at home, or in an ambulance). Point-of-care testing is a practical solution to provide fast and reliable tests—it bypasses the need for a clinical laboratory, which may entail longer wait times and logistical requirements.

(86) (D) PT/INR tests.

A coagulation profile assessment is done with PT/INR assays. These tests are mostly performed to evaluate the blood's clotting capacity and to track the effects of anticoagulant medication, such as warfarin.

(87) (B) Monitor warfarin therapy.

A point-of-care test called a urine dipstick is used to screen for and assess many urinary system-related diseases. A healthcare worker dips a specially made strip (dipstick) into a urine sample and notes how the color of the strip changes on the various pads. The dipstick can identify abnormalities in urine, such as blood, protein, glucose, ketones, nitrites, and pH levels. This information can be used to make preliminary diagnoses of kidney problems, urinary tract infections, and other urinary illnesses.

(88) (C) CT scan.

Imaging tests are not usually regarded as point-of-care testing. The most commonly ordered imaging tests include computed tomography (CT) scans, magnetic resonance imaging (MRI), ultrasound, and X-rays. They are carried out in specialist imaging departments or facilities and provide detailed images of inside body structures.

(89) (D) Fecal occult blood.

One point-of-care test that can be used to screen for colorectal cancer is the fecal occult blood test (FOBT). It finds stains of blood hidden in the stool, which could be a sign of cancer or colorectal polyps. FOBT is a non-invasive, reasonably easy test that can be carried out at home or in a medical facility to help in the early detection of colorectal cancer.

(90) (C) Both healthcare workers and laypeople.

Some point-of-care tests can be performed by both healthcare workers and laypeople. Point-of-care tests are less complex than their laboratory counterparts and generally very reliable. However, the incorrect use of techniques or a misinterpreted result may give rise to adverse situations (for example, the use of hemoglobin A1c tests to diagnose diabetes or misinterpreting a PT/INR test at home and wrongfully modifying a warfarin dose). Therefore, these tests must be used responsibly—it is of utmost importance to adequately educate a patient who will use point-of-care testing at home and provide clear instructions.

(91) (A) A document with information for a laboratory test.

A laboratory requisition is required whenever a lab test must be performed outside a medical office. It is a document that contains all the information needed for a laboratory to adequately perform the desired test on the patient's specimen (e.g., a microbiological culture of Mr. Doe's urine sample).

(92) (B) Patient's financial information.

A complete laboratory requisition includes many informational details, such as

- Healthcare provider's identification: full name, address, and contact information like a phone number.
- Patient's identification: full name, address, social security number, age, date of birth, gender, and insurance information.
- Specimen details: the source, date, and time of specimen collection.
- Testing details: the specific test to be performed and the provisional diagnosis.

(93) (B) Urine collected at any time of the day in a clean container.

Urine specimens may be collected using various techniques for different purposes. In most cases, urine samples require a random specimen, which is simply urine collected in a clean container at any time of the day. For most purposes, at least 12 mL of urine is necessary (half the container is usually enough). Although urine samples can be refrigerated, they should be processed within one hour after collection.

(94) (C) To quantify the twenty-four-hour protein clearance.

An early morning or first-morning urine specimen is collected early in the morning after the patient wakes up, and it may be used during the assessment of proteins like Bence Jones proteins (proteins present in patients with multiple myeloma) or pregnancy. Three early morning samples may be ordered to test for tuberculosis.

(95) (A) Urine collected after cleaning the genitals and discarding the first stream.

A patient must clean their genitals (to clean the distal portion of the urethra) and discard the first stream of urine to provide a clean-catch midstream urine specimen. This technique is commonly used to diagnose urinary tract infections. Catheterization can also collect samples for a urine culture, as they have a lower chance of contamination.

(96) (A) Bilirubin analysis.

Medical specimens require varying types of care and handling. Therefore, the appropriate guidelines must be considered during the management of each specimen. Some processing requirements include

- **Temperature**, e.g., urine specimens require refrigeration when not processed right away.
- **Light protection**, e.g., specimens for bilirubin analysis.
- **Sterility**, e.g., any specimen for a culture must be contained in a sterile container.

(97) (C) Refrigerated (2-8°C).

Stool collection is usually achieved with the help of a special kit. Some kits come with a plastic spoon or spatula, a specimen container, and a plastic potty or similar container to avoid contact with toilet water. However, any clean and empty container will work. The spoon is used to fill the specimen container, which is closed and sealed in a plastic bag. Instruct the patient to include stool samples with diarrhea/liquid, blood, ova (eggs), mucus, or any finding that may be considered abnormal. A stool sample can be refrigerated (2-8°C) but should be taken to the laboratory as soon as possible. Stool specimens are used to evaluate medical conditions, such as infections (especially by parasites or bacteria) or gastrointestinal neoplasms like colon cancer or polyps.

(98) (C) CSF.

Cerebrospinal fluid (CSF) is the transparent, colorless fluid that envelops the brain and spinal cord in the central nervous system (CNS). It differs from whole blood and plays important roles in the CNS's hydration and defense.

(99) (A) To transport oxygen.

Red blood cells are mature cells with hemoglobin that carry oxygen from the lungs to the rest of the body. They also carry carbon dioxide back to the lungs.

(100) (D) Immature red blood cells.

The bloodstream contains immature red blood cells called reticulocytes. They have a reticular (mesh-like) look because they still contain ribosome fragments. A reticulocyte count measures bone marrow activity and analyzes blood loss, anemia, and treatment response.

(101) (C) To stop bleeding.

Platelets are small clotting cells without a nucleus. They are fragments from megakaryocytes, which are bigger cells with a nucleus found in the bone marrow (rarely present in the blood). Platelets gather at the site of an injury or damage to a blood vessel to form a plug and start the clotting process, which helps halt bleeding.

(102) (C) Add anticoagulants and then centrifuge.

In order to extract plasma, anticoagulants are added to whole blood to stop it from clotting. After that, the blood sample is centrifuged to extract the liquid component, called plasma, from the formed elements, which include platelets, red blood cells, and white blood cells.

(103) (D) Lymphocytes.

White blood cells are a group of mature cells that protect the body from infections. Unlike red blood cells, they are colorless and have a nucleus. They can be divided into

- Granulocytes: neutrophils, basophils, and eosinophils.
- Agranulocytes: lymphocytes and monocytes.

(104) (C) It does not have clotting factors.

Serum is the liquid portion of clotted blood. It is obtained when the clotting factors are naturally activated after the specimen is collected. During the blood clotting process, the serum and clotting factors are separated. Serum is collected when the clot is removed from a blood sample.

(105) (C) Red blood cells.

Plasma is the liquid portion of blood and contains water, antibodies, albumin, globulins, coagulation factors, and other substances. However, as red blood cells are components of the blood's cellular makeup, they are not a part of plasma.

(106) (B) Anemia.

Reticulocytes are usually found within the bone marrow. However, bone marrow can release these slightly immature cells into the peripheral blood in patients with anemia. They show that the bone marrow has produced more red blood cells in response to the body's increased requirement for oxygen-carrying capacity.

(107) (D) They have a nucleus.

Red blood cells do not contain a nucleus, which is removed throughout development. This makes more room for hemoglobin, which is the molecule that carries oxygen. Red blood cells have a distinct form and function as a result.

(108) (C) 55%.

Plasma is the liquid portion of the blood and represents approximately fifty-five percent of the whole blood volume. Plasma is mostly water (ninety-one percent) with various substances like clotting factors, antibodies, albumin, globulins, lipids, carbohydrates, and hormones. Anticoagulants must be added to the sample to avoid activation of clotting factors and obtain plasma.

(109) (C) During sexual contact.

Sexual contact is the main way that the hepatitis B virus (HBV) spreads, although it can also be spread through various other means. Individuals who share contaminated syringes or needles, as well as direct transmission from an infected mother to her infant during birth, can result in the transmission of HBV.

(110) (A) Respiratory droplets.

The hepatitis B virus (HBV) is mainly spread through sexual contact, contaminated needles or sharps, and vertical transmission from infected mothers. Although respiratory droplets are not a frequent means of HBV transmission, respiratory infections can still be avoided by adhering to respiratory hygiene precautions.

(111) (B) 10%.

Ten percent of those who have acute hepatitis B may go on to acquire chronic hepatitis B. Chronic hepatitis B is defined as an infection that lasts longer than six months. The majority of people with acute hepatitis B infection recover fully without any long-term effects in a matter of months. Nevertheless, a tiny fraction of infections develop into chronic diseases that can cause persistent liver inflammation and other complications.

(112) (C) Lung cancer.

Long-term effects of a persistent hepatitis B infection might include portal hypertension, liver cancer, and cirrhosis of the liver. However, it is not directly linked to lung cancer. The formation of abnormal cells in the lungs is the main cause of lung cancer, and risk factors include smoking and exposure to specific environmental chemicals like asbestos.

(113) (A) The risk of chronic HCV infection is higher than chronic HBV infection.

Hepatitis C virus (HCV), similar to the hepatitis B virus, causes inflammation of the liver and can be transmitted via blood. However, HCV is predominantly present in patients who receive unsafe blood transfusions or share syringes when using intravenous drugs. Additionally, the majority of patients who become infected with the hepatitis C virus will develop chronic hepatitis C, which has no cure and cannot be prevented with vaccines.

(114) (B) Patient's last successful collection site.

In order to choose the right vein for the current phlebotomy procedure, medical assistants should identify the patient's most recent successful collection site.

(115) (C) Administer sedatives to help the patient relax.

Once the patient enters the room, the healthcare worker must present themself and verify that the patient's identity matches the order. A medical record, date of birth, or government-issued photo identification can be used. It is not uncommon for a patient to feel uncomfortable or anxious during this process, and it is important to be respectful and help them to relax. Explain the procedure to the patient and ask for verbal consent. Talk to them to help them shift their focus away from the procedure when possible. If the patient is visibly anxious, ask them what would make them feel more comfortable. Other ways to help the patient with their fear or anxiety include lying down in a supine position or counting.

(116) (D) The patient's insurance information.

Before the procedure can begin, the patient's healthcare provider must formally request a phlebotomy procedure. This can be achieved with a requisition or laboratory form. The Clinical Laboratory Improvement Amendments (CLIA) establishes the regulations to order laboratory tests, which include the laboratory form requirements. The requisition should contain the following information:

- Identification and contact information of the person who requested the test, usually the patient's healthcare provider.
- Patient identification information, which includes at least one unique identifier (social security number or healthcare record number), name, and date of birth.
- Specimen information, such as time and date of specimen collection.
- Test to be performed.
- Any other relevant information related to the sample or test, such as timing details, patient fasting, use of medications, or presence of fever.

(117) (B) Lidocaine.

To collect blood for laboratory assessment, a medical assistant needs to assemble the required equipment. This includes the following items.

- Patient's health record (and other appropriate means to correctly identify the patient).
- Phlebotomy order.
- Gauze.
- Tourniquet.
- Bandages or hypoallergenic tape.
- Alcohol pads (70% isopropyl alcohol).
- Safe disposal method (sharps and biohazard waste containers).
- Required blood collection devices (vacuum tubes, needles, tubes, syringes).

Specific items may vary for special collections (such as blood cultures or glucose tolerance tests).

(118) (A) When the child is fearful or anxious.

Phlebotomy in the pediatric population can be particularly difficult, and it should be performed by trained healthcare workers. It is normal for children of most ages to feel fearful during the procedure, and healthcare workers may need to employ various techniques to help their patients feel safer and cooperative.

(119) (A) Remove the needle before removing the tourniquet.

Hematomas are one of the most common problems associated with a phlebotomy procedure. Strategies to avoid this result include the following.

- Remove the tourniquet before removing the needle.
- Prioritize straight, superficial, and clearly visible veins.
- Avoid the intersection of veins.
- Apply pressure after removing the needle.

(120) (D) Serum cortisol level.

The circadian rhythm causes fluctuations in the level of serum cortisol. This hormone exhibits a diurnal rhythm, which peaks in the morning and drops in the evening. The circadian rhythm is the body's internal clock and controls this pattern. Numerous physiological functions are influenced by cortisol, such as metabolism, the stress response, and the sleep-wake cycle.

(121) (C) Diagnose colorectal cancer.

Electrocardiography is a diagnostic process that creates a graphical pattern based on the changes in electrical charge generated by cardiac activity. The instrument employed is an electrocardiograph, which produces a record called an electrocardiogram (ECG or EKG). Electrocardiography assesses arrhythmias, cardiovascular conditions like myocardial infarction, and other medical conditions like electrolyte imbalances (e.g., altered serum potassium).

(122) (A) Voltage.

Voltage is represented on the electrocardiograph via the y-axis. The voltage axis measures the electrical potential difference or amplitude of the electrical impulses obtained from the heart. Each square on the vertical grid usually corresponds to one millivolt (mV) of voltage.

(123) (A) 1 mm represents 0.04 seconds.

An electrocardiograph is a graphic recording of a patient's electrical cardiac activity. It contains vertical and horizontal lines at 1 mm intervals where the x-axis represents time (1 mm represents 0.04 seconds) and the y-axis represents voltage (10 mm represents 1 mV).

(124) (D) Ten electrodes.

There are ten electrodes or sensors (four for the limbs and six for the chest). They are used to record the heart's electrical activity from various angles. Electrodes are usually available as self-adhesive and disposable pads.

(125) (D) It is sometimes required if the chest has excess hair.

During an EKG, a disposable razor may be needed if the patient has excess hair on their chest. Hair can get in the way of the electrodes attaching correctly, which makes it more difficult to capture the heart's electrical activity accurately. The electrodes can more easily adhere to the skin by shaving off extra hair. This ensures excellent signal capture and enhances the quality of the EKG recording.

(126) (A) P wave.

The P wave on an EKG shows the depolarization of the atria. This tiny upward waveform appears before the QRS complex. The heart muscle's electrical activation or contraction is called depolarization. The propagation of electrical impulses across the atria starts atrial contraction and makes it easier for blood to enter the ventricles.

(127) (A) Depolarization of the ventricles.

The QRS complex is the combination of the Q, R, and S waves that represent the ventricles' depolarization. It is responsible for the contraction of the ventricles and the pumping of blood to the body.

(128) (C) T wave.

The T wave on an EKG shows the ventricles' repolarization. Repolarization follows the ventricles' depolarization and contraction (indicated by the QRS complex), which enables the ventricles to relax and prepare for the subsequent heartbeat. The T wave represents the ventricular muscle's electrical recovery and relaxation.

(129) (D) U wave.

Patients with hypokalemia (low serum potassium levels) may show the U wave, a little upward waveform, on an EKG. The slow repolarization of the Purkinje fibers in the ventricles is represented by the U wave, which usually appears after the T wave. It is thought to be connected to the ventricles' delayed repolarization, especially when electrolyte abnormalities are present.

(130) (D) Time the electrical impulse travels from the SA node to the AV node.

The PR interval begins with the P wave and ends with a point that connects the isoelectric line with the QRS complex. The PR interval represents the time the electrical impulse travels from the sinoatrial (SA) node to the auriculoventricular (AV) node.

(131) (C) ST segment.

The ST segment is an interval that begins at the end of the QRS complex and ends at the start of the T wave. It represents the time between the end of ventricular depolarization and repolarization.

(132) (D) Athletes.

A slower heart rate (less than sixty beats per minute) that arises from the sinus node, the heart's natural pacemaker, is referred to as sinus bradycardia. Although sinus bradycardia may occasionally be a sign of an underlying medical issue, it may also be deemed normal in some people. Due to their high degree of athleticism, athletes are frequently known to display sinus bradycardia as a physiological adaptation. Lowering one's resting heart rate is a normal result of regular exercise and athletic training for physically active people.

(133) (C) HR >100 beats per minute.

Sinus arrhythmias are characterized by an increased or decreased fire rate of the SA node, which results in tachycardia (more than 100 beats per minute) and bradycardia (less than sixty beats per minute). Sinus tachycardia can be a normal occurrence during exercise and extreme emotions. Sinus bradycardia can be a normal occurrence in some athletes. In other situations, these findings may be pathologic. Sinus arrhythmias may appear as a relatively normal EKG but with a faster or slower frequency.

(134) (C) After the age of fifty.

A colonoscopy is a screening test that looks for cancer or polyps in the colon. It is generally advised for anyone with a family history of colon polyps or cancer to get a colonoscopy after the age of fifty. The age recommendation is based on the increased risk of colorectal cancer with aging. For those with a significant family history or other risk factors, screening may begin sooner.

(135) (A) To diagnose specific diseases at an early stage.

Medical screenings are a valuable tool employed in preventive medicine. These diagnostic interventions aim to identify specific conditions at an early stage. In many cases, screenings take specific risk factors into consideration. For example, patients between fifty and eighty years old with a significant history of smoking should be screened for lung cancer. However, universal screenings encompass a broader population. For example, all patients older than forty-five years should be screened for diabetes and prediabetes, which includes those who are not overweight or obese.

(136) (B) Women below the age of sixty-five.

The Papanicolaou test is also known as a Pap smear or cervical cytology. It is a cytological sample taken from the cervix. The screening is done in women below the age of sixty-five to help detect cervical cancer.

(137) (A) After the age of forty.

Mammography is performed as a screening test for breast cancer in women after reaching the age of forty since the breast tissue becomes less dense after that age. It should be performed every one or two years.

(138) (C) They may result in overdiagnosis and extra medical costs for unnecessary treatment.

Prostate-specific antigen (PSA) screens were previously a common tool to help detect prostate cancer. However, the United States Preventive Services Task Force (USPSTF) now opposes the use of this screening due to overdiagnosis (PSA may be elevated in patients with non-malignant conditions, such as benign prostatic hyperplasia).

(139) (A) Physician.

Physicians manage many aspects of patient care, especially for those with complex conditions. They examine patients, diagnose the disease process, and develop effective treatment plans.

(140) (C) Social or community health worker.

Social or community health workers are in charge of coordinating care for high-risk patients. These individuals may require the service with recurrence or have complex and difficult-to-treat conditions.

(141) (C) Restoring blood flow.

The main concern when a patient presents with torsion of a limb is restoring blood flow. Torsion can cut off circulation and cause tissue damage or necrosis if not treated promptly.

(142) (B) Immobilize the affected area.

The initial step a medical assistant should take when a patient presents with a suspected bone fracture is to immobilize the affected area. This prevents further injury and reduces pain while awaiting further medical evaluation and treatment.

(143) (C) Pharmacist.

Pharmacists manage medication and related resources. They have extensive training with a focus on drugs and how to use them appropriately. They work in tandem with other medical professionals to promote patient safety and optimize pharmaceutical therapy. They are responsible for the following tasks.

- Review prescriptions.
- Provide pharmacological information.
- Identify any possible interactions or adverse effects.
- Ensure patients are given the correct prescriptions in the right quantities.

(144) (B) Health record.

A health record is a legal document that notes clinical findings, the progress of treatments, and a patient's medical and family history. It helps healthcare providers communicate with each other by recording relevant information and serves as a research document.

(145) (C) Can only be used by one person at a time.

Numerous healthcare personnel participating in a patient's care can access and use an EHR simultaneously, which is one of the significant advantages of this technology. Thanks to this, healthcare team members may now collaborate and communicate efficiently.

(146) (B) Can be used by multiple persons at a time.

Records can be electronic (electronic health records or EHRs) or paper-based. Each has its benefits and disadvantages. However, EHRs now dominate medical documentation. Paper documentation is harder to share, requires more physical space, is easier to misfile or lose, can only be used by one person at a time, and can be difficult to read. Conversely, EHRs are very efficient and versatile, can be shared when required, and are easy to read and update. In addition, EHR software often has other practical features, such as scheduling and billing systems.

(147) (B) Chief complaint.

A chief complaint is an accurate and concise chronology and description of the patient's condition. It includes any treatment the patient has received and its success or failure.

(148) (C) Progress notes.

As patients continue to be seen by their healthcare team, their progress and the evolution of disease are recorded in the progress notes. This section documents various new findings, orders, and events.

(149) (B) Consent forms.

Patients (or legal representatives) may be required to sign consent forms before certain procedures, especially those that carry some risk, such as surgical procedures or when the patient must agree to or refuse treatment. Before a signature is obtained, the provider must explain the procedure or treatment, which includes the consequences of accepting or refusing the recommendation.

(150) (D) Consent form.

Consent forms do not directly contribute to a patient's diagnosis. They are mainly used to record a patient's approval for particular operations, therapies, or interventions.

(151) (A) Clinical findings.

Clinical and paraclinical findings include objective discoveries from the physical exam and laboratory or imaging reports. The findings are recorded in this section and include measurements and observations such as abnormalities, physical indicators, or clinical manifestations.

(152) (A) New patient visit.

A new patient visit is a patient's first appointment with their new healthcare provider. It focuses on a thorough assessment of their personal and family medical history. It may also include additional testing. If a patient comes for a specific condition, it may also be discussed. A patient may again be considered a new patient after three or more years without a visit.

(153) (B) Follow-up visit.

Follow-up visits are scheduled right after a standard office visit in order to review the progress of a condition. The healthcare provider may analyze the patient's diagnostic results to develop a treatment plan or check the patient's response to treatment.

(154) (D) Preventive health exam.

Preventive health exams are also known as physicals or annual exams. They are yearly routine exams to check overall health, schedule screening tests, order immunizations, and identify risk factors.

(155) (C) Urgent visit.

An urgent visit allows patients to see their provider as soon as possible without going to urgent care or an emergency room. In these cases, it is important to determine the severity of the situation (triage) and schedule the next available appointment to ensure timely treatment.

(156) (A) Telehealth visit.

Telehealth visits allow patients to receive care via phone or video. Many types of visits can be safely arranged as telehealth visits unless a physical exam is required (e.g., the yearly preventive health exam or physical).

(157) (D) Screening visit.

Screening visits can be arranged after a standard visit as a part of a personalized screening or prevention plan. They involve the preventive study of a patient with or without risk factors for a specific condition (e.g., screening for diabetes in a fifty-year-old patient).

(158) (B) Specialty visit.

Patients who require a specialty visit must make an appointment with a specialist. A primary care physician often provides a referral for patients who need special care (e.g., a specific diagnosis, treatment, or procedure that a specialist must oversee).

(159) (A) Follow-up visits usually require more time than new patient visits.

The scheduling process may vary from patient to patient and between different types of visits. New patient visits usually require more time to discuss medical history and fill out forms. Patients who require fasting before a procedure should be seen early in the morning. Patients who require frequent visits should be seen at the same location (day or hour) to increase patient compliance. It is important to verify that a specialist accepts a patient's insurance when providing a referral.

(160) (C) HIPAA forms.

The Health Insurance Portability and Accountability Act (HIPAA) protects patient health information. The patient or their legal representative must sign HIPAA forms to allow their health information or photographs to be disclosed for research or shared with a third party.

(161) (A) Concept of *face*.

Holistic considerations in healthcare delivery include cultural, religious, psychosocial, and economic factors. These are necessary in many instances to maximize care in inpatient and outpatient settings. Cultural factors shape the way patients view health, drugs, diseases, and the healing process. For example, an important consideration in Asian cultures is the concept of *face*. This references the need to preserve dignity and prestige throughout the diagnosis and treatment process. Latin American patients, on the other hand, tend to favor the use of home remedies alongside traditional medicine and rely on familial support.

(162) (A) Blood transfusions.

Jehovah's Witnesses are against receiving blood transfusions. They regard it as a transgression of their religious beliefs since they think the Bible forbids consuming or introducing blood into the body. When this procedure is recommended, Jehovah's Witnesses seek out and prefer alternate treatments that do not entail blood transfusions.

(163) (C) They impair compliance.

Mental health can impact the effectiveness of medical treatments for physical conditions. Anxiety and depression are both relatively common during disease and may impair patient compliance and result in worse outcomes.

(164) (B) Christian evangelical groups.

Various Christian evangelical groups reject the use of vaccines. Certain religious groups may also have dietary restrictions or may require accommodations for prayer as an inpatient.

(165) (D) Affect psychosocial well-being.

Financial worries about the expense of healthcare and insurance can significantly impact the psychological state of patients. It may adversely affect their general well-being, which can raise stress, anxiety, and uncertainty. Anxiety about not having enough money for prescription drugs or necessary therapies can be upsetting and detrimental to a patient's mental health.

(166) (A) Biological.

A patient's condition or disability may affect their capacity to engage meaningfully in a conversation, which limits their understanding and involvement in their care when not considered. Examples include patients with dementia, stroke, and hearing loss. Biological barriers also include age and developmental stages. For example, pediatric patients may have difficulty understanding and expressing their symptoms and concerns.

(167) (B) Language.

Sometimes, patients and healthcare providers do not speak the same language. However, language barriers may go beyond that. Patients may not have health literacy and can misinterpret certain words. It is essential to speak clearly and avoid excessive use of medical terms.

(168) (C) Introduce problems.

The advent of telehealth has reduced the issue of geographical distance for various medical services. However, poor technological infrastructure may introduce new problems during virtual visits, such as poor internet connection or lack of proper equipment.

(169) (D) Hearing loss.

Depression, fear, anxiety, and other psychological factors may affect how patients understand and transmit information to their healthcare providers.

(170) (B) The inner sense of gender, which may align with being male, female, both, or neither.

Gender identity is the inner sense of gender, which may align with being male, female, both, or neither. This group of characteristics is associated with and determined by several psychosocial, cultural, and behavioral factors.

(171) (C) Ask the patient about their preferred pronouns.

Pronouns are words used to replace a noun. Examples of pronouns include I, me, he, she, him, her, they, them, theirs, myself, and herself. Pronouns denote someone's gender, which may or may not align with the person's biological gender. In the majority of cases, if the pronouns a healthcare worker uses do not align with a patient's gender identity, they will correct them. To avoid such situations, MAs can ask their patients about their preferred pronouns or use gender-neutral pronouns like the singular form of *they* (they, them, theirs).

(172) (B) Assume based on appearance.

It is improper for medical assistants to infer someone's gender identity from their exterior appearance. Healthcare workers who assume a patient's gender identity without their confirmation can misgender or discomfort them. To ensure courteous and inclusive communication, medical assistants should instead ask patients about their preferred pronouns or use gender-neutral ones.

(173) (B) Pronouns should be avoided altogether.

Gender may or may not align with the person's sex assigned at birth. As a result, it is important to know how to use pronouns as a courtesy to patients. It is a way to connect with them and provide the best care possible.

(174) (D) 21st Century Cures Act.

The National Institutes of Health (NIH) is given resources and funds by the 21st Century Cures Act to support biomedical science research. The act was passed to hasten the creation and authorization of novel medical therapies, such as medications and medical equipment. It seeks to boost patient access to novel medicines, encourage innovation, and increase the effectiveness of the healthcare system.

(175) (C) Social Security Act.

The Social Security Act established a federal benefit system to provide general welfare to retired, jobless, and disabled people. It created Social Security retirement benefits, Supplemental Security Income (SSI), and Social Security Disability Insurance (SSDI).

(176) (A) Health Information Technology for Economic and Clinical Health (HITECH) Act.

The Health Information Technology for Economic and Clinical Health (HITECH) Act aims to promote the use of technology and EHRs to increase efficiency, privacy, and safety in the healthcare system.

(177) (B) Public Readiness and Emergency Preparedness (PREP) Act.

The Public Readiness and Emergency Preparedness (PREP) Act authorizes the Secretary of HHS to provide liability protection through a PREP Act declaration to individuals or groups in relation to the administration of medical countermeasures.

(178) (C) HHS Acquisition Regulation (HHSAR).

The Department of Health and Human Services (HHS) Acquisition Regulation (HHSAR) creates procurement and acquisition procedures. The Federal Acquisition Regulation (FAR) applies and supplements this body of regulations.

(179) (A) Health Insurance Portability and Accountability Act (HIPAA).

The Health Insurance Portability and Accountability Act (HIPAA) is a privacy rule that addresses the disclosure and use of protected health information. It regulates how health plans, healthcare providers, and other organizations that manage patient data disclose and use protected health information (PHI). HIPAA establishes guidelines and rules to safeguard the confidentiality and integrity of personal health information.

(180) (B) Patient.

In most cases, the patient has the power to grant consent. This action is necessary for healthcare workers to touch or treat patients or disclose any information about them.

Test 2

(181) Which type of drug is used to treat certain health conditions?

(A) Therapeutic.

(B) Diagnostic.

(C) Palliative.

(D) Preventive.

(182) Which type of drug is used to treat certain symptoms of severe or fatal disease processes and provide relief?

(A) Therapeutic.

(B) Diagnostic.

(C) Palliative.

(D) Preventive.

(183) Knowledge of pharmacology is necessary for medical assistants for all the following reasons except:

(A) To understand the effects of prescribed medications.

(B) To learn administration methods.

(C) To be aware of possible adverse effects.

(D) To understand the manufacture of medications.

(184) Which class of drugs is used to relieve and control pain?

(A) Analgesics.

(B) Antacids.

(C) Antiarrhythmics.

(D) Antibiotics.

(185) Which drug classification is used to treat irregular or abnormal heartbeats?

(A) Antacids.

(B) Antiarrhythmics.

(C) Antibiotics.

(D) Anticoagulants.

(186) Which drug classification is used to prevent the formation of blood clots?

(A) Analgesics.

(B) Antiarrhythmics.

(C) Antibiotics.

(D) Anticoagulants.

(187) Which drug class is used to treat hypertension, tachycardia, and arrhythmias?

(A) Beta-blockers.

(B) Bronchodilators.

(C) Corticosteroids.

(D) Cytotoxics.

(188) Which drug class represents synthetic analogs of adrenal gland hormones and treats conditions like rheumatoid arthritis?

(A) Beta-blockers.

(B) Bronchodilators.

(C) Corticosteroids.

(D) Cytotoxics.

(189) What is the main role of expectorants in the field of medicine?

(A) To induce and prolong sleep.

(B) To reduce blood glucose levels.

(C) To treat constipation.

(D) To clear mucus from the respiratory airways.

(190) What is the main role of antihistamines in the field of medicine?

(A) To treat allergic conditions.

(B) To treat various types of cancer.

(C) To treat hypertension.

(D) To treat psychiatric conditions.

(191) Which regulatory body oversees the safety and labeling of over the counter medications in the United States?

(A) Food and Drug Administration (FDA).

(B) Drug Enforcement Administration (DEA).

(C) National Institutes of Health (NIH).

(D) World Health Organization (WHO).

(192) Which type of medication can be sold to the general public without a prescription?

(A) Prescription medications.

(B) Over the counter medications.

(C) Controlled substance.

(D) Vaccines.

(193) Which OTC medication is commonly used for motion sickness?

(A) Acetaminophen.

(B) Dimenhydrinate.

(C) Hydrocortisone.

(D) Pyrithione zinc.

(194) Which of the following substances is classified as a Schedule II controlled substance?

(A) Morphine.

(B) Ketamine.

(C) Tramadol.

(D) Pregabalin.

(195) Which schedule of controlled substances has the lowest potential for abuse?

(A) Schedule II.

(B) Schedule III.

(C) Schedule IV.

(D) Schedule V.

(196) Which of the following statements is not correct regarding side effects and adverse reactions?

(A) Adverse reactions are inherently negative.

(B) Side effects can be positive (but unintended) or negative (but manageable).

(C) Side effects are usually more predictable than adverse reactions.

(D) Drowsiness is an adverse reaction that may occur in patients using antihistamines.

(197) What is the general term used to describe valid clinical reasons for using a drug to treat specific conditions?

(A) Indications.

(B) Off-label indications.

(C) Relative contraindications.

(D) Absolute contraindications.

(198) What is the general term that refers to a valid reason to avoid the use of a drug?

(A) Indications.

(B) Contraindications.

(C) Off-label indications.

(D) Relative contraindications.

(199) What is the key difference between absolute and relative contraindications?

(A) Absolute contraindications are life-threatening and relative contraindications require caution and risk-benefit analysis.

(B) Absolute contraindications can be resolved and relative contraindications cannot.

(C) Absolute contraindications are more common than relative contraindications.

(D) Absolute contraindications are specific to dosage and presentation and relative contraindications are not.

(200) What is the enclosure usually made of in a capsule medication form?

(A) Gelatin.

(B) Cocoa butter.

(C) Polyethylene glycol.

(D) Oily solution.

(201) Which medication form is a flat tablet that dissolves inside the mouth?

(A) Tablet.

(B) Capsule.

(C) Powder.

(D) Lozenge.

(202) Which medication form involves the drug being suspended in a liquid solution for oral administration?

(A) Suspension.

(B) Syrup.

(C) Emulsion.

(D) Elixir.

(203) Which medication form requires shaking before use due to the presence of a lipid suspended in water?

(A) Suspension.

(B) Syrup.

(C) Emulsion.

(D) Elixir.

(204) Which defense mechanism involves transforming a negative response or feeling into something positive or productive?

(A) Undoing.

(B) Sublimation.

(C) Projection.

(D) Compensation.

(205) Which condition is characterized by chest pain related to decreased blood flow to the heart?

(A) Appendicitis.

(B) Alzheimer's disease.

(C) Angina.

(D) Acute cholecystitis.

(206) Which condition is characterized by inflammation of the airways and presents with wheezing and coughing?

(A) Asthma.

(B) Atrial fibrillation.

(C) Bacterial vaginosis.

(D) Breast cancer.

(207) Which condition is characterized by chronic inflammation of the digestive tract and presents with symptoms like diarrhea, weight loss, and pain?

(A) Crohn's disease.

(B) Deep vein thrombosis.

(C) Otitis.

(D) Hepatitis.

(208) What is a common symptom of food poisoning?

(A) Diarrhea.

(B) Vertigo.

(C) Iron deficiency anemia.

(D) Pneumonia.

(209) Which condition is characterized by infection of the gastrointestinal tract and presents with symptoms like diarrhea and nausea?

(A) Appendicitis.

(B) Gastroenteritis.

(C) Urinary tract infection.

(D) Prostate cancer.

(210) What is the sensation experienced in vertigo?

(A) Sensation of motion or spinning.

(B) Chest pain and inflammation.

(C) Low hemoglobin levels.

(D) Dysuria and frequent urination.

(211) Which laboratory test is used to assess blood cells and can help diagnose conditions like anemia and infections?

(A) Stool analysis.

(B) Blood chemistry.

(C) Urinalysis.

(D) Complete blood count (CBC).

(212) Which of the following conditions is not assessed by a urinalysis?

(A) Urine thyroid hormone levels.

(B) Urine PH levels.

(C) Urine glucose levels.

(D) Urinary tract infections and kidney disease.

(213) Which laboratory test measures oxygen, carbon dioxide, bicarbonate, and pH levels in the blood?

(A) Urinalysis.

(B) Blood gas analysis.

(C) Hormone levels.

(D) Oximetry.

(214) Which imaging technique uses X-rays to visualize tissues based on their degree of X-ray absorption?

(A) Radiography.

(B) MRI scan.

(C) PET scan.

(D) Ultrasonography.

(215) Which imaging technique employs magnets and radio waves to create a computerized image without X-ray radiation?

(A) Radiography.

(B) CT scan.

(C) MRI scan.

(D) PET scan.

(216) Which of the following is not a symptom associated with orthostatic hypotension?

(A) Vertigo.

(B) Lightheadedness.

(C) Blurred vision.

(D) Abdominal cramp.

(217) Which term is used to describe a sudden drop in blood pressure after changes in position?

(A) Orthostatic hypotension.

(B) Vertigo.

(C) Hypertension.

(D) Syncope.

(218) Where is the cuff placed to measure blood pressure in the arm with a sphygmomanometer?

(A) 1 inch below the antecubital fossa.

(B) 1 inch above the antecubital fossa.

(C) 1 inch below the popliteal fossa.

(D) 1 inch above the popliteal fossa.

(219) Which of the following is not a unit of measurement commonly used for temperature?

(A) Fahrenheit (°F).

(B) Celsius (°C).

(C) Kelvin (K).

(D) Ohm (O).

(220) What is the average temperature range for an adult across the day?

(A) 96.6°F to 98.6°F.

(B) 97.6°F to 99°F.

(C) 98.6°F to 100°F.

(D) 99°F to 101°F.

(221) What temperature reading is considered febrile?

(A) Higher than 99.6°F.

(B) Higher than 100.4°F.

(C) Higher than 102°F.

(D) Higher than 105.8°F.

(222) What is the term for extremely low temperatures that are potentially lethal?

(A) Hypothermia.

(B) Hyperpyrexia.

(C) Febrile.

(D) Hyperthermia.

(223) Which site of temperature measurement tends to have readings 1°F or 0.6°C lower than oral readings?

(A) Axillary.

(B) Tympanic.

(C) Temporal artery.

(D) Oral.

(224) Which of the following is the most reliable noninvasive method for temperature measurement?

(A) Tympanic thermometer.

(B) Digital thermometer.

(C) Temporal artery scanner.

(D) Oral thermometer.

(225) Which of the following arteries is not commonly used to measure the pulse?

(A) Carotid.

(B) Temporal.

(C) Aorta.

(D) Brachial.

(226) How can the heart rate be determined at the apex of the heart?

(A) Palpating the radial artery.

(B) Palpating the carotid artery.

(C) Auscultating with a stethoscope.

(D) Observing the dorsalis pedis artery.

(227) What is the normal range for pulse rate in healthy adults?

(A) 30-60 beats per minute.

(B) 60-100 beats per minute.

(C) 100-140 beats per minute.

(D) 140-180 beats per minute.

(228) What is an abnormal rhythm of the pulse called?

(A) Tachycardia.

(B) Bradycardia.

(C) Arrhythmia.

(D) Amplitude.

(229) What does the amplitude of the pulse mainly refer to?

(A) The number of pulsations measured in one minute.

(B) The regularity of time between pulsations.

(C) The strength of the heart contractions.

(D) The condition of the artery.

(230) How should the patient's head be positioned during eye instillation?

(A) Tilted forward.

(B) Tilted backward and looking up.

(C) Turned to the left side.

(D) Turned to the right side.

(231) How should ointment be administered during eye instillation?

(A) Squeeze from the outer to the inner canthus.

(B) Squeeze from the inner to the outer canthus.

(C) Apply in a circular motion.

(D) Apply with a gentle patting motion.

(232) What is the correct method for performing ear irrigation on a patient?

(A) Use cold water to minimize discomfort.

(B) Direct the irrigation solution towards the eardrum.

(C) Pull the ear upward and back to straighten the ear canal.

(D) Use a high-pressure stream to ensure thorough cleaning.

(233) How should drops be administered during ear instillation?

(A) Place the tip in the meatus and instill drops.

(B) Apply drops to the outer earlobe.

(C) Apply drops to the back of the ear.

(D) Squeeze drops onto a cotton swab and insert into the ear canal.

(234) What type of wound is characterized by straight and clean cuts?

(A) Incisions.

(B) Lacerations.

(C) Abrasions.

(D) Contusions.

(235) What are lacerations characterized by?

(A) Straight and clean cuts.

(B) Irregular edges.

(C) Superficial scrapes.

(D) Rupture of small blood vessels.

(236) How can abrasions be treated?

(A) Closure with sutures or Steri-Strips.

(B) Cleaning and covering with a sterile dressing.

(C) Cold packs and suturing.

(D) With systemic antibiotics.

(237) What is a contusion?

(A) A tear characterized by irregular edges.

(B) A superficial scrape of the skin.

(C) A non-penetrating injury that damages the skin and deeper tissues without laceration.

(D) A wound that requires closure with sutures or Steri-Strips.

(238) Which drugs are commonly administered subcutaneously?

(A) Opioids.

(B) Heparin.

(C) Antibiotics.

(D) Vaccines.

(239) What is the recommended angle for inserting subcutaneous injections?

(A) 30 degrees.

(B) 45 degrees.

(C) 60 degrees.

(D) 90 degrees.

(240) Which of the following body parts is not commonly used for administering subcutaneous injections?

(A) Upper arm.

(B) Abdomen.

(C) Thighs.

(D) Buttocks.

(241) When faster absorption of medication is required, which route of administration is preferred?

(A) Oral.

(B) Intramuscular.

(C) Subcutaneous.

(D) Topical.

(242) All of the following muscles are commonly used for intramuscular injections except:

(A) Biceps brachii.

(B) Gluteus medius.

(C) Vastus lateralis.

(D) Deltoid.

(243) What is the recommended angle for inserting intramuscular injections?

(A) 30 degrees.

(B) 45 degrees.

(C) 60 degrees.

(D) 90 degrees.

(244) Which type of suture material absorbs or dissolves after the healing process is completed?

(A) Catgut.

(B) Nylon.

(C) Silk.

(D) Polyester.

(245) Which type of suture material requires manual removal after the healing process is complete?

(A) Catgut.

(B) Nylon.

(C) Vicryl.

(D) PDS.

(246) What are the type of sutures suitable for suturing inner or deep layers of tissue known as?

(A) Absorbable sutures.

(B) Nonabsorbable sutures.

(C) Catgut sutures.

(D) Silk sutures.

(247) What are the type of sutures suitable for suturing superficial skin wounds known as?

(A) Absorbable sutures.

(B) Nonabsorbable sutures.

(C) Catgut sutures.

(D) Silk sutures.

(248) When should a sample for a culture be taken during suture removal?

(A) If the wound is red.

(B) If the wound presents discharge.

(C) If the patient requests it.

(D) If the sutures are difficult to remove.

(249) What instrument is used to cut sutures during removal?

(A) Suture removal scissors.

(B) Surgical staple remover.

(C) Dressing forceps.

(D) Steri-Strips.

(250) How should surgical staples be removed?

(A) Using suture removal scissors.

(B) Using a staple remover.

(C) Using dressing forceps.

(D) Using Steri-Strips.

(251) Which direction should the gauze be used to clean the eyelid and eyelashes?

(A) From outer canthus to inner canthus.

(B) From inner canthus to outer canthus.

(C) From bottom to top.

(D) From top to bottom.

(252) What is the recommended first-line treatment for anaphylaxis?

(A) Intravenous antihistamines.

(B) Glucocorticoids.

(C) Intramuscular epinephrine.

(D) Diphenhydramine.

(253) A severe and generalized allergic reaction is known as what?

(A) Anaphylaxis.

(B) Anaphylactic shock.

(C) Urticaria.

(D) Angioedema.

(254) What is the most common sterilization technique that uses steam, pressure, temperature, and time?

(A) Steam sterilization.

(B) Flash sterilization.

(C) Low-temperature sterilization.

(D) Peracetic acid sterilization.

(255) Which sterilization method does not require heat and includes ethylene oxide, hydrogen peroxide, and hydrogen peroxide/ozone?

(A) Steam sterilization.

(B) Flash sterilization.

(C) Low-temperature sterilization.

(D) Peracetic acid sterilization.

(256) Which method of sterilization is commonly employed to sterilize endoscopic tubing?

(A) Steam sterilization.

(B) Flash sterilization.

(C) Low-temperature sterilization.

(D) Peracetic acid sterilization.

(257) What is the purpose of decontamination (pre-cleaning) in the sterilization process?

(A) To remove visible traces of tissues, soil, or fluids.

(B) To sterilize the items.

(C) To arrange the items properly.

(D) To monitor the sterilization parameters.

(258) How should the items be arranged for sterilization?

(A) In a random order.

(B) In a way that ensures all surfaces come into contact with the sterilizing agent.

(C) In separate sterilization cycles.

(D) In a way that minimizes contact with the sterilizing agent.

(259) What should be avoided while unfolding the sterile kit?

(A) Touching the inside portion or the content.

(B) Opening the lowermost flap first.

(C) Placing the kit on a non-sterile surface.

(D) Skipping the step of checking the indicator tape.

(260) Which stage of cleaning involves cleaning products and warmer water?

(A) Pre-cleaning.

(B) Main cleaning.

(C) Rinsing.

(D) Disinfection.

(261) Which of the following signs indicates an infection of a wound?

(A) Dryness and peeling around the wound.

(B) Redness, swelling, and pus.

(C) Light scabbing over the wound.

(D) Wound edges closing together.

(262) During which stage of cleaning is a disinfectant used on the item or surface?

(A) Rinsing.

(B) Disinfection.

(C) Final rinse.

(D) Drying.

(263) What is a potential risk of dog saliva contacting an open wound?

(A) Immediate healing.

(B) Reduction in swelling.

(C) Increased risk of infection.

(D) Faster clotting.

(264) What should be done before turning on the water for handwashing?

(A) Remove any jewelry.

(B) Use a paper towel to touch the faucet.

(C) Use warm or lukewarm water.

(D) Place hands into the water.

(265) What is the normal range for specific gravity in urinalysis?

(A) 1.010 to 1.015.

(B) 1.015 to 1.020.

(C) 1.010 to 1.025.

(D) 1.025 to 1.030.

(266) All of the following should be absolutely negative in a urinalysis except:

(A) Blood.

(B) WBC.

(C) Leukocyte esterase.

(D) Ketones.

(267) What is the normal range for pH in urinalysis?

(A) 3.0 to 5.0.

(B) 4.5 to 7.8.

(C) 7.8 to 8.5.

(D) 8.5 to 10.0.

(268) How many red blood cells per high-power field are considered within the normal range in urinalysis?

(A) 0 to 2 cells per high-power field.

(B) 0 to 4 cells per high-power field.

(C) 4 to 8 cells per high-power field.

(D) 8 to 12 cells per high-power field.

(269) What is the primary function of epithelial cells in the human body?

(A) Energy production.

(B) Protein synthesis.

(C) Protection and regulation of substance flow.

(D) Muscle contraction.

(270) What is the primary function of red blood cells (RBCs) in the human body?

(A) Immune response.

(B) Blood clotting.

(C) Oxygen transport.

(D) Hormone regulation.

(271) What is the normal range for pH in a basic stool analysis?

(A) 6.0 to 6.5.

(B) 6.5 to 7.0.

(C) 7.0 to 7.5.

(D) 7.5 to 8.0.

(272) What is the normal range for osmolality in a basic stool analysis?

(A) 200 to 250 mOsmol/kg.

(B) 250 to 280 mOsmol/kg.

(C) 280 to 325 mOsmol/kg.

(D) 325 to 350 mOsmol/kg.

(273) What is the maximum permissible amount of fat in a basic stool analysis?

(A) 7 g/d.

(B) 10 g/d.

(C) 15 g/d.

(D) 20 g/d.

(274) What is the normal range for alpha-1-antitrypsin in a basic stool analysis?

(A) Less than 400 mg/L.

(B) Less than 540 mg/L.

(C) 540 to 600 mg/L.

(D) Greater than 600 mg/L.

(275) What is the expected total lung capacity for a 40-year-old female?

(A) 6.9 L.

(B) 4.9 L.

(C) 3.3 L.

(D) 2.6 L.

(276) How soon should a sputum specimen be taken to the laboratory?

(A) Within 24 hours.

(B) Within 48 hours.

(C) Within 1-2 hours.

(D) Within 3-4 hours.

(277) Which of the following does not require a patient reminder when collecting a sputum specimen?

(A) Spit into the container.

(B) Perform hand washing to reduce the chances of contaminating the specimen.

(C) Container is sterile and should not be opened until ready to use.

(D) Close the container tightly.

(278) Which of the following substances may not present higher levels during stressful conditions?

(A) Cortisol.

(B) Catecholamines.

(C) White blood cells.

(D) Insulin.

(279) Which of the following best describes the significance of a platelet count in a complete blood count (CBC)?

(A) Determines oxygen-carrying capacity.

(B) Measures blood clotting ability.

(C) Assesses immune function.

(D) Evaluates kidney function.

(280) What is the normal upper limit for serum total cholesterol (TC) in a healthy adult?

(A) <150 mg/dL.

(B) <200 mg/dL.

(C) <250 mg/dL.

(D) <300 mg/dL.

(281) What is the recommended range for high-density lipoprotein (HDL)?

(A) <40 mg/dL.

(B) ≥60 mg/dL.

(C) ≥100 mg/dL.

(D) <120 mg/dL.

(282) What is the normal upper limit for serum triglycerides (TG) in a healthy adult?

(A) <100 mg/dL.

(B) <130 mg/dL.

(C) <150 mg/dL.

(D) <180 mg/dL.

(283) Which of the following statements best describes the significance of high-density lipoprotein (HDL) levels in a lipid panel?

(A) High HDL levels are associated with an increased risk of cardiovascular disease.

(B) HDL helps remove cholesterol from the bloodstream.

(C) Low HDL levels indicate better cardiovascular health.

(D) HDL levels are irrelevant to heart disease risk.

(284) What is the normal range for serum bicarbonate (HCO3) in arterial blood?

(A) 15-20 mEq/L.

(B) 21-26 mEq/L.

(C) 27-32 mEq/L.

(D) 33-38 mEq/L.

(285) What is the preferred location for phlebotomy?

(A) Back of the hand.

(B) Foot.

(C) Antecubital fossa.

(D) Popliteal fossa.

(286) What should be done if there is a presence of infection at a potential phlebotomy site?

(A) Use povidone-iodine for disinfection.

(B) Proceed with venipuncture carefully.

(C) Select another site.

(D) Apply a tourniquet for longer than 2 minutes.

(287) Why should the side of a mastectomy be avoided for phlebotomy?

(A) Increased risk of infection.

(B) Impaired lymphatic flow altering the test results.

(C) Difficulty in finding a visible vein.

(D) Higher probability of hematoma formation.

(288) What is the recommended disinfectant for preparing the phlebotomy site?

(A) 70% isopropyl alcohol.

(B) Povidone-iodine.

(C) Hydrogen peroxide.

(D) Chlorhexidine.

(289) What is the recommended disinfectant for preparing the phlebotomy site when collecting a blood sample for blood culture?

(A) 70% isopropyl alcohol.

(B) Povidone-iodine.

(C) Hydrogen peroxide.

(D) Chlorhexidine.

(290) What should be done if there is a presence of hematoma at a potential phlebotomy site?

(A) Apply cold compresses before proceeding.

(B) Proceed with venipuncture carefully.

(C) Select another site.

(D) Apply a tourniquet for longer than 2 minutes.

(291) Which tube is used for coagulation tests such as PT, PTT, and INR?

(A) Gray.

(B) Lavender.

(C) Light blue.

(D) Royal blue.

(292) Which tube is used to study trace elements like aluminum, mercury, and selenium?

(A) Gray.

(B) Lavender.

(C) Light blue.

(D) Royal blue.

(293) Which tube is used for chemistry tests and particularly for glucose levels?

(A) Gray.

(B) Lavender.

(C) Light blue.

(D) Royal blue.

(294) Which tube is used for hematology tests that include complete blood count and hemoglobin?

(A) Gray.

(B) Lavender.

(C) Light blue.

(D) Royal blue.

(295) How far should a tourniquet be placed after selecting a vein for a phlebotomy?

(A) 4 fingers below the site.

(B) 4 fingers above the site.

(C) 8 fingers below the site.

(D) 8 fingers above the site.

(296) Which step should be performed first in the vacuum tube venipuncture method?

(A) Position the patient.

(B) Verify the order.

(C) Gather equipment and supplies.

(D) Perform hand washing.

(297) What is the purpose of applying a tourniquet in the vacuum tube venipuncture method?

(A) To anchor the vein.

(B) To remove the needle.

(C) To mix the blood and additives.

(D) To improve vein visibility.

(298) What is the correct procedure to follow after withdrawing the needle during venipuncture?

(A) Immediately discard the needle in a sharps container.

(B) Apply ice to the venipuncture site.

(C) Apply pressure over the venipuncture site with a clean gauze pad.

(D) Instruct the patient to hold their arm above their head.

(299) What should be done to the tubes after they are filled with blood and additives in the vacuum tube venipuncture method?

(A) Remove the tourniquet.

(B) Apply pressure over the venipuncture site.

(C) Invert the tubes to mix the blood and additives.

(D) Label the tubes with the required information.

(300) How should contaminated materials be disposed of in a medical setting?

(A) Place them in a regular trash bin.

(B) Disinfect them before disposal.

(C) Place them in a designated biohazard container.

(D) Incinerate them immediately.

(301) Which method of EKG recording involves patient participation in an exercise challenge?

(A) Holter monitor.

(B) Cardiac stress test.

(C) Event monitor.

(D) 12-lead EKG.

(302) What is the main purpose of an event monitor?

(A) To monitor cardiac activity for prolonged periods of time.

(B) To record cardiac activity during a period of cardiovascular stress.

(C) To diagnose conditions that may need more than 24 hours to appear.

(D) To determine if the patient presents an arrhythmia during exercise.

(303) Which leads are part of the precordial leads in a 12-lead EKG?

(A) I, II, III.

(B) aVR, aVL, aVF.

(C) V1, V2, V3, V4, V5, V6.

(D) A1, A2, A3.

(304) Which leads are part of the augmented leads in a 12-lead EKG?

(A) I, II, III.

(B) aVR, aVL, aVF.

(C) V1, V2, V3, V4, V5, V6.

(D) A1, A2, A3.

(305) What is a portable EKG recording device that a patient carries for 24 hours or more known as?

(A) Holter monitor.

(B) Cardiac stress test.

(C) Event monitor.

(D) 12-lead EKG.

(306) What is the cause of somatic tremor artifacts in an EKG?

(A) Patient anxiety and discomfort.

(B) Muscle movement.

(C) Talking during the procedure.

(D) Medical conditions causing tremors.

(307) When are pacemaker spikes artifacts usually seen in an EKG?

(A) Patients with a pacemaker.

(B) Patients with high blood pressure.

(C) Patients experiencing dyspnea.

(D) Patients with a history of anxiety.

(308) An EKG artifact that is characterized by the isoelectric line shifting up or down is known as what?

(A) Alternating current interference.

(B) Somatic tremor.

(C) Wandering baseline.

(D) Interrupted baseline.

(309) Which EKG artifact can be corrected by unplugging any other unnecessary electronic devices?

(A) Alternating current interference.

(B) Somatic tremor.

(C) Wandering baseline.

(D) Interrupted baseline.

(310) An EKG artifact that is characterized by breaks in the isoelectric line is known as what?

(A) Alternating current interference.

(B) Somatic tremor.

(C) Wandering baseline.

(D) Interrupted baseline.

(311) Where should the EKG test be performed to minimize external interference?
(A) Near other electrical devices.
(B) In a quiet and well-lit room.
(C) Close to X-ray machines.
(D) In a laboratory setting.

(312) How should the patient be positioned for the EKG test?
(A) Semi-Fowler position.
(B) Sitting position.
(C) Supine position.
(D) Prone position.

(313) How should a patient with orthopnea be positioned for the EKG test?
(A) Semi-Fowler position.
(B) Sitting position.
(C) Supine position.
(D) Prone position.

(314) What is the most appropriate initial treatment for a twisted ankle?
(A) Apply heat to the affected area.
(B) Rest, ice, compression, and elevation (RICE).
(C) Immediately resume physical activity.
(D) Massage the ankle vigorously.

(315) How do provider-level barriers impact access to care?
(A) Patients may not trust their provider.
(B) Patients worry about the cost of care.
(C) Patients have difficulty with transportation.
(D) Patients do not know their coverage.

(316) What is the main goal of physiotherapy?

(A) To perform surgical interventions.

(B) To diagnose medical conditions.

(C) To improve mobility and function through physical methods.

(D) To prescribe medications for pain relief.

(317) Tools that are used to determine, quantify, and document the safe, competent, appropriate, and timely delivery of care are known as what?

(A) Clinical quality measures.

(B) Evidence based medicine.

(C) Document assessment.

(D) Quality of care.

(318) What is the main role of medical assistants in the provision of patient education?

(A) Their role is only restricted to education regarding proper intake of medications.

(B) Primary source of medical education for the patients.

(C) Reinforce and complement the information provided by the physician.

(D) They don't play any role in patient education.

(319) Which of the following statements regarding the inclusion of family members in patient education is not true?

(A) It improves patient compliance.

(B) It creates lack of motivation both in the patient and the family members in the majority of cases.

(C) It helps the family comprehend the patient's condition much better.

(D) It will allow the family members to support the patients in a meaningful and understanding manner.

(320) Which patients may need B12 vitamin supplementation?

(A) Patients with limited consumption of animal products.

(B) Patients with iron deficiency anemia.

(C) Patients with obesity.

(D) Patients with heart failure.

(321) Who needs a daily folic acid supplementation?

(A) Menstruating woman.

(B) Pregnant woman.

(C) Patients with pneumonia.

(D) Patients with heart failure.

(322) Which one of the following foods increases the risks of thromboembolism when taken with warfarin?

(A) Meat.

(B) Leafy vegetables.

(C) Fish.

(D) Egg.

(323) Which one of the following drugs interacts with foods that contain tyrame and may result in a hypertensive crisis?

(A) Oral hypoglycemic.

(B) NSAIDs.

(C) Monoamine oxidase inhibitors.

(D) Ciprofloxacin.

(324) Which one of the following is a limitation associated with the use of EHR systems?

(A) They require a stable electrical energy source.

(B) They cannot be tailored to specific medical practices.

(C) They lack appointment management features.

(D) They do not support medical billing.

(325) All of the following meet the eligibility criteria for Medicare coverage except which group?

(A) Patients who are ≤ 15 years old.

(B) Patients with blindness.

(C) Patients with severe disabilities.

(D) Patients who are ≥65 years old.

(326) All of the following are covered by Medicare Part A except what?

(A) Inpatient care in hospitals.

(B) Skilled nursing facility care.

(C) Immunization.

(D) Hospice care.

(327) All of the following are covered by Medicare Part B except what?

(A) Outpatient care.

(B) Skilled nursing facility care.

(C) Durable medical equipment.

(D) Screening.

(328) Which Medicare provides prescription drug coverage in outpatient settings?

(A) Medicare Part A.

(B) Medicare Part B.

(C) Medicare Part C.

(D) Medicare Part D.

(329) What is the document called that describes the determination of the amount of the benefit from an insurance plan?

(A) Insurance claim.

(B) Subscriber.

(C) Explanation of benefits.

(D) Patient encounter form.

(330) What is the notice issued by health care providers to Medicare beneficiaries when a medical service may not be covered by Medicare?

(A) Advanced Beneficiary Notice (ABN).

(B) Carrier.

(C) Disallowed charge.

(D) Utilization.

(331) What is the term for the coverage cost of a health insurance plan or policy?

(A) Premium.

(B) Coinsurance.

(C) Cost sharing.

(D) Deductible.

(332) Which term refers to the fixed percentage of costs paid by the patient after paying a deductible?

(A) Premium.

(B) Coinsurance.

(C) Cost sharing.

(D) Deductible.

(333) What is the term for the share of costs paid out of pocket by the patient for covered services?

(A) Premium.

(B) Coinsurance.

(C) Cost sharing.

(D) Deductible.

(334) What is the amount paid by the patient for a covered service before the insurer pays the rest?

(A) Premium.

(B) Coinsurance.

(C) Cost sharing.

(D) Deductible.

(335) What is the term for the fixed amount paid by the consumer for a covered service after the deductible?

(A) Premium.

(B) Coinsurance.

(C) Cost sharing.

(D) Copayment or copay.

(336) Which of the following is not an example of nonverbal cue for communication?

(A) Eye contact.

(B) Hand gestures.

(C) Saying "next."

(D) Nodding.

(337) All of the following are ways in which nonverbal cues can be used to enhance patient care during in-person visits except what?

(A) Comforting the patient.

(B) Transmitting anger.

(C) Enhancing patient safety.

(D) Establishing rapport.

(338) What role do camera positioning and lighting play in virtual visits?

(A) They are not important.

(B) They affect the effectiveness of nonverbal communication.

(C) They do not impact communication at all.

(D) They only matter for in-person visits.

(339) What is the purpose of the communication cycle between patient and health care provider?

(A) To exchange information.

(B) To establish dominance.

(C) To ignore nonverbal cues.

(D) To create noise.

(340) Which of the following are key components of therapeutic communication?

(A) Active listening.

(B) Leading questions.

(C) Closed-ended questions.

(D) Uncontrolled emotions.

(341) Why is it important to avoid using leading questions in therapeutic communication?

(A) They limit the patient's response.

(B) They encourage open dialogue.

(C) They provide detailed information.

(D) They show empathy.

(342) When should closed-ended questions be used in interviewing and questioning techniques?

(A) To encourage patients to elaborate.

(B) To limit the patient's response.

(C) To prompt specific responses.

(D) To show cultural sensitivity.

(343) What role does cultural and religious context play in effective communication with patients?

(A) It is not important.

(B) It helps build rapport and trust.

(C) It limits communication options.

(D) It encourages closed-ended questions.

(344) When should open-ended questions be used in therapeutic communication?

(A) When you need specific information.

(B) When you want the patient to elaborate their responses.

(C) When you want a "yes" or "no" answer.

(D) When you want to control the conversation.

(345) What should be done when clarification or additional information is needed during therapeutic communication?

(A) Return to the patient and ask for more information.

(B) Ignore the need for clarification.

(C) Assume the information provided is accurate.

(D) Conclude the conversation.

(346) How can medical assistants ensure that patients feel comfortable and respected when asked sensitive questions?

(A) By using leading questions.

(B) By avoiding providing context.

(C) By explaining the reason for the question.

(D) By judging the patient's responses.

(347) What is the main task of an active listener?

(A) To interrupt the patient.

(B) To understand what the patient is trying to say.

(C) To talk more than listen.

(D) To provide solutions immediately.

(348) How does active listening differ from passive listening?

(A) Active listening is bidirectional and passive listening is unidirectional.

(B) Active listening involves interrupting the speaker.

(C) Passive listening encourages the speaker to elaborate.

(D) Passive listening involves asking questions.

(349) What is the purpose of using clarification as an active listening technique?

(A) To confuse the patient.

(B) To avoid understanding the patient's message.

(C) To encourage the patient to elaborate.

(D) To provide immediate solutions.

(350) How can restatement be helpful in active listening?

(A) By ignoring what the patient is saying.

(B) By paraphrasing the patient's message.

(C) By interrupting the patient.

(D) By talking about unrelated topics.

(351) Why is reflection an important tool in active listening?

(A) To dismiss the patient's feelings.

(B) To avoid acknowledging the patient's emotions.

(C) To show understanding and empathy towards the patient.

(D) To provide quick solutions.

(352) What type of diagram is commonly used in cause and effect analysis?

(A) Fishbone diagram.

(B) Incident diagram.

(C) Bar diagram.

(D) Pie chart.

(353) What is the main goal of cause and effect analysis (root cause analysis)?

(A) Assign blame for the problem.

(B) Identify the most important causes of a problem.

(C) Provide opinions on the event.

(D) Ignore potential causes.

(354) Which type of consent is formally granted by a mentally competent person after receiving adequate information about the treatment or procedure?

(A) Informed consent.

(B) Implied consent.

(C) Expressed consent.

(D) Formal consent.

(355) What is an advanced directive?

(A) A legal document specifying a person's health wishes in advance.

(B) A document appointing a legal guardian.

(C) A document granting power of attorney.

(D) A document outlining financial decisions for the future.

(356) What is the main difference between legal guardianship and power of attorney?

(A) Legal guardianship requires a hearing before being effective, power of attorney does not.

(B) Legal guardianship is appointed by a court and can be contested, power of attorney is requested by the person.

(C) Legal guardianship is for managing health care and finance decisions, power of attorney is for acting on someone's behalf.

(D) Legal guardianship is temporary, power of attorney is permanent.

(357) When does a power of attorney become nullified?

(A) When a person becomes incapacitated.

(B) When a person grants the power to act on their behalf.

(C) When a person contests the appointment.

(D) When a person reaches a certain age.

(358) A person or guardian appointed by a court to manage health care and finance decisions for someone who is unable to make said decisions is known as what?

(A) Health care proxy.

(B) Power of attorney holder.

(C) Legal guardian.

(D) Court-appointed advocate.

(359) Which one of the following statements is not correct regarding the maintenance, storage, and disposal of records?

(A) Maintenance of records may vary between states.

(B) Health information must be safely stored and protected from natural damage, theft, and accidental disclosure.

(C) Destruction of paper records must render the information permanently indecipherable.

(D) Deleted information in digital storage devices can be restored but it is not recommended to destroy the device carrying this information.

(360) All of the following factors guarantee whether patient information can be shared with family members and friends according to HIPAA except what?

(A) Express permission from the patient.

(B) Implied consent from the patient.

(C) Professional judgment by the provider.

(D) Permission from the family members.

Test 2 Answers and Explanations

(181) (A) Therapeutic.

Therapeutic medications are essential to treat a wide range of illnesses and health conditions. With the intention to restore health or reduce symptoms, they are made to target and alter the underlying illness processes or symptoms. Health care providers prescribe these medications based on the patient's medical needs and diagnosis. Therapeutic medications can generate desired therapeutic effects, such as lower blood pressure, prevent infections, control inflammation, manage pain, or regulate hormone levels. They act on particular receptors, enzymes, or pathways in the body. To achieve favorable patient results, their appropriate use and administration are essential.

(182) (C) Palliative.

Palliative medications play a significant role to relieve symptoms and enhance the quality of life for those who suffer from severe or fatal illnesses. These medications are intended to treat and lessen symptoms such as pain, nausea, dyspnea, and anxiety. Medications used in palliative care may include sedatives, antiemetics, analgesics, and anxiolytics. Palliative medications help patients maintain dignity, lessen suffering, and improve their general well-being. They efficiently regulate symptoms and foster comfort.

(183) (D) To understand the manufacture of medications.

Medical assistants will work with pharmacologic agents in their day-to-day practice. Therefore, basic knowledge of pharmacology is needed to understand the effects of prescribed medications, administration methods, possible adverse effects, and other functions. It is not necessary to understand the manufacture of medications.

(184) (A) Analgesics.

Analgesics are also known as painkillers. These drugs help to relieve and control pain. They are usually divided into opioid and non-opioid analgesics. Opioids are used to treat severe pain (such as post-surgical pain or cancer) and include morphine (Avinza®), tramadol (Ultram®), and oxymorphone (Opana®). Non-opioids can be used to treat various types of pain and include nonsteroidal anti-inflammatory drugs (NSAIDs such as ibuprofen [Advil®], naproxen [Aleve®], and diclofenac [Cataflam®]) and acetaminophen (Tylenol®).

(185) (B) Antiarrhythmics.

Antiarrhythmic medications are essential to the medical profession because they aid in the management and treatment of arrhythmias. Arrhythmias are irregular or abnormal cardiac rhythms. These medications bring the heart's electrical activity under control, reestablish a regular heartbeat, and halt the development of potentially harmful arrhythmias. Antiarrhythmic medications can help enhance cardiac function, lessen symptoms, and lower the risk of arrhythmia-related problems through management and regulation of the heart's electrical signals. This improves cardiovascular health.

(186) (D) Anticoagulants.

Anticoagulant medications are essential because they stop blood clots from forming. They are prescribed to patients who are at risk of thromboembolic events, such as stroke or deep vein thrombosis. Anticoagulants contribute to the maintenance of blood fluidity and lower the risk of clot formation by blocking the clotting factors in the blood. This lessens the possibility of blood vessel obstructions and averts dangerous situations like pulmonary embolism. Anticoagulants are necessary to treat atrial fibrillation, deep vein thrombosis, and specific defects of the heart valve.

(187) (A) Beta-blockers.

Beta-blockers act on beta-adrenergic receptors. This helps treat hypertension, tachycardia, arrhythmias, glaucoma, hyperthyroidism, and heart failure.

(188) (C) Corticosteroids.

Corticosteroids are synthetic analogs of the steroid hormones produced by the adrenal gland (glucocorticoids and mineralocorticoids). These drugs are commonly employed in most medical fields to treat asthma, chronic obstructive pulmonary disease, rheumatoid arthritis, and systemic lupus erythematosus.

(189) (D) To clear mucus from the respiratory airways.

Expectorant helps to clear mucus from the respiratory airways. Expectorants may come present alongside cough suppressants.

(190) (A) To treat allergic conditions.

Antihistamines are commonly used to treat various types of allergic conditions. Some antihistamines are employed to treat peptic ulcer and gastroesophageal reflux disease, such as cimetidine (Tagamet®).

(191) (A) Food and Drug Administration (FDA).

Over the counter (OTC) medications are also known as nonprescription medications. They are drugs that can be sold to the general public without the requirement of a prescription by a health care professional. In the United States, OTC drugs are regulated by the Food and Drug Administration (FDA). They must include a "Drug Facts" label to educate the consumer. These drugs are safe to use when directions on the label or those dictated by a health care professional are adequately followed.

(192) (B) Over the counter medications.

Drugs that can be obtained over the counter (OTC) do not require a prescription from a medical expert. They are widely used for self-treatment of common illnesses and symptoms and are easily accessible to the general public. OTC drugs include antipyretics (fever reducers), cough suppressants, analgesics (pain relievers), and antihistamines. They are governed by relevant authorities and usually have labeled instructions to guarantee safe and correct use.

(193) (B) Dimenhydrinate.

Dimenhydrinate is used to treat motion sickness symptoms like nausea, vomiting, and lightheadedness. It is categorized as an antiemetic and antihistamine medication. By inhibiting the body's production of histamine, dimenhydrinate helps lessen the symptoms of motion sickness. It can be found in many different over the counter forms, including liquid, chewable pills, and tablets.

(194) (A) Morphine.

Schedule II (C-II) substances such as morphine have a high abuse potential but clinical applications as well. Prescriptions for these substances must be written or electronic. Oral or fax prescriptions are not allowed. No refills are allowed.

(195) (D) Schedule V.

Schedule V (C-V) substances have the lowest potential for abuse. Prescriptions may be oral, written, or electronic. Examples include products that contain less than 200 milligrams of codeine per 100 milliliters, pregabalin, promethazine, attapulgite, and lomotil (diphenoxylate/atropine).

(196) (D) Drowsiness is an adverse reaction that may occur in patients using antihistamines.

The terms "side effects" and "adverse reactions" are usually considered interchangeable among health care professionals and organizations. However, this is not entirely correct. Although both are unintended responses to substances, there is an important distinction. Adverse reactions are inherently negative. Side effects can be positive (but unintended) or negative (but manageable). They are usually more predictable than adverse reactions. Drowsiness is a side effect that may occur in patients using antihistamines for an allergic reaction. In most cases, patients do not have to stop the medication as they may mitigate the drowsiness side effect by taking the medication in the evening. Adverse reactions are always negative and unintended.

(197) (A) Indications.

All drugs used in medicine have specific use for a particular clinical indication. Indications are valid clinical reasons to use a drug to treat one or more conditions. In the United States, the FDA oversees the approval process. The indication can be found in the Prescribing Information label. Health care professionals may prescribe medications for indications that have not been approved by the FDA.

(198) (B) Contraindications.

A contraindication is a term used in medicine to describe a particular disease or factor that provides a valid reason not to use a certain medication, therapy, or procedure. It suggests that for certain patients the intervention's possible dangers or negative consequences exceed its possible advantages. There are two types of contraindications. Absolute contraindications denote risk to life. Relative contraindications call for prudence and a thorough assessment of the risk-benefit ratio before implementation of the intervention.

(199) (A) Absolute contraindications are life-threatening and relative contraindications require caution and risk-benefit analysis.

A relative contraindication demands caution and a risk-benefit analysis. In these situations, a temporary or potentially manageable factor may need to be resolved before use of the drug. An absolute contraindication means that the use of the drug may result in a life-threatening event. Truly absolute contraindications cannot be resolved but they are not very common.

(200) (A) Gelatin.

A capsule pharmaceutical type usually has an enclosure composed of gelatin or a similar material. The active ingredients of the drug are encapsulated in gelatin capsules. These are made up of two halves linked together. Gelatin is derived from animal products. It provides a handy and easily digested capsule shell that holds the liquid or powdered contents inside. This containcr aids in protection of the drug and makes it easier to administer and absorb within the body.

(201) (D) Lozenge.

A lozenge is a term used in medicine to describe a flat tablet-shaped drug that dissolves gradually in the mouth. Lozenges are frequently used to administer active substances that relieve localized discomfort in the mouth, throat, and surrounding tissues. They are frequently used to treat mouth dryness, control coughs, and soothe sore throats. Compared to other oral drug forms, the lozenge's delayed breakdown allows the medication to be released gradually and has a longer-lasting effect.

(202) (A) Suspension.

A suspension in medicine is a type of liquid medication in which the substance is dissolved or suspended in a liquid. The medication particles stay suspended in the liquid rather than dissolving entirely. Suspensions are frequently employed oral administration. The fluid must be thoroughly shaken prior to administration to guarantee that the medication particles are distributed evenly. Suspensions are frequently utilized when a drug's solubility or stability in a liquid solution is restricted because they enable precise dosage.

(203) (C) Emulsion.

A drug preparation called an emulsion is made up of a lipid suspended or distributed in water. Emulsions are distinguished by their two-phase structure in which tiny lipid droplets are dispersed uniformly across the aqueous base. Emulsions usually need to be shaken or mixed before use to guarantee adequate dispersion. Emulsions are frequently employed in topical treatments where they can transfer drugs to the skin or mucous membranes with a smooth, spreadable consistency.

(204) (B) Sublimation.

In medicine, sublimation is a defensive strategy that entails the direction of unpleasant or negative feelings into constructive or uplifting endeavors. Patients may sublimate in a medical setting by taking part in advocacy work, support groups, or other activities that aid in their recovery. Sublimation can improve coping strategies and general well-being by converting unpleasant emotions into positive behaviors. Health care professionals should advise patients to investigate and apply sublimation as a beneficial coping strategy for the difficulties posed by their illness.

(205) (C) Angina.

A partial blockage in the coronary arteries which lower blood flow to the heart muscle can cause angina. Angina is a condition marked by discomfort or pain in the chest. Usually, physical activity or emotional tension sets it off. The discomfort that radiates to the left shoulder, jaw, or arm may feel like pressure, squeezing, or tightness in the chest. Medications like nitroglycerin in addition to rest are frequently used to treat angina and increase cardiac blood flow.

(206) (A) Asthma.

Asthma is a chronic lung condition that is characterized by the inflammation of the airways. This is usually related to allergic reactions. Clinical findings include wheezing, coughing, and dyspnea.

(207) (A) Crohn's disease.

Crohn's disease is a type of chronic bowel disease that results in inflammation of the digestive tract. This further results in chronic diarrhea, pain, bloating, and weight loss. It is a very important risk factor for colorectal cancer.

(208) (A) Diarrhea.

Food poisoning is a condition caused by consumption of foods contaminated by bacteria, viruses, or other toxins. Clinical findings include diarrhea, pain, bloating, and dehydration.

(209) (B) Gastroenteritis.

An infection or inflammation of the gastrointestinal tract is called gastroenteritis. It is usually brought on by bacteria, viruses, or parasites and manifests as fever, vomiting, diarrhea, and stomach pain. Person-to-person contact, tainted food or drink, and inadequate hygiene standards can all spread gastroenteritis. The main goals of treatment are symptom alleviation, rest, and rehydration. Medical intervention may be required in extreme cases to avoid consequences such as dehydration.

(210) (A) Sensation of motion or spinning.

A disconcerting symptom of vertigo is a false sense of motion or spinning. This can be felt either in one's own body or in the environment around them. It frequently coexists with inner ear conditions such vestibular neuritis, Ménière's disease, and benign paroxysmal positional vertigo (BPPV). Vertigo can be characterized by nausea, dizziness, imbalance, and concentration trouble. Vertigo can be treated with medication, exercises in vestibular rehabilitation, or techniques to realign misplaced inner ear crystals depending on the underlying reason.

(211) (D) Complete blood count (CBC).

A common blood test used in medicine to assess the blood's cellular components is known as the complete blood count (CBC). It provides insightful details about platelets, white blood cells, and red blood cells. Factors including hemoglobin, hematocrit, red and white blood cell counts, and platelet counts are also measured by the complete blood count (CBC). It aids in the detection and monitoring of illnesses such as anemia, infections, bleeding issues, and some types of cancer. The results of CBC help medical practitioners accurately assess patients and choose the best course of treatment for them.

(212) (A) Urine thyroid hormone levels.

A urine sample is analyzed as part of a diagnostic procedure called a urinalysis. It provides important details about the condition and operation of the kidneys, urinary tract, and other body systems. Urinalysis evaluates the presence of cells, chemicals, pH, specific gravity, and other properties of urine. Diagnosis of kidney disorders, diabetes, and urinary tract infections is a common use urinalysis. Urinalysis aids medical practitioners in patient diagnosis, monitoring, therapy planning, and general health assessment. Urinalysis doesn't assess urine thyroid hormone levels.

(213) (B) Blood gas analysis.

A diagnostic procedure called blood gas analysis checks the oxygen, bicarbonate, pH, and carbon dioxide levels in venous or arterial blood. It provides important details regarding general blood oxygenation, acid-base equilibrium, and respiratory function. Blood gas analysis is used to evaluate and treat patients with respiratory conditions including asthma, acute respiratory distress syndrome, or chronic obstructive pulmonary disease (COPD). It supports medical practitioners in choosing the best course of action and keeping track of how well respiratory treatments are working.

(214) (A) Radiography.

Radiography is an imaging technique that employs X-rays to visualize various tissues according to the degree of X-ray absorption. Dense tissues like the bones absorb the X-rays and are visualized as white. Tissues filled with air like the lungs are seen as black.

(215) (C) MRI scan.

MRI scan is an imaging technique that employs magnets and radio waves to create a computerized image without X-ray radiation. It provides a more detailed image of soft tissues, which includes muscle tissues and the brain.

(216) (D) Abdominal cramp.

Orthostatic hypotension is also known as postural hypotension. It is a specific type of hypotension characterized by a sudden drop in blood pressure after changes in position such as lying down to sitting up. Symptoms associated with orthostatic hypotension include vertigo, lightheadedness, blurred vision, and syncope. It is relatively common in older patients.

(217) (A) Orthostatic hypotension.

An abrupt drop in blood pressure following a change in posture is referred to as orthostatic hypotension or postural hypotension. When standing up from a seated or lying posture, there is a considerable drop in blood pressure. This causes symptoms including lightheadedness, dizziness, and even fainting. This is a frequent condition, especially in the elderly.

(218) (B) 1 inch above the antecubital fossa.

Blood pressure is frequently measured with a sphygmomanometer and a stethoscope. In most cases, blood pressure is measured in the arm and the cuff should be 1 inch above the antecubital fossa. It should cover two-thirds of the surface of the arm.

(219) (D) Ohm (O).

Fahrenheit (°F) and Celsius (°C) are the general measurement units for temperature. Many countries use Celsius as the official unit of measurement though Fahrenheit is more common in the United States. These units stand for several temperature measurement scales. There are less widely used units that are employed in specialist and scientific contexts such as Kelvin (K) and Rankine (°R). Ohm measures electrical resistance.

(220) (B) 97.6°F to 99°F.

The temperature of an adult varies between 97.6°F to 99°F (or 36.4°C to 37.2°C) across the day. From early in the morning to late afternoon, adults have an average temperature of 98.6°F (37°C).

(221) (B) Higher than 100.4°F.

A reading higher than 100.4°F or 38°C is considered to be febrile. Fever is a common response to infection. Patterns include continuous fever, intermittent fever (fever with periods of normal temperature), and remittent fever (a continuous fever with significant fluctuations). An extremely high-temperature reading (105.8°F or 41°C) is known as hyperpyrexia and temperatures above this level are potentially lethal.

(222) (A) Hypothermia.

Extremely low temperatures (97°F or 36°C) are known as hypothermia. This happens when the body cools more quickly than it can heat itself and causes the core temperature to plummet. Shivering, disorientation, a slower heart rate, and loss of coordination are some of the signs of hypothermia. It can be fatal if left untreated and lead to cardiac arrest and organ failure.

(223) (A) Axillary.

It is important to consider that temperature readings vary depending on the measurement site. Axillary temperatures are 1°F or 0.6°C lower than oral readings. Always document the site of temperature measurement unless it is unnecessary for oral readings.

(224) (C) Temporal artery scanner.

Temporal artery scanner is the most reliable noninvasive method for temperature measurement. The application process consists of placing the device in the middle of the forehead and pressing the button. After hearing a beep continue by placing it behind the ear lobe without releasing the button. The highest recorded temperature is the one documented.

(225) (C) Aorta.

Pulse can be felt and measured in various parts of the body. The most common and reliable arteries are those pressed against a bone or solid structures. These include the carotid, temporal, femoral, brachial, radial, popliteal, and dorsalis pedis arteries. The aorta is not accessible externally for palpation.

(226) (C) Auscultating with a stethoscope.

Auscultation with a stethoscope can reveal the heart rate at the heart's peak. The apex of the heart is often located at the fifth intercostal space or midclavicular line. This is where the stethoscope is placed on the chest. The lub-dub sound of the heart valves closing can be heard by the health care professional when listening closely to the patient's heart contractions. These sounds have a frequency that relates to heart rate and make it possible to determine pulse.

(227) (B) 60-100 beats per minute.

Rate is the number of pulsations measured in one minute. A normal pulse rate is 60-100 pulsations or beats per minute in healthy adults. A higher rate is known as tachycardia and a slower rate is known as bradycardia.

(228) (C) Arrhythmia.

Rhythm is the regularity of time between pulsations. Normal pulsations have a constant frequency in which the time between pulsations is the same. However, abnormal rhythms are known as arrhythmias and can be found in certain cardiovascular diseases. Healthy patients may present arrhythmias during exercise.

(229) (C) The strength of the heart contractions.

Amplitude refers to the strength of the heart contractions and how it is felt during the assessment of the pulse. It depends on both the force of contraction and the condition of the artery (hardened or softened).

(230) (B) Tilted backward and looking up.

The patient should gaze up and have their head turned backward during eye instillation. The inferior conjunctival sac where the drug is delivered is better exposed in this position. The patient creates a better angle for putting the drops or ointment into the eye by leaning their head back and looking up. In addition to facilitating appropriate absorption and distribution within the eye, this position guarantees that the drug reaches the intended area.

(231) (B) Squeeze from the inner to the outer canthus.

Carefully squeeze the ointment from the inner to the outside canthus during eye instillation. Near the inner corner of the eye is where the ointment tube or applicator should be placed. Slide the applicator or tube along the lower eyelid and toward the outer corner of the eye and apply light pressure as you go. This makes the ointment's dispersion across the conjunctival sac smooth and uniform. Prevent injury or irritation by avoiding direct contact with the eye.

(232) (C) Pull the ear upward and back to straighten the ear canal.

The correct method for performing ear irrigation involves pulling the ear upward and back to straighten the ear canal. This technique helps the irrigation solution reach the affected area effectively without causing damage to the eardrum.

(233) (A) Place the tip in the meatus and instill drops.

The recommended method for administration of drops during ear instillation is to insert the drug bottle's tip into the meatus (ear canal) and then instill the necessary amount of drops. Hold the pill bottle in your dominant hand and then use your other hand to gently pull the earlobe down and back (for kids under three years old) or the pinna up and back (for patients over three years old). To ensure that the drops effectively reach their intended site, make sure to squeeze them into the ear canal.

(234) (A) Incisions.

A wound that has precise, linear cuts is referred to as an incision. Usually incisions are formed on purpose with the use of sharp surgical equipment such as scalpels or knives. These wounds frequently result from surgical treatments or other medical interventions and have well lined edges. Sutures or Steri-Strips may be needed to close incisions to promote healing and reduce the chance of infection. Precise wound care and sterile procedures are essential to promote the best possible recovery.

(235) (B) Irregular edges.

The edges of lacerations are not uniform. Lacerations feature ragged or fractured edges in contrast to neat, linear cuts. Sharp objects, blunt force trauma, and accidents are some of the causes of these injuries. Due to the unevenness of the wound margins, cuts would need to be carefully positioned and sealed with stitches or Steri-Strips in order to encourage healing and reduce scarring. It is frequently essential to seek immediate medical attention to evaluate the extent of the laceration and choose the best course of action.

(236) (B) Cleaning and covering with a sterile dressing.

Cleaning the wound well with water and mild soap can help treat abrasions and remove any dirt or debris. To shield the wound from further infection, a sterile dressing can be applied after cleansing. It is critical to keep the dressing dry, clean, and changed on a frequent basis.

(237) (C) A non-penetrating injury that damages the skin and deeper tissues without laceration.

Contusion is a type of non-penetrating injury that damages the skin and deeper tissues without laceration. The rupture of small blood vessels results in a hematoma. It can be treated with cold packs and oral analgesics.

(238) (B) Heparin.

Heparin and insulin are two common subcutaneous medication administrations. Diabetes is commonly treated using insulin which enables blood sugar levels to be regulated. Heparin is an anticoagulant that is often injected subcutaneously to stop blood clots from forming. Because it allows for absorption into the adipose tissue beneath the skin, subcutaneous injection of these drugs provides a practical and efficient method of delivery.

(239) (B) 45 degrees.

These injections are usually inserted at a 45-degree angle. They may be inserted at a 90-degree angle depending on the length of the needle or the amount of adipose tissue. The adequate technique includes pinching the skin before the insertion to create an accessible skinfold.

(240) (D) Buttocks.

Subcutaneous injections can be administered in various parts of the body, such as the upper arm, abdomen, and thighs. In the case of patients who require multiple or frequent injections, an injection log may be used to rotate injection sites.

(241) (B) Intramuscular.

The intramuscular route is preferred when faster absorption of medication is required because muscles have a rich blood supply, which allows the medication to be absorbed more quickly into the bloodstream compared to subcutaneous or oral routes.

(242) (A) Biceps brachii.

The most common muscles are the deltoid, the gluteus medius, and the vastus lateralis. The deltoid muscle holds up to 2 mL of medication in adults, and the gluteus medius and vastus lateralis are viable up to 3 mL.

(243) (D) 90 degrees.

It is advised to place intramuscular injections at an angle of 90 degrees. A straight angle should be formed when the needle is inserted, perpendicular to the skin. This angle makes it possible for the drug to enter the muscle tissue properly and provide its effects. To guarantee precise and secure intramuscular injection delivery, it is important to adhere to this recommendation.

(244) (A) Catgut.

One kind of suture material that is frequently utilized in surgical procedures is catgut. It comes from the submucosal layer of the intestines of sheep or goats, not from cats. Because catgut sutures are absorbable, the body will gradually break them down and absorb them. They are frequently used to suture inner or deep layers of tissue. Once the healing process is finished, they dissolve by enzymatic action and negate the need for human removal.

(245) (B) Nylon.

One kind of nonabsorbable suture material that is frequently utilized in surgical procedures is nylon. Polyamide is a synthetic polymer used to make them. After the healing process, nylon sutures must be manually removed because they do not absorb or dissolve in the body. They are frequently used to suture skin closures and other superficial wounds. Because of their strength and flexibility, nylon sutures can be used in a variety of surgical procedures.

(246) (A) Absorbable sutures.

Absorbable sutures include catgut, polyglactin 910 (Vicryl), polydioxanone (PDS), and poliglecaprone 25 (Monocryl). These sutures absorb or dissolve via enzymatic action after the healing process is completed. As a result, they can be used to suture inner or deep layers of tissue without requiring manual removal.

(247) (B) Nonabsorbable sutures.

Nonabsorbable sutures include nylon, silk, polyester, polypropylene (Prolene), and surgical steel. These sutures do not dissolve and they must be removed after the healing process is complete. Nonabsorbable sutures are employed in superficial wounds such as those on the skin.

(248) (B) If the wound presents discharge.

If there is drainage from the site, a sample for a culture should be obtained while the sutures are being removed. It's critical to gather a sample for culture study if there are any signs of infection such as pus or an unusual odor. This makes it possible to identify any possible microbial or bacterial growth and helps in choosing the best course of action. If an infection is detected, the wound discharge can be cultured to help inform the selection of medications if needed.

(249) (A) Suture removal scissors.

Suture removal scissors are the tool used to cut sutures during removal. The lower blade of suture removal scissors is blunt and the upper blade is sharp. They make it possible to precisely cut the suture material near the skin's surface without endangering the surrounding tissue. The lower blade provides a firm cutting surface and the pointed upper blade facilitates easy slipping under the suture.

(250) (B) Using a staple remover.

A staple remover should be used to extract surgical staples. Put the staple remover's bottom jaw under a staple and gently press down on the mechanism to close it all the way. After closing, remove the tool. The staple is simple to extract and throw away within a sharps container. Until every staple is extracted from the incision site the procedure is repeated.

(251) (B) From inner canthus to outer canthus.

Pour solution into a gauze and use it to clean the eyelid and eyelashes. Begin near the nose and clean laterally from the inner canthus to the outer canthus. Dispose of the gauze after each wipe.

(252) (C) Intramuscular epinephrine.

The treatment of anaphylaxis is based on early intervention with epinephrine and complementary use of steroids and antihistamines. It is recommended to use intramuscular epinephrine (0.01 mg/kg up to 0.5 mg in adults) within the first 20 minutes after the onset of symptoms. The use of glucocorticoids and intravenous antihistamines is complementary. It does not replace intramuscular epinephrine as these drugs do not effectively treat acute symptoms, especially life-threatening signs related to acute hypotension and bronchospasm.

(253) (A) Anaphylaxis.

A severe and generalized allergic reaction is known as anaphylaxis. This type of systemic reaction is potentially life-threatening and may occur within seconds or minutes of exposure to an allergen. An episode of anaphylaxis is most commonly uniphasic. Approximately 10% of cases may be biphasic in which symptoms may return one hour after resolution. Anaphylaxis may result in difficulty breathing, palpitations, wheezing, nausea and vomiting, abdominal pain, urticarial, flushing, swelling of the face, lips, or tongue, hoarseness or stridor, and angioedema.

(254) (A) Steam sterilization.

Steam is the most common sterilization technique. It is usually the best choice if available and appropriate to use with the item that requires sterilization. Steam employs an autoclave and relies on the use of steam, pressure, temperature, and time.

(255) (C) Low-temperature sterilization.

Low-temperature sterilization includes various other methods that, unlike steam sterilization, do not require heat. Examples include ethylene oxide, hydrogen peroxide, and hydrogen peroxide/ozone. If an item cannot be sterilized with high heat or moisture then low-temperature sterilization is commonly employed.

(256) (D) Peracetic acid sterilization.

Peracetic acid sterilization is a method of sterilization that employs concentrated peracetic acid as a sterilizer. It is most commonly used to sterilize endoscopic tubing.

(257) (A) To remove visible traces of tissues, soil, or fluids.

All sterilization techniques require decontamination prior to sterilization. This can be achieved by manually pre-cleaning the item to eliminate visible traces of tissues, soil, or fluids.

(258) (B) In a way that ensures all surfaces come into contact with the sterilizing agent.

The items that require sterilization should be arranged in such a way that all the surfaces come into contact with the sterilizing agent. This allows complete sterilization and adequate circulation of the agent.

(259) (A) Touching the inside portion or the content.

To establish a sterile field, a medical assistant will need a Mayo stand or a countertop and a sterilized instrument kit wrapped with autoclave paper. If required, clean the Mayo stand or countertop and allow it to dry. Then perform hand washing and allow to dry. Place the sterile kit on the Mayo stand or countertop and check the indicator tape. Finally position the kit so the uppermost flap opens towards your body. Then open the uppermost flap and unfold the kit without touching the inside portion or the content.

(260) (B) Main cleaning.

The second step in the cleaning procedure is main cleaning. It entails cleaning agents and hotter water to get rid of filth, grime, and stains from objects or surfaces. Scrubbing, wiping, and other cleaning methods are used at this stage to guarantee a thorough cleaning. The primary cleaning phase is essential for getting rid of obvious impurities and setting up the surface or object for next processes like rinsing and disinfection.

(261) (B) Redness, swelling, and pus.

Infection of a wound is indicated by redness, swelling, and the presence of pus. These signs suggest that the body is responding to a bacterial invasion, which requires medical attention to prevent further complications.

(262) (B) Disinfection.

The object or surface is treated with an appropriate disinfectant during this step based on the disinfectant's efficacy against particular germs. To eliminate or render inactive any pathogens present, they must remain in contact with the surface for the necessary duration.

(263) (C) Increased risk of infection.

Dog saliva contains various bacteria that can lead to infections if it comes into contact with an open wound. This can result in conditions such as cellulitis or more severe systemic infections if not properly cleaned and treated.

(264) (A) Remove any jewelry.

Remove any jewelry that can get in the way of your hand washing routine before you turn on the water. This includes watches, bracelets, and rings. Jewelry removal ensures that there are no obstacles to prevent you from cleaning your hands completely.

(265) (C) 1.010 to 1.025.

Urine solute concentration is measured by specific gravity. This also aids in assessing the kidneys' capacity to concentrate urine. Specific gravity ranges of 1.010 to 1.025 is normal. Urine that is diluted may have values below this range. Urine that is concentrated may have values above this range.

(266) (B) WBC.

A few white blood cells (WBCs) per high-power field that usually range from 0 to 5 cells can be regarded as normal. If the WBC count is noticeably higher than usual or if there are further aberrant findings, it can point to a urinary tract infection or inflammation that needs to be further assessed and treated. WBCs in urine should be interpreted in light of the patient's symptoms and other clinical considerations.

(267) (B) 4.5 to 7.8.

Urine's acidity or alkalinity is determined by its pH. A urinalysis's normal pH range is between 4.5 and 7.8. Urine with a value of less than 4.5 might be acidic. Urine with a value more than 7.8 might be alkaline. pH variations can reveal details about specific metabolic and renal conditions.

(268) (B) 0 to 4 cells per high-power field.

Red blood cells (RBCs) in the urine can be a sign of diseases that include kidney stones, bladder tumors, and urinary tract infections. Red blood cell counts in a normal urinalysis usually vary from 0 to 4 per high-power field. Increased RBC counts could be an indication of bleeding or other medical issues.

(269) (C) Protection and regulation of substance flow.

Epithelial cells form protective barriers on surfaces throughout the body, including the skin, glands, and various internal organs. They help regulate the flow of substances into and out of these areas.

(270) (C) Oxygen transport.

Red blood cells are responsible for transporting oxygen from the lungs to the body's tissues and organs. They contain hemoglobin, which is a protein that enables efficient oxygen delivery and carbon dioxide removal from the body.

(271) (C) 7.0 to 7.5.

In a basic stool analysis, the pH usually ranges from 7.0 to 7.5. pH values outside of this range could be a sign of an unbalanced gut environment. Alkaline stool pH (over 7.5) may be connected to bacterial overgrowth or specific drugs. Acidic stool pH (below 7.0) may be linked to disorders like malabsorption or diarrhea.

(272) (C) 280 to 325 mOsmol/kg.

The solute concentration in stools is measured by osmolality. The usual range for osmolality in a simple stool analysis is normally between 280 and 325 mOsmol/kg. Values outside of this range could point to gastrointestinal tract osmotic imbalances or malabsorption issues.

(273) (A) 7 g/d.

The greatest amount of fat that is generally regarded safe in a basic stool analysis is 7 grams per day (g/d). Increases in fat could be a sign of problems with fat absorption or digestion. This could be related to disorders like pancreatic insufficiency or malabsorption syndromes.

(274) (B) Less than 540 mg/L

One protein that can be tested in stool and used to gauge gastrointestinal protein loss is alpha-1-antitrypsin. Alpha-1-antitrypsin has a normal range of less than 540 mg/L.

Increased alpha-1-antitrypsin levels can indicate protein-losing enteropathy. This is linked to illnesses such intestinal infections and inflammatory bowel disease.

(275) (B) 4.9 L.

A 40-year-old woman's total lung capacity is estimated to be 4.9 liters. This figure indicates the total amount of air that her lungs can contain and includes the inspiratory reserve volume, tidal volume, expiratory reserve volume, and residual volume.

(276) (C) Within 1-2 hours.

After collection, it is imperative to get the sputum specimen to the lab as quickly as possible. It is advised to do it within one to two hours. The specimen's viability and integrity are preserved for reliable testing due to this timely delivery. The sample composition may alter as a result of delayed delivery. This could have an impact on the validity of the test findings.

(277) (A) Spit into the container.

The sample should be sputum which comes from the lung. Remind the patient to not spit into the container. Also remind the patient that the container is sterile and must not be opened until ready to use. In the case of tuberculosis assessment, the health care provider may request three samples across three consecutive days.

(278) (D) Insulin.

The body responds to stress by releasing various kinds of substances and hormones. This may result in higher levels of cortisol, catecholamines, and white blood cells. The level of insulin in the blood is not raised.

(279) (B) Measures blood clotting ability.

Platelet count is a critical component of a complete blood count as it measures the number of platelets in the blood. Adequate platelet levels are necessary to prevent excessive bleeding and to facilitate wound healing.

(280) (B) <200 mg/dL.

Less than 200 mg/dL is the recommended range for total cholesterol (TC). It is widely recognized that maintaining total cholesterol levels below 200 mg/dL is ideal for heart health and lowers the risk of cardiovascular illnesses.

(281) (B) ≥60 mg/dL.

High-density lipoprotein (HDL) levels should be 60 mg/dL or above. Because it assists in removing excess cholesterol from the bloodstream and transports it back to the liver for processing, HDL is frequently referred to as "good cholesterol." Reduced risk of heart disease has been associated with higher HDL levels.

(282) (C) <150 mg/dL.

Triglycerides (TG) should be within the acceptable range of less than 150 mg/dL. The blood contains a form of fat called triglycerides. An increased risk of heart disease is linked to elevated triglyceride levels. For general cardiovascular health, triglyceride levels under 150 mg/dL are usually regarded as ideal.

(283) (B) HDL helps remove cholesterol from the bloodstream.

High-density lipoprotein (HDL) is often referred to as "good" cholesterol because it helps remove cholesterol from the bloodstream as it transports it to the liver for excretion or reuse. Higher levels of HDL are associated with a lower risk of cardiovascular disease, as HDL can help prevent the buildup of plaque in the arteries.

(284) (B) 21-26 mEq/L.

In arterial blood, the typical range for serum bicarbonate (HCO3) is 21–26 mEq/L. The body's acid-base equilibrium is preserved in part by HCO3. This is an important buffer and essential for controlling blood pH. Appropriate acid-base equilibrium and regular physiological functioning are ensured by maintaining serum bicarbonate levels within this range.

(285) (C) Antecubital fossa.

Phlebotomy is best performed in the antecubital fossa. It's the region where the elbow bends and makes the veins easier to see and reach. The median cubital vein is located in the antecubital fossa and is frequently chosen for venipuncture due to its straight, conspicuous nature. There is also a lack of nearby arteries or nerves which makes it appropriate for blood collection.

(286) (C) Select another site.

It is essential to choose an alternative location for blood collection if an infection is detected at a possible phlebotomy site. Cellulitis and erysipelas are two infections that can make the process more difficult and raise the possibility of introducing bacteria into the circulatory system. Selecting an alternative, infection-free spot is important to preserve patient safety and avert more issues.

(287) (B) Impaired lymphatic flow altering the test results.

Phlebotomy shouldn't be done on the side of a mastectomy. A mastectomy is a clinical surgery in which lymph nodes and breast tissue are removed. On the afflicted side, lymphatic flow may be compromised as a result. Variations in lymphatic flow can impact test results and cause alterations in blood composition. Venipuncture on the side of the mastectomy is not advised in order to guarantee precise and reliable laboratory results.

(288) (A) 70% isopropyl alcohol.

70% isopropyl alcohol is the recommended disinfection for getting the phlebotomy site ready. In hospital environments, isopropyl alcohol is often utilized as a disinfectant. By efficiently eliminating a variety of skin-surface pathogens, it lowers the possibility of venipuncture-related bacterial bloodstream introduction.

(289) (B) Povidone-iodine.

The phlebotomy site should be prepared with povidone-iodine before a blood sample is taken especially for blood culture. Povidone-iodine is efficient against a variety of pathogens such as bacteria, fungus, and viruses. It possesses broad-spectrum antibacterial characteristics. To acquire precise and trustworthy blood culture findings, it helps lower the chance of introducing contaminants during the blood collection process.

(290) (C) Select another site.

A hematoma is a localized accumulation of blood outside of blood vessels that frequently happens as a result of a blood vessel rupture or leakage during or after venipuncture. Selecting a different location for blood collection is advised if a hematoma is found at a possible phlebotomy site. When a hematoma is present during phlebotomy, blood samples may be contaminated or changed. This could have an impact on test findings.

(291) (C) Light blue.

Prothrombin time (PT), partial thromboplastin time (PTT), international normalized ratio (INR), D-dimer, and other coagulation-related analyses are among the coagulation tests that are performed using the light blue tube. Because it contains sodium citrate which binds calcium, it acts as an anticoagulant and prevents blood clotting.

(292) (D) Royal blue.

The analysis of trace elements in blood, including aluminum, mercury, lead, selenium, and other elements, is done using the royal blue tube. Sodium heparin is an anticoagulant that is present in this tube.

(293) (A) Gray.

For chemistry tests, the gray tube is particularly useful for measuring glucose levels. Potassium oxalate and sodium fluoride are present as additions. Sodium fluoride inhibits glycolysis and keeps the blood sample's glucose from breaking down while it is being stored.

(294) (B) Lavender.

Hematology assays that include a complete blood count (CBC), hemoglobin, hematocrit, and other analyses pertaining to blood cells are performed with the lavender tube. As an anticoagulant, it contains ethylenediaminetetraacetic acid or EDTA. Because it inhibits clotting and maintains cell shape, EDTA aids in the preservation of the blood sample.

(295) (B) 4 fingers above the site.

Once the vein has been selected, place a tourniquet 4 fingers above the site. After cleaning and gloving, use 70% isopropyl alcohol to disinfect the area. Povidone-iodine is used instead when collecting blood for a blood culture. Wait for approximately 30 seconds for the area to dry.

(296) (B) Verify the order.

Verify the order before starting the blood collection procedure to make sure the right tests are being performed on the right patient. In this phase, the requisition form or electronic order must be matched with the patient's identifying information.

(297) (D) To improve vein visibility.

A tourniquet placed usually four fingers above the inner elbow area or antecubital fossa helps to temporarily stop blood flow. This makes the nearby veins more noticeable and simpler to find. The veins easier to see and makes venipuncture more successful.

(298) (C) Apply pressure over the venipuncture site with a clean gauze pad.

After withdrawing the needle during venipuncture, it is important to apply pressure over the site with a clean gauze pad. This helps to stop the bleeding and prevents the formation of a hematoma (a localized collection of blood outside the blood vessels). Proper pressure application ensures quick and effective healing of the puncture site.

(299) (C) Invert the tubes to mix the blood and additives.

The tubes must be gently inverted to guarantee that the blood and any additives in the vacuum tubes are mixed properly. Repeatedly inverting the tubes facilitates a complete blending of the blood with any anticoagulants or additives. This guarantees precise outcomes in the lab tests that follow.

(300) (C) Place them in a designated biohazard container.

Contaminated materials should be disposed of in a designated biohazard container. This ensures that potentially infectious materials are handled safely and in compliance with health regulations.

(301) (B) Cardiac stress test.

Cardiac stress test is a specialized test performed to record cardiac activity during a period of cardiovascular stress. The patient participates in an exercise challenge such as running on a treadmill. The cardiologist can use this EKG study to determine if the patient presents an arrhythmia during exercise or other relevant cardiovascular findings.

(302) (C) To diagnose conditions that may need more than 24 hours to appear.

Event monitor is a small cardiac monitor that records the activity of the heart for various days and usually up to 30 days. They are used to diagnose conditions that may need more than 24 hours to appear and cannot be accurately determined with a Holter monitor.

(303) (C) V1, V2, V3, V4, V5, V6.

Chest electrodes positioned at precise points on the patient's chest represent the precordial leads in a 12-lead EKG. From a frontal plane perspective, these leads provide important information regarding the electrical activity of the heart. The leads V1, V2, V3, V4, V5, and V6 are the precordial leads. These leads are positioned on the chest in a certain way so that electrical activity from various heart areas may be recorded.

(304) (B) aVR, aVL, aVF.

A 12-lead EKG's augmented leads are obtained from the limb electrodes and provide an alternative view of the electrical activity of the heart. aVR (augmented vector right), aVL (augmented vector left), and aVF (augmented vector foot) are the three augmented leads. The electrical potential difference between two limb electrodes and a central reference point is measured by these leads.

(305) (A) Holter monitor.

Holter monitor is a portable EKG recording device that a patient carries for 24 hours or more. It is used to monitor a patient's cardiac activity for prolonged periods of time. It can also be activated periodically such as when the patient presents symptoms. The patient is instructed to keep a journal and record any stressful or symptomatic events. They should describe the event and report the time and duration of the occurrence.

(306) (B) Muscle movement.

Somatic tremor is simply the electrical activity of muscle movement that affects the tracing of the EKG. This makes it look jagged. Tremors may occur when the patient is anxious, uncomfortable, talking, or moving. The patient may also have a condition that causes tremors. Talk with the patient to calm them down and try to make them feel comfortable.

(307) (A) Patients with a pacemaker.

Pacemaker spikes are artifacts in the form of spikes. These spikes are vertical and short signals that are normally found in patients with a pacemaker. Medical devices called pacemakers are made to control the electrical activity of the heart and guarantee healthy cardiac function.

(308) (C) Wandering baseline.

Wandering baseline is when the isoelectric line shifts up or down instead of presenting horizontally. It may occur when the patient moves or an electrode is not positioned correctly. Ask the patients to stay still and check the electrodes.

(309) (A) Alternating current interference.

Alternating current interference are interferences created by other electrical devices. Check that the electrocardiograph is connected to a grounded outlet and verify the wires do not cross each other. Unplug any other unnecessary devices. This interference is seen as spikes in the EKG.

(310) (D) Interrupted baseline.

Interrupted baseline is the interruption of the isoelectric line. This may take place when the stylus of the electrocardiograph moves up and down erratically. The electrodes may not be placed correctly or the wires may be damaged.

(311) (B) In a quiet and well-lit room.

Minimizing external interference during the EKG exam can be achieved by conducting it in a well-lit, quiet environment. This is important since X-ray machines, lab equipment, and external electrical devices can all add interference or electrical noise into the EKG signal. This can cause readings to be off. The likelihood of signal distortion or artifacts from outside sources is decreased when the test is conducted in a quiet setting. This provides more accurate and trustworthy results.

(312) (C) Supine position.

For the EKG test, the patient should be placed in a supine posture. This entails resting their arms and legs apart while lying flat on their back. The supine position guarantees a stable and comfortable posture during the procedure and facilitates easy access to the patient's chest for the placement of electrodes.

(313) (A) Semi-Fowler position.

The semi-Fowler position may be used for patients with dyspnea. In this case, inform and discuss the positioning with the physician.

(314) (B) Rest, ice, compression, and elevation (RICE).

The RICE method is the most appropriate initial treatment for a twisted ankle. Resting the ankle prevents further injury, applying ice reduces swelling and pain, using compression helps control swelling, and elevating the ankle reduces blood flow to the injured area to decrease swelling.

(315) (A) Patients may not trust their provider.

Providers may impose barriers on patients if they do not speak the patient's language or do not understand their culture or religion. In some cases, the patient may not trust their provider or perceive discrimination due to their gender, race, ethnicity, nationality, ability to pay, or as a beneficiary of a public health care program.

(316) (C) To improve mobility and function through physical methods.

The main goal of physiotherapy is to improve mobility and function through physical methods such as exercises, manual therapy, and education. Physiotherapists work to help patients recover from injuries, manage chronic conditions, and prevent future injuries.

(317) (A) Clinical quality measures.

Clinical quality measures (CQMs) are tools to determine, quantify, and document the safe, competent, appropriate, and timely delivery of care. Ideally, CQMs are included in the electronic health record. They are used to measure health care performance, identify weaknesses, and find ways to improve.

(318) (C) Reinforce and complement the information provided by the physician.

Patient education should include high-quality and accurate information about the patient's condition, medications, procedures, quality of life, and required medical equipment or supplies. In many cases, medical assistants will reinforce and complement the information provided by the physician. It may occur in the office or during virtual visits.

(319) (B) It creates lack of motivation both in the patient and the family members in the majority of cases.

In many cases, the participation of family members in the learning process improves patient compliance. The inclusion of the patient's family may directly help the patient in their learning. This helps the family comprehend the patient's condition much better and allows them to provide support in a meaningful and understanding manner.

(320) (A) Patients with limited consumption of animal products.

People with diet restrictions or specific conditions may need to use supplements. For example, B12 vitamin supplementation may be needed in patients who have a limited consumption of animal products. Similarly, some patients may need to use supplements after a bariatric surgery.

(321) (B) Pregnant woman.

Pregnant patients or those planning to get pregnant should receive folic acid supplementation daily. Increased folic acid consumption is necessary for pregnant women to promote the fetus's growth and development. Sufficient folate intake is essential during pregnancy to avoid neural tube abnormalities in the fetus. Pregnant women are often advised to consume foods high in folate and to take a daily dosage of folic acid.

(322) (B) Leafy vegetables.

Warfarin is an anticoagulant that interacts with multiple foods. Leafy greens increase the risk of thromboembolism, cooked onions increase warfarin activity, charbroiled decreases it, and cranberry juice increases the international normalized ratio (INR) without increasing the risk of bleeding in older patients.

(323) (C) Monoamine oxidase inhibitors.

Antidepressants (monoamine oxidase inhibitors) interact with foods that contain tyramine (ripened bananas, matured cheese, salami, yogurt), which may result in a hypertensive crisis.

(324) (A) They require a stable electrical energy source.

An electronic health record (EHR) is a system that allows health care providers and institutions to optimize their work and save time and money. These computer programs can be tailored to the needs of specific types of medical practice, such as medical and surgical specialties. EHR software usually includes an appointment management system to schedule, remind, and confirm visits, which is especially useful for medical offices. Finally, the software may also allow the management of laboratory tests, imaging, referrals, and medical billing. EHR systems will not work without electrical energy which may be affected by natural events or infrastructural issues.

(325) (A) Patients who are ≤ 15 years old.

Medicare provides the Original plan, which provides insurance to patients who are ≥65 years old or to younger patients with blindness, severe disabilities, or widowed. Patients who are ≤ 15 years old are not eligible for Medicare coverage because of their age.

(326) (C) Immunization.

Medicare Part A helps to cover inpatient care in hospitals and skilled nursing facilities. It may also help to cover hospice and home health care in some cases. Immunization is covered by Medicare Part B.

(327) (B) Skilled nursing facility care.

Medicare Part B helps to cover outpatient care, home health care, services from physicians, durable medical equipment such as walkers, beds, wheelchairs, and certain preventive services including screenings, immunization, IPPE, and AWVs. It does not cover skilled nursing facility care.

(328) (D) Medicarc Part D.

Medicare Part D provides prescription drug coverage in outpatient settings. It is provided by private insurance companies approved by Medicare. Helping beneficiaries get inexpensive access to critical prescription drugs is the goal of Medicare Part D.

(329) (C) Explanation of benefits.

An insurance company will provide an Explanation of Benefits (EOB), which is a document that summarizes the specifics of a claim and explains how the benefit amount is determined. It gives details on the services provided, the amount the health care provider charged, the amount the insurance plan covered, and any amount that may still be the patient's responsibility.

(330) (A) Advanced Beneficiary Notice (ABN).

Advanced Beneficiary Notice is a notice issued by health care providers to Medicare beneficiaries when a medical service or item may not be covered or paid for by Medicare. If the patient wants to receive the medical service or item, the health care provider may ask the patient to pay upfront and bill Medicare. If Medicare accepts the claim then the patient receives a refund. If Medicare denies the claim then the patient may appeal the decision.

(331) (A) Premium.

The price that a person or organization must pay for a health insurance plan or policy is known as the premium. To keep coverage, it is usually paid on a regular basis such as monthly or annual. The type of plan, degree of coverage, age, region, and number of people covered by the insurance are just a few of the variables that may affect the premium amount.

(332) (B) Coinsurance.

A cost-sharing agreement known as coinsurance exists between the patient or consumer and the insurance company. It is stated as a set proportion of the price of an item or service that is covered. The patient bears the cost of the coinsurance after they have paid the deductible and the insurance company pays the remaining portion.

(333) (C) Cost sharing.

The amount that the patient or consumer must pay out-of-pocket for covered services or goods is referred to as cost sharing. Costs like deductibles, coinsurance, and copayments may be included in this. By distributing the financial burden between the patient and the insurance company, cost sharing makes sure that everyone pays a portion of the total cost of health care.

(334) (D) Deductible.

A deductible is the amount a patient or consumer must pay for services or goods before their insurance starts to pay the rest of the costs. For instance, before insurance coverage begins, a patient with a $1,000 deductible on their health insurance plan must pay $1,000 out of cash for approved services.

(335) (D) Copayment or copay.

A copayment is sometimes known as a copay. It is a set sum that the patient or customer must pay for a service or good that is covered. Copayments usually follow the payment of the deductible.

(336) (C) Saying "next."

Nonverbal communication refers to communication without linguistic content. It includes eye contact, facial expressions, posture, hand gestures, and voice characteristics (pitch, rate, loudness). These cues are relevant for both in-person and virtual visits. MAs may need to consider certain factors to apply them effectively in each setting. Saying "next" reflects linguistic content.

(337) (B) Transmitting anger.

Nonverbal cues during in-person visits can be used to comfort a patient, transmit empathy, and enhance the patient's sense of safety. They can also create rapport. Transmitting anger is not used.

(338) (B) They affect the effectiveness of nonverbal communication.

Most strategies used during in-person visits can also be used during virtual visits. Camera positioning, camera angle, and lighting play an important role in the process. There is no physical proximity with the patient. Nonverbal cues like nodding and eye contact can be used to let the patient feel heard. Remember that looking at the camera emulates eye contact during video communication.

(339) (A) To exchange information.

The communication cycle represents the interactions between patient and health care provider with the purpose of exchanging information. Both participants are responsible for receiving and transmitting information. An important consideration is noise which may affect how the information is transmitted or interpreted. Noise can literally be loud or distracting sounds but can also include pain, anxiety, fear, and other feelings.

(340) (A) Active listening.

Therapeutic communication is paying close attention, expressing empathy, and giving verbal and nonverbal clues to indicate understanding while actively listening to the patient. In addition to facilitating successful communication and helping to build trust, active listening affirms the patient's experiences and feelings.

(341) (A) They limit the patient's response.

Leading questions are those that imply a certain course of action or demand a certain kind of response from the patient. Leading inquiries impede the patient's capacity to fully express themselves and give a thorough response in this way.

(342) (C) To prompt specific responses.

Closed-ended queries are used to get precise information from the patient or elicit succinct responses. They frequently ask for succinct, factual replies or elicit "yes" or "no" responses. When precise information or clarification is required, closed-ended questions might be useful. Open-ended questions tend to encourage patients to elaborate and express their thoughts and experiences more thoroughly in therapeutic discussion.

(343) (B) It helps build rapport and trust.

Cultural and religious context plays an important role in effective communication with patients. Understanding and respecting a patient's cultural and religious beliefs, values, and practices allows health care professionals to establish rapport and trust. It helps create a supportive environment where patients feel understood, validated, and respected. Cultural and religious context should be considered when selecting appropriate communication strategies, terminology, and nonverbal cues to ensure effective and culturally sensitive interactions.

(344) (B) When you want the patient to elaborate their responses.

Open-ended questions are valuable in therapeutic communication as they encourage patients to provide detailed and comprehensive responses. These questions prompt the patient to share their thoughts, feelings, and experiences in their own words. They allow for a deeper understanding of their perspective. Open-ended questions promote patient-centered communication, active engagement, and the exploration of complex issues.

(345) (A) Return to the patient and ask for more information.

Ensuring clarity and understanding is important in therapeutic communication. Health care providers should go back to the patient and request more details or explanations if more information is required.

(346) (C) By explaining the reason for the question.

By providing an explanation for their inquiries, medical assistants may guarantee that patients feel appreciated and at ease when they pose delicate queries. Patients are better able to comprehend the significance of the information being sought when context is provided and the rationale behind particular queries is clarified. Patients are reassured by this clarity that the questions are being asked only for health care purposes and in their best interest.

(347) (B) To understand what the patient is trying to say.

Understanding what the patient is attempting to convey is the primary responsibility of an active listener. To actively listen to a patient, one must actively engage in their speech, give their whole attention, and make an effort to understand their viewpoints, feelings, and thoughts.

(348) (A) Active listening is bidirectional and passive listening is unidirectional.

Active listening does not only involve hearing what the patient is saying since it is bidirectional. The active listener asks questions and encourages the patient to elaborate. This is in contrast with unidirectional passive listening which only involves listening.

(349) (C) To encourage the patient to elaborate.

To gain a deeper comprehension of the patient's message and to seek out further information, clarification is an important technique in active listening. The active listener invites the patient to provide more details, clarify any unclear areas, or elaborate on their ideas and experiences by employing expressions and inquiries.

(350) (B) By paraphrasing the patient's message.

Part of an active listening method called restatement shows that you understand the patient by paraphrasing or summarizing what they have said. Restating the patient's message gives the active listener a chance to make sure they've understood it and gives the patient a chance to clear up any confusion.

(351) (C) To show understanding and empathy towards the patient.

Reflection is a strategy for active listening in which the patient's feelings, emotions, or experiences are acknowledged and reflected back to them. It shows that the active listener is sensitive to the patient's feelings and has the capacity to understand their point of view. The active listener supports the patient's feelings and experiences by employing reflection techniques. This creates a secure and encouraging environment in which the patient can express themselves.

(352) (A) Fishbone diagram.

Diagrams are frequently used during this analysis. The fishbone diagram resembles a fishbone with a head and spine. It consists of writing the problem on the right side (head) and a central line to the left (spine) with diagonal lines (bones). Each diagonal line contains a group (equipment, patient, provider, environment) and possible causes. Each cause is analyzed and discussed among professionals. This helps to identify the most important causes and find a solution.

(353) (B) Identify the most important causes of a problem.

Cause and effect analysis aims to pinpoint the fundamental reasons behind a problem or unfavorable occurrence. By examining and comprehending the elements that led to the problem's or occurrence, specialists can address the underlying causes of issues instead of merely treating the symptoms.

(354) (A) Informed consent.

Informed consent is a consent that is formally granted by a mentally competent person after receiving adequate information about the treatment or procedure. This includes a description of the procedure as well as its risks and benefits.

(355) (A) A legal document specifying a person's health wishes in advance.

An advanced directive is also known as a living will or advance decision. It is a legal document that specifies in advance a person's wishes and preferences in relation to their health. This is in case they are no longer capable of deciding for themselves in the future due to an illness. Furthermore, one or more people may serve as spokespersons on behalf of the patient in such circumstances.

(356) (B) Legal guardianship is appointed by a court and can be contested, power of attorney is requested by the person.

Legal guardianship requires a hearing before being effective and power of attorney does not. On the other hand, legal guardianship is appointed by a court and can be contested and power of attorney is requested by the person that desires to appoint an agent.

(357) (A) When a person becomes incapacitated.

Power of attorney is a legal document in which a person grants another person the power to act on their behalf. However, power of attorney is nullified once a person becomes incapacitated for any reason. The exception is for a durable power of attorney.

(358) (C) Legal guardian.

Legal guardianship is a person (guardian) appointed by a court that oversees management of health care and finance decisions for someone who is unable to make said decisions.

(359) (D) Deleted information in digital storage devices can be restored but it is not recommended to destroy the device carrying this information.

The disposal or destruction of records according to the HIPAA Medical Records Destruction Rules requires an assessment to consider potential privacy risks associated with the destruction process. Destruction of paper records must render the information permanently indecipherable through shredding. In some instances, deleted information in digital storage devices can be restored. Therefore, the device carrying this information should be destroyed via pulverization, melting, or incineration. If unsure in relation to the maintenance, storage, and destruction of records, seek professional advice on compliance.

(360) (D) Permission from the family members.

The release of patient information is a process regulated by the HIPAA Privacy Rule. According to HIPAA, information can be shared with family members and friends if the patient gives express permission, if the patient implies consent (inviting their friend or family member into the room), or if the provider determines through professional judgment that sharing the information is in the best interest of the patient.

Test 3

(361) How does the drug dissolve in the sublingual route of administration?

(A) Under the tongue.

(B) In the nasal cavity.

(C) On the skin.

(D) In the eye.

(362) In which route of administration is the drug applied onto the skin?

(A) Urethral route.

(B) Rectal route.

(C) Topical route.

(D) Intra-arterial route.

(363) Which route of administration is used for drugs that require bypassing the gastrointestinal tract?

(A) Parenteral route.

(B) Inhalation route.

(C) Otic route.

(D) Vaginal route.

(364) Which organization, in addition to the FDA, recommends the use of tall man lettering to differentiate between similar drug names?

(A) ISMP.

(B) LASA.

(C) Orthographic.

(D) Spelling and Pronunciation Committee.

(365) What general term is used to describe medications that have similar spelling or pronunciation, which may cause medication errors?

(A) Look-alike medications.

(B) Sound-alike medications.

(C) Orthographic medications.

(D) LASA medications.

(366) What is drug bioavailability?

(A) The fraction of the administered drug that reaches systemic circulation.

(B) The rate of gastrointestinal absorption.

(C) The inactivation of drugs by digestive enzymes.

(D) The binding of drugs to proteins or other molecules.

(367) Which administration route usually results in 100% bioavailability?

(A) Oral administration.

(B) Intravenous administration.

(C) Topical administration.

(D) Inhalation administration.

(368) Which organ is mainly responsible for the excretion of most drugs?

(A) Kidneys.

(B) Lungs.

(C) Intestines.

(D) Pancreas.

(369) What are the two main groups into which nutrients are commonly divided?

(A) Vitamins and electrolytes.

(B) Carbohydrates and fats.

(C) Macronutrients and micronutrients.

(D) Proteins and minerals.

(370) Which type of carbohydrate is not broken down into simple sugars but aids in digestion?

(A) Monosaccharides.

(B) Disaccharides.

(C) Oligosaccharides.

(D) Dietary fiber.

(371) Which label includes information about the order of ingredients by weight?

(A) Nutrition Facts Labels.

(B) Front-of-package labels.

(C) Side or back labels.

(D) Warning labels.

(372) What are public health advocates recommending be incorporated into front-of-package labels?

(A) Positive nutritional qualities.

(B) Warning labels.

(C) Serving information.

(D) Nutrient percentages.

(373) Which foods should be avoided by individuals with celiac disease?

(A) Foods containing gluten.

(B) Foods high in saturated fats.

(C) Foods with added sugar.

(D) Foods with high sodium content.

(374) Which of the following should not be limited in the diet of someone with kidney disease?

(A) Carbohydrate.

(B) Sodium.

(C) Potassium.

(D) Phosphorus.

(375) Which eating disorder is characterized by episodes of excessive or uncontrolled eating without purging behaviors?

(A) Binge-eating disorder.

(B) Anorexia nervosa.

(C) Bulimia nervosa.

(D) Avoidant restrictive food intake disorder (ARFID).

(376) Which eating disorder is characterized by binge-eating episodes followed by behaviors aimed at preventing weight gain?

(A) Binge-eating disorder.

(B) Anorexia nervosa.

(C) Bulimia nervosa.

(D) Avoidant restrictive food intake disorder (ARFID).

(377) Which eating disorder is characterized by excessive selectivity with the amount and type of food consumed, without body image issues or fear of weight gain?

(A) Binge-eating disorder.

(B) Anorexia nervosa.

(C) Bulimia nervosa.

(D) Avoidant restrictive food intake disorder (ARFID).

(378) Which stage of psychosocial development occurs during infancy to one year?

(A) Stage 1 (trust vs. mistrust).

(B) Stage 2 (autonomy vs. shame and doubt).

(C) Stage 3 (initiative vs. guilt).

(D) Stage 4 (competence vs. inferiority).

(379) During which stage do young adults develop their interpersonal skills and seek intimate relationships?

(A) Stage 5 (identity vs. role confusion).

(B) Stage 6 (intimacy vs. isolation).

(C) Stage 7 (generativity vs. stagnation).

(D) Stage 8 (integrity vs. despair).

(380) Which mental health condition is characterized by a persistent feeling of sadness and lack of pleasure, along with symptoms like changes in appetite and thoughts of death?

(A) Generalized anxiety.

(B) Panic attacks.

(C) Depression.

(D) ADHD.

(381) Which mental health condition is characterized by disorganized, excessive, and impulsive activity?

(A) PTSD.

(B) ADHD.

(C) Autism spectrum disorder.

(D) Depression.

(382) Which defense mechanism involves rejecting information or denying its existence?

(A) Denial.

(B) Regression.

(C) Repression.

(D) Rationalization.

(383) Which defense mechanism involves unconsciously erasing a traumatic experience?

(A) Denial.

(B) Regression.

(C) Repression.

(D) Rationalization.

(384) What defense mechanism involves trying to find explanations or justifications for a result or outcome?

(A) Denial.

(B) Regression.

(C) Repression.

(D) Rationalization.

(385) What is the primary purpose of a PET scan?

(A) Visualizing bones and dense tissues.

(B) Creating 3D images of tissues.

(C) Studying soft tissues like muscles and the brain.

(D) Assessing blood flow, cancer, and neurological conditions.

(386) What is the main purpose of a biopsy?

A) To analyze tissue or cell samples.

B) To remove tumors.

C) To guide surgical interventions.

D) To administer medication.

(387) Which type of biopsy involves removing the tissue sample by excision?

(A) Needle biopsy.

(B) Punch biopsy.

(C) Excisional biopsy.

(D) Perioperative biopsy.

(388) What imaging technique is most commonly used to guide a needle biopsy?

(A) Ultrasound.

(B) X-ray.

(C) MRI.

(D) CT scan.

(389) During which type of procedure is an endoscopic biopsy performed?

(A) Biopsy surgery.

(B) Perioperative biopsy.

(C) Colonoscopy.

(D) Needle biopsy.

(390) Which treatment modality employs medication to treat or manage a medical condition?

(A) Pharmacological therapy.

(B) Surgical treatment.

(C) Chemotherapy.

(D) Radiation therapy.

(391) Which treatment modality modulates the body's immune response in order to help destroy cancer cells?

(A) Pharmacological therapy.

(B) Surgical treatment.

(C) Immunotherapy.

(D) Blood transfusion.

(392) What does incidence measure in epidemiology?

(A) Number of death cases during a period of time.

(B) Number of existing cases during a period of time.

(C) Number of cases with comorbidities.

(D) Number of new-onset cases during a period of time.

(393) What do risk factors indicate in epidemiology?

(A) Decreased risk of developing a specific condition.

(B) Increased risk of developing a specific condition.

(C) Number of cases during a period of time.

(D) Number of death cases during a period of time.

(394) What is an outbreak in the field of epidemiology?

(A) Increase in the incidence of a specific infectious disease within a specific facility.

(B) Number of death cases during a period of time.

(C) Outbreak with a global threat to the health of the general population.

(D) Number of all cases during a period of time.

(395) What is a pandemic in the field of epidemiology?

(A) Increase in the incidence of a specific infectious disease within a specific facility.

(B) Number of death cases during a period of time.

(C) Outbreak with a global threat to the health of the general population.

(D) Number of all cases during a period of time.

(396) What is the normal range for respiratory rate in healthy adults?

(A) 6-12 respirations per minute.

(B) 12-20 respirations per minute.

(C) 20-30 respirations per minute.

(D) 30-40 respirations per minute.

(397) What is the correct term for the cessation of respiration?

(A) Tachypnea.

(B) Bradypnea.

(C) Apnea.

(D) Hyperpnea.

(398) What is the characteristic sound heard in patients when the small airways are partially obstructed?

(A) Dyspnea.

(B) Orthopnea.

(C) Wheezing.

(D) Hyperpnea.

(399) What is the correct term for shortness of breath?

(A) Tachypnea.

(B) Bradypnea.

(C) Dyspnea.

(D) Hypopnea.

(400) During which states is orthopnea commonly experienced by patients?

(A) When lying down.

(B) During exercise.

(C) After eating.

(D) When standing up.

(401) Which of the following is not true of the purpose of measuring a patient's respiratory rate without them noticing?

(A) To ensure accurate measurement.

(B) To avoid altering the respiratory rate.

(C) To prevent the patient from consciously controlling their breathing.

(D) There is no point in doing that.

(402) What does pulse oximetry measure?

(A) Respiratory rate.

(B) Oxygen saturation.

(C) Blood pressure.

(D) Heart rate.

(403) All of the following body parts are commonly used for pulse oximetry measurements except:

(A) Finger.

(B) Earlobe.

(C) Toes.

(D) Throat.

(404) What is the correct term for the numerical scale used to measure pain, ranging from zero to ten?

(A) Visual analog scale.

(B) Pain severity scale.

(C) Pain assessment scale.

(D) Numeric pain scale.

(405) What is the term for the first menstruation in females?

(A) Menstruation.

(B) Menarche.

(C) Ovulation.

(D) Fecundation.

(406) What does LMP stand for in relation to menstrual status?

(A) Last Menstrual Period.

(B) Last Menstrual Phase.

(C) Late Menstrual Process.

(D) Long Menstrual Cycle.

(407) What is the recommended attire for small children during height measurement?

(A) Diaper and a shirt.

(B) Naked.

(C) Diaper only.

(D) Any clothing is acceptable.

(408) What is the correct way to measure a baby's head circumference?

(A) Place the tape measure around the baby's neck.

(B) Place the tape measure just above the ears and eyebrows.

(C) Measure from the chin to the top of the head.

(D) Measure around the baby's chest.

(409) How many people are recommended to participate in the measurement of height for small children?

(A) One person.

(B) Two people.

(C) Three people.

(D) It can be done with or without assistance.

(410) Which stage of wound infection involves the presence of microorganisms but no proliferation or host reaction?

(A) Contamination.

(B) Colonization.

(C) Local wound infection.

(D) Spreading infection.

(411) What characterizes the stage of colonization in wound infection?

(A) Limited proliferation without host reaction.

(B) Hypergranulation, exudate, bleeding, and delayed healing.

(C) The presence of microorganisms but no proliferation or host reaction.

(D) Systemic symptoms such as malaise, fever, and asthenia.

(412) What are the signs of local wound infection in covert cases?

(A) Inflammation extension and wound dehiscence.

(B) Limited proliferation without host reaction.

(C) Hypergranulation, exudate, bleeding, and delayed healing.

(D) Systemic symptoms such as malaise, fever, and asthenia.

(413) What is characteristic of the spreading infection stage in wound infection?

(A) Limited proliferation without host reaction.

(B) Hypergranulation, exudate, bleeding, and delayed healing.

(C) Inflammation extension and wound dehiscence.

(D) Systemic symptoms such as malaise, fever, and asthenia.

(414) What are the systemic symptoms associated with systemic infection in wound infection?

(A) Hypergranulation, exudate, bleeding, and delayed healing.

(B) Signs of inflammation and purulent exudate.

(C) Inflammation extension and wound dehiscence.

(D) Malaise, fever, and sepsis.

(415) What is the purpose of a breast biopsy?

(A) To remove the breast tissue.

(B) To take a sample of breast tissue for study under a microscope.

(C) To treat breast infections.

(D) To increase milk production.

(416) What does cataract surgery involve?

(A) Correcting refractive errors in the eye.

(B) Removing foreign bodies from the eye.

(C) Replacing the clouded lens of the eye with an artificial lens.

(D) Correcting strabismus.

(417) When is a cholecystectomy usually performed?

(A) To treat acute hepatitis.

(B) To rule out malignancy of the gallbladder.

(C) To remove gallbladder stones.

(D) When the gallbladder becomes infected or in the treatment of gallbladder cancer.

(418) What is the purpose of a hysterectomy?

(A) To remove the uterus.

(B) To repair uterine rupture.

(C) To study the uterus with an ultrasound.

(D) To perform a cesarean delivery.

(419) What is the purpose of debridement in wound care?

(A) To instill antibiotics into the infected site.

(B) Providing cold compresses.

(C) Suturing lacerations.

(D) To remove infected and nonviable tissue from wounds.

(420) What is the difference between an urgency and an emergency?

(A) An urgency requires immediate examination and/or treatment within twenty-four hours, while an emergency requires immediate examination and/or treatment in the emergency department.

(B) An urgency is a severe or life-threatening condition, while an emergency is a less severe condition.

(C) An urgency can be treated in an outpatient setting, while an emergency requires hospitalization.

(D) An urgency is a medical condition, while an emergency is an injury.

(421) All of the following are precautions that should be taken before using an AED except:

(A) Ensure there is no water in the area.

(B) Remove the patient's clothing and dry their chest.

(C) Announce the use of the defibrillator and ensure no one is touching the patient.

(D) Make sure somebody holds the hands and legs of the patient.

(422) What is the recommended rate of compressions per minute during CPR in adults?

(A) 60-80 compressions per minute.

(B) 80-100 compressions per minute.

(C) 100-120 compressions per minute.

(D) 120-140 compressions per minute.

(423) How far should the chest be compressed during high-quality CPR?

(A) One inch.

(B) Two inches.

(C) Three inches.

(D) Four inches.

(424) What is the first step to take when providing Basic Life Support (BLS) to an unresponsive adult patient?

(A) Call for help and activate the emergency response system.

(B) Begin chest compressions immediately.

(C) Check the patient's blood pressure.

(D) Administer a rescue breath.

(425) All of the following information is usually recorded in a medication log except:

(A) Name of the drug.

(B) Patient name.

(C) Birth year of the patient.

(D) Date and time of administration.

(426) What do specialty pharmacies mainly handle?

(A) Specialty drugs.

(B) Over-the-counter medications.

(C) Generic drugs.

(D) Prescription medications.

(427) All of the following patients may require services from a specialty pharmacy except:

(A) Patients with multiple sclerosis.

(B) Patients with rheumatoid arthritis.

(C) Patients with asthma.

(D) Patients with Crohn's disease.

(428) How often should the progress note of a patient be updated?

(A) Every twelve hours.

(B) Daily.

(C) Weekly.

(D) Every time the patient is evaluated.

(429) All of the following are the roles of telehealth care except:

(A) To replace traditional in-person care.

(B) To provide remote monitoring and chat-based care.

(C) To extend benefits of traditional care visits to e-visits.

(D) To integrate with in-person care for patient compliance and communication.

(430) What should a medical assistant do if a patient requires emergency care during a telehealth call?

(A) Hang up and call the emergency medical service.

(B) Put the call on hold and call the emergency medical service.

(C) Stay on line with the patient and call the emergency medical service.

(D) Hang up and advise the patient to call the emergency medical service.

(431) The electronic generation, transmission, and filling of medical prescriptions with the help of computer-based applications is known as:

(A) CPOE.

(B) DME.

(C) Electronic prescribing.

(D) E order.

(432) What is the potential life-threatening complication of anaphylaxis characterized by a sharp decrease in blood pressure and insufficient blood supply to essential organs?

(A) Difficulty breathing.

(B) Urticaria.

(C) Anaphylactic shock.

(D) Angioedema.

(433) All of the following are clinical findings commonly associated with anaphylaxis except:

(A) Difficulty breathing.

(B) Palpitations.

(C) Urticaria.

(D) Fever.

(434) What should be used to dispose of needles and sharps?

(A) Red bags.

(B) Yellow bags.

(C) Sharps containers.

(D) Black bags.

(435) Which type of waste is disposed of in red bags?

(A) Contaminated gloves.

(B) IV bags and tubing.

(C) Mercury-containing items.

(D) Batteries containing cadmium, lead, or silver.

(436) How should soiled dressings and bandages be disposed of in a healthcare setting?

(A) In regular trash bins.

(B) In yellow biohazard bags.

(C) In sharps containers.

(D) In recycling bins.

(437) What should be the first thing you do before using a chemical product?

(A) Review the product's safety data sheet.

(B) Use protective equipment.

(C) Perform hand washing afterward.

(D) Follow the facility's plan in case of an accident or injury.

(438) All of the following statements regarding correct handling of chemicals are true except:

(A) Verify that the product inside the container is the correct one, as stated by the label.

(B) Keep the chemical products stored in a tight container.

(C) Perform hand washing after handling chemical products.

(D) Do not consume foods or drinks when handling chemical products.

(439) What is the purpose of the source or reservoir in the chain of infection?

(A) To provide a pathway for the pathogen to exit.

(B) To provide an environment for the microorganism to multiply.

(C) To facilitate direct transmission to the susceptible host.

(D) To act as a barrier against the pathogen's entry.

(440) Which of the following is the most common sign of an infectious disease?

(A) Asthenia.

(B) Cough.

(C) Nausea, vomiting.

(D) Fever.

(441) What is an important tool for the prevention and response to epidemics and pandemics?

(A) Vaccines and immunizations.

(B) Recapping or bending needles.

(C) Disposal of needles after use.

(D) Use of non-sterile instruments.

(442) All of the following are considered vulnerable populations during outbreaks, epidemics, and pandemics except:

(A) Elderly individuals.

(B) Pregnant women.

(C) Children.

(D) Adults.

(443) All of the following are considered a susceptible host in the chain of infection except:

(A) Individuals with no underlying health conditions.

(B) Individuals with immunodeficiency.

(C) Individuals with poor nutrition.

(D) Individuals using medication that affects the immune system.

(444) Which pH range do acidophilic bacteria prefer?

(A) pH below 5.5.

(B) pH above 5.5 to 7.5.

(C) pH from 7.5 to 9.5.

(D) pH from 9.5 to 11.

(445) What is the main purpose of an audiometer in hearing testing?

(A) Diagnosing middle ear infection.

(B) Diagnosing TM perforation.

(C) Measure hearing threshold.

(D) Assessing the patency of the ear canal.

(446) Which test can be clinically performed with a tuning fork?

(A) Inner ear visualization.

(B) Middle ear visualization.

(C) Rhinoscopy.

(D) Rinne test.

(447) What does peak flow rate measure in respiratory testing?

(A) Forced expiratory volume in one second.

(B) Forced vital capacity.

(C) Tidal volume.

(D) Flow rate during forced expiration after deep inspiration.

(448) What is the purpose of spirometry in respiratory testing?

(A) Measure sound intensity.

(B) Measure hearing threshold.

(C) Measure lung function.

(D) Measure peak flow rate.

(449) Which respiratory conditions can be diagnosed using spirometry?

(A) Pneumonia.

(B) Asthma.

(C) Common cold.

(D) Pulmonary tuberculosis.

(450) Which chart is commonly used for visual acuity testing?

(A) Ishihara charts.

(B) Snellen charts.

(C) Weber charts.

(D) Rhine charts.

(451) Which chart is commonly utilized to diagnose color blindness?

(A) Ishihara charts.

(B) Snellen charts.

(C) LogMAR charts.

(D) Refractor charts.

(452) How far should the person stand from the chart when assessing visual acuity using the Snellen chart?

(A) The patient stands ten feet away from the chart.

(B) The patient stands twenty feet away from the chart.

(C) The patient stands thirty feet away from the chart.

(D) The patient stands forty feet away from the chart.

(453) Which of the following is an error that can occur in the preanalytical stage of quality assurance?

(A) Calibration errors.

(B) Reagent errors.

(C) Collection errors.

(D) Reporting errors.

(454) What type of errors can happen during the analytical stage of quality assurance?

(A) Disposal errors.

(B) Reporting errors.

(C) Calibration errors.

(D) Delivery errors.

(455) Which stage of quality assurance involves variables related to the reporting and delivery of results?

(A) Preanalytical stage.

(B) Analytical stage.

(C) Postanalytical stage.

(D) Calibration stage.

(456) Which error is associated with the postanalytical stage of quality assurance?

(A) Collection errors.

(B) Processing errors.

(C) Interpretation error.

(D) Storage errors.

(457) Which stage of quality assurance includes variables related to specimen ordering, collection, storage, transport, and preanalytical processing?

(A) Preanalytical stage.

(B) Analytical stage.

(C) Postanalytical stage.

(D) Calibration stage.

(458) Which one of the following is the correct reference value for hemoglobin (Hgb) in a healthy adult man?

(A) 10-14 g/dL.

(B) 14-18 g/dL.

(C) 18-22 g/dL.

(D) 22-26 g/dL.

(459) What is the normal reference range for hematocrit (Hct) in a healthy adult man?

(A) 16%-25%.

(B) 26%-35%.

(C) 36%-45%.

(D) 46%-55%.

(460) Which one of the following is the correct reference value for mean corpuscular volume (MCV)?

(A) 20-40 fL/cell.

(B) 40-60 fL/cell.

(C) 60-80 fL/cell.

(D) 80-100 fL/cell.

(461) Which one of the following is the normal reference value for white blood cell count (WBC)?

(A) 4.5-11.0 x 10^3 cells/mm^3.

(B) 11.0-17.6 x 10^3 cells/mm^3.

(C) 22.0-27.0 x 10^3 cells/mm^3.

(D) 42.0-51.0 x 10^3 cells/mm^3.

(462) Which one of the following is the normal reference value for platelet count (Plt)?

(A) 50,000-150,000 cells/mm^3.

(B) 150,000-350,000 cells/mm^3.

(C) 350,000-500,000 cells/mm^3.

(D) 500,000-700,000 cells/mm^3.

(463) Which of the following is the normal reference value for international normalized ratio (INR)?

(A) 0.9-1.1.

(B) 1.2-1.5.

(C) 1.6-2.0.

(D) 2.1-2.3.

(464) Which of the following are reference values for prothrombin time (PT)?

(A) 4-9 seconds.

(B) 10-13 seconds.

(C) 14-17 seconds.

(D) 18-21 seconds.

(465) All of the following tests require protection from light except:

(A) CBC.

(B) Bilirubin.

(C) Riboflavin.

(D) Vitamin E.

(466) What is the recommended storage temperature for most whole blood samples?

(A) Room temperature (around 25°C).

(B) 4-8°C without freezing.

(C) -20°C.

(D) -80°C.

(467) How should blood samples requiring protection from light be handled?

(A) Wrapped with aluminum foil.

(B) Stored in a cold room.

(C) Placed in the freezer.

(D) Exposed to direct sunlight.

(468) How are remaining blood samples usually disposed of in the majority of cases?

(A) Recycling.

(B) Autoclaving.

(C) Incineration.

(D) Disposal in regular trash bins.

(469) At what angle should the needle be inserted during venipuncture?

(A) 45-degree angle.

(B) 90-degree angle.

(C) 15-degree angle.

(D) 70-degree angle.

(470) What is the normal range for albumin in adults?

(A) 3.5-5 g/dL.

(B) 2.0-3.2 g/dL.

(C) 6.0-7.5 g/dL.

(D) 3.4-4.2 g/dL.

(471) What is the normal range for blood urea nitrogen (BUN) in adults?

(A) 8-23 mg/dL.

(B) 0.1-0.3 mg/dL.

(C) 10-30 mg/dL.

(D) 15-45 mg/dL.

(472) What is the normal range for total serum calcium?

(A) 3.8-5 mg/dL.

(B) 0.3-1.2 mg/dL.

(C) 8.2-10.2 mg/dL.

(D) 27-131 mg/dL.

(473) What is the normal range for total bilirubin in adults?

(A) 0.1-0.3 mg/dL.

(B) 0.3-1.2 mg/dL.

(C) 6.2-7.2 mg/dL.

(D) 3.5-5 g/dL.

(474) Which vacuum tube contains lithium heparin and gel for plasma separation?

(A) Plain red.

(B) Red-gray/Gold.

(C) Green.

(D) Light green.

(475) What action should be taken when blood is visible inside the hub of the syringe during a phlebotomy?

(A) Pull the plunger with the dominant hand.

(B) Pull the plunger with the non-dominant hand.

(C) Push the plunger with the dominant hand.

(D) Push the plunger with the non-dominant hand.

(476) What is the normal range for serum glucose in adults?

(A) 40-70 mg/dL.

(B) 70-110 mg/dL.

(C) 110-150 mg/dL.

(D) 150-200 mg/dL.

(477) What is the normal range for potassium in adults?

(A) 0.6-1.2 mEq/L.

(B) 2.4-3.4 mEq/L.

(C) 3.5-5.0 mEq/L.

(D) 1.3-2.1 mEq/L.

(478) What is the normal range for hemoglobin A1C in adults?

(A) 4%-7%.

(B) 7%-10%.

(C) 10%-13%.

(D) 13%-16%.

(479) What is the normal range for sodium in adults?

(A) 128-136 mEq/L.

(B) 136-142 mEq/L.

(C) 142-148 mEq/L.

(D) 148-154 mEq/L.

(480) What is the normal range for uric acid in adults?

(A) 4-8 mg/dL.

(B) 42-68 mg/dL.

(C) 75-95 mg/dL.

(D) 80-120 mg/dL.

(481) Where should the precordial electrode V4 be placed?

(A) Second intercostal space (right parasternal line).

(B) Fourth intercostal space (left parasternal line).

(C) Fifth intercostal space (left mid-clavicular line).

(D) Sixth intercostal space (right mid-axillary line).

(482) What is the correct lead wire color coding for the right arm?

(A) White.

(B) Black.

(C) Green.

(D) Red.

(483) What is the correct lead wire color coding for the left leg?

(A) White.

(B) Black.

(C) Green.

(D) Red.

(484) Where should the precordial electrode V2 be placed?

(A) Second intercostal space (right parasternal line).

(B) Fourth intercostal space (left parasternal line).

(C) Fifth intercostal space (left mid-clavicular line).

(D) Sixth intercostal space (right mid-axillary line).

(485) What is the correct lead wire color coding for the precordial electrode V6?

(A) Red.

(B) Yellow.

(C) Green.

(D) Purple.

(486) Where should the precordial electrode V6 be placed?

(A) Second intercostal space (right parasternal line).

(B) Fourth intercostal space (left parasternal line).

(C) First intercostal space.

(D) Fifth intercostal space (left mid-axillary line).

(487) Where should electrodes be placed for an ECG test if the patient has an amputated limb?

(A) Just above the site of amputation.

(B) Directly on the site of amputation.

(C) On the opposite limb.

(D) Well above the site of amputation.

(488) What modification should be made when placing precordial electrodes for patients with dextrocardia/situs inversus?

(A) Place them on the left side of the chest.

(B) Place them on the right side of the chest.

(C) Place them on the back instead of the chest.

(D) Do not use precordial electrodes in these cases.

(489) Where should electrodes be placed in relation to injuries or incisions?

(A) Directly on the injury or incision.

(B) Close to the injury or incision.

(C) EKG is contraindicated during such conditions.

(D) Apply additional adhesive to secure electrodes on injuries or incisions.

(490) What modification can be made for electrode placement in children?

(A) Move V3 to the left side of the chest.

(B) Move V3 to the right side of the chest.

(C) Remove V3 from the precordial electrode placement.

(D) Place electrodes closer together on the chest.

(491) Which arrhythmia is characterized by an extremely fast heartbeat and a sawtooth pattern?

(A) Sinus arrhythmia.

(B) Atrial fibrillation.

(C) Atrial flutter.

(D) Ventricular tachycardia.

(492) What is the defining feature of ventricular tachycardia?

(A) Increased heart rate with irregular and wide QRS complexes.

(B) Sawtooth pattern of P waves.

(C) Ectopic foci in the atria.

(D) Erratic and unidentifiable waves.

(493) All of the following can cause metabolic arrhythmias except:

(A) Increased potassium levels.

(B) Decreased potassium levels.

(C) Toxicity from digoxin.

(D) Valvular disorders.

(494) What is the standard speed of an electrocardiograph?

(A) 10 mm per second.

(B) 20 mm per second.

(C) 25 mm per second.

(D) 50 mm per second.

(495) Who is responsible for managing the referral process by scheduling the visit with the required specialist?

(A) Medical assistant.

(B) Referral coordinator.

(C) Specialist doctors.

(D) The ambulance drivers.

(496) Which one of the following statements is not correct regarding the referral process?

(A) An efficient referral process requires organization.

(B) The exchange of information with the specialist is very important.

(C) The specialist cannot ask for extra information besides the one mentioned on the referral paper.

(D) Current diagnosis is usually incorporated on the referral paper.

(497) All of the following should be ideally incorporated in to the referral paper except:

(A) Date of the appointment.

(B) Name of the primary care provider.

(C) Unapproved acronyms.

(D) Urgency.

(498) Which one of the following statements is incorrect regarding the benefits of nutrition?

(A) Nutrition goes beyond losing weight.

(B) There is ample evidence that supports a ketogenic diet.

(C) Whole grains are important components of a healthy diet.

(D) The risks of diseases like diabetes can be prevented with proper nutritional arrangements.

(499) All of the following are considered unhealthy and should be avoided as much as possible except:

(A) Processed foods.

(B) Fiber.

(C) Saturated fats.

(D) Processed meats.

(500) Who is in charge of patient registration, verification of information, and managing calls, emails, and appointments?

(A) Nurse.

(B) Receptionist.

(C) Physician assistant.

(D) Pharmacist.

(501) Which team member is responsible for coordinating the office workflow in a patient-centered medical home?

(A) Nurse.

(B) Physician assistant.

(C) Office manager.

(D) Social or community health worker.

(502) Which one of the following drugs has an increased risk of gastric bleeding and hepatic damage when taken together with alcohol?

(A) Oral hypoglycemic.

(B) NSAIDs.

(C) Monoamine oxidase inhibitors.

(D) Ciprofloxacin.

(503) The absorption of which of the following drugs decreases when taken together with milk?

(A) Oral hypoglycemic.

(B) NSAIDs.

(C) Monoamine oxidase inhibitors.

(D) Ciprofloxacin.

(504) What do telehealth apps like Teladoc and MDLIVE provide?

(A) Medical consultation for patients.

(B) Education for health care students.

(C) Clinical and drug information for health care providers.

(D) Remote monitoring services.

(505) All of the following statements are correct regarding telehealth software and apps except:

(A) Health care providers may not have the knowledge required to manage telehealth software and apps.

(B) It is possible to perform a throughout physical exam during a virtual visit.

(C) Poor internet connection is one of the challenges encountered.

(D) Patient and the health care provider not speaking the same language is one of the barriers that can hinder visual visits.

(506) Which event mainly contributed to the increased prevalence of telehealth?

(A) COVID-19 pandemic.

(B) Introduction of wearable devices.

(C) Advancements in physical examination equipment.

(D) Expansion of in-person appointments.

(507) Which of the following is an example of video communication software used in telehealth?

(A) Teladoc.

(B) Epocrates.

(C) Lecturio.

(D) Zoom.

(508) Which one of the following instruments requires a relatively frequent inspection when compared with the others?

(A) Stethoscope.

(B) Wheelchair.

(C) Sterilization equipment.

(D) Chairs.

(509) What is the primary purpose of medical coding in healthcare?

(A) To enhance patient-physician communication.

(B) To standardize and simplify the reporting of medical services for billing purposes.

(C) To provide detailed descriptions of medical procedures for research purposes.

(D) To ensure patient confidentiality.

(510) Which classification system is commonly used in the United States for diagnostic codes?

(A) ICD-11.

(B) ICD-10-CM.

(C) ICD-10-PCS.

(D) HCPCS.

(511) What is the purpose of the Current Procedural Terminology (CPT)?

(A) To provide diagnostic codes for physicians.

(B) To standardize procedure codes for outpatient settings.

(C) To report medical services for Medicare patients.

(D) To disseminate laboratory results for patients.

(512) Which term refers to the detailed itemized bill that lists all the services and procedures performed during a patient visit?

(A) Explanation of Benefits (EOB).

(B) Superbill.

(C) Invoice.

(D) Claim form.

(513) What are the three levels of HCPCS codes used to report medical services for Medicare patients?

(A) Level I, Level II, Level III.

(B) ICD-10-CM, ICD-10-PCS, CPT.

(C) Diagnostic, Procedural, Local.

(D) ICD 1, ICD 2, ICD 3.

(514) Why is it important for MAs to be compliant with HIPAA regulations when handling patient information?

(A) To sell patient information for profit.

(B) To ensure patient confidentiality and privacy.

(C) To make data entry more challenging.

(D) To avoid following guidelines.

(515) Why do some equipment in health care facilities require more frequent inspections than others?

(A) To waste time.

(B) To ensure patient safety.

(C) To increase costs.

(D) To avoid compliance with regulations.

(516) What is the primary dietary consideration for diabetic patients to help manage their blood sugar levels?

(A) Consuming high amounts of protein.

(B) Avoiding all carbohydrates.

(C) Monitoring carbohydrate intake.

(D) Increasing fat consumption.

(517) What is an important aspect of telephone etiquette for medical assistants?

(A) Avoid greeting the caller.

(B) Treat everyone with attention and respect.

(C) Ask for personal information immediately.

(D) Disclose all patient information.

(518) What should medical assistants do when answering phone calls?

(A) Disclose protected health information.

(B) Greet the caller and introduce themselves.

(C) Ignore the caller's questions.

(D) Hang up if it is a sales call.

(519) What is the primary goal of coaching in patient care?

(A) To focus on past actions.

(B) To discourage patient participation.

(C) To enhance patient development for the future.

(D) To promote patient compliance.

(520) What is the main purpose of feedback for medical assistants in patient care?

(A) To reflect on past actions.

(B) To predict future outcomes.

(C) To discourage patients.

(D) To ignore positive behaviors.

(521) What type of communication should emails be used for?

(A) For urgent communication.

(B) For formal business letters.

(C) For non-urgent communication.

(D) For handwritten notes.

(522) What should a well-structured email have in terms of its subject line?

(A) A concise description of the email contents.

(B) A vague and unclear title.

(C) A long and detailed description.

(D) No subject line at all.

(523) How should an email usually start and end to maintain proper etiquette?

(A) Start with a closing, end with a salutation.

(B) Start with a closing, end with contact information.

(C) Start without any greeting or salutation.

(D) Start with a salutation, end with a closing and contact information.

(524) What is the purpose of patient satisfaction surveys in healthcare facilities?

(A) To assess the quality of care provided.

(B) To evaluate the financial performance of the facility.

(C) To determine the number of staff members needed.

(D) To track patient demographics.

(525) What standardized survey is commonly used by hospitals to evaluate and compare care quality?

(A) Patient Demographics Survey.

(B) Hospital Consumer Assessment of Healthcare Providers and Systems Survey (HCAHPS).

(C) Financial Performance Survey.

(D) Staff Satisfaction Survey.

(526) What does the Dix and Page model for de-escalation in healthcare settings consist of?

(A) Assessment, Communication, Tactics.

(B) Assessment, Medication, Restraint.

(C) Diagnosis, Treatment, Follow-up.

(D) Observation, Intervention, Monitoring.

(527) What are some strategies to de-escalate aggressive behavior in healthcare settings?

(A) Ignoring the patient's behavior.

(B) Providing solutions and gaining the patient's trust.

(C) Avoiding communication with the patient.

(D) Using physical force to restrain the patient.

(528) What does the CUS method stand for when it comes to escalating problematic situations in healthcare settings?

(A) Concern-Uncomfortable-Safety Issue.

(B) Calm-Understanding-Solution.

(C) Careful-Understanding-Support.

(D) Calm-Understanding-Support.

(529) When should a healthcare professional declare that there is a safety issue in place according to the CUS method?

(A) As soon as they feel uncomfortable.

(B) After stating they are concerned and why.

(C) If the concern remains unresolved.

(D) Whenever they want to.

(530) What is the main purpose of an Unusual Occurrence Report (Incident Report/Event Report)?

(A) To document and report unwanted or unexpected events.

(B) To identify the causes of a problem.

(C) To provide a subjective and biased summary of the event.

(D) To notify individuals affected by the event.

(531) Which one of the following statements is not correct regarding professional presence?

(A) It inspires and transmits respect.

(B) It results in jealousy among coworkers.

(C) It Improves integrity.

(D) It results in improved self-esteem.

(532) Which one of the following variables is not an appropriate component of professional presence?

(A) Being an active listener.

(B) Grooming formally.

(C) Acting in self-interest.

(D) Honesty.

(533) All of the following are reasons why appearance is important in professional presence for healthcare providers except:

(A) Patients prefer formal attire or scrubs.

(B) Hygiene and grooming reflect professionalism.

(C) It inspires respect and confidence.

(D) It will attract more clients than your colleagues.

(534) Failure to perform a required act such as failure to call a physician during an emergency is known as:

(A) Misfeasance.

(B) Malfeasance.

(C) Nonfeasance.

(D) Disintegrity.

(535) Performance of an illegal act such as a medical assistant prescribing a medication is known as:

(A) Misfeasance.

(B) Malfeasance.

(C) Nonfeasance.

(D) Disintegrity.

(536) Inappropriate execution of a legal act such as the inadequate use of a non-sterile instrument during a sterile procedure is known as:

(A) Misfeasance.

(B) Malfeasance.

(C) Nonfeasance.

(D) Dis integrity.

(537) All of the following are populations that are generally protected under mandatory reporting laws except:

(A) Children.

(B) People with disabilities.

(C) The elderly.

(D) Women.

(538) All of the following conditions prohibit the legal guardian or parents of a minor from access to the information of the minor except:

(A) Whenever the healthcare professional wishes to.

(B) The minor is able to consent.

(C) Care is authorized by a court.

(D) Whenever the minor, provider, parents agree that the minor and the provider can have a confidential relationship.

(539) All of the following are primary causes of medical malpractice except:

(A) Negligence.

(B) Lack of knowledge.

(C) Lack of experience.

(D) Being young.

(540) How should paper records be rendered during the destruction process?

(A) Shredding.

(B) Pulverization.

(C) Melting.

(D) Throwing them away.

Test 3 Answers and Explanations

(361) (A) Under the tongue.

When taking a medication sublingually, it dissolves beneath the tongue. Because of their great vascularization, the mucous membranes beneath the tongue enable the medication to enter the bloodstream quickly. Usually, the medication is made in a form that dissolves or disintegrates quickly beneath the tongue, like a tablet or film. This enables the medication to be directly absorbed through the thin mucous membranes, avoiding first-pass metabolism in the liver and the gastrointestinal system.

(362) (C) Topical route.

The topical route is the method of administration in which the medication is delivered topically. Medications are prepared as lotions, creams, ointments, gels, or patches in this method, and they are applied directly to the skin's surface. The substance is absorbed via the epidermal layers and enters the bloodstream, where it may have systemic or localized effects, based on the particular prescription. Topical treatment is frequently utilized for transdermal drug delivery, pain control, and dermatological problems.

(363) (A) Parenteral route.

Parenteral administration is the method used to administer medications that need to avoid the gastrointestinal system. When drugs are administered parenterally, they are injected into the body through a different route than the digestive system. This covers a range of techniques, including intrathecal, intramuscular, subcutaneous, intravenous, and intradermal routes. Parenteral administration circumvents the gastrointestinal route, which enables quick and accurate drug delivery, immediate systemic effects, and the avoidance of problems like insufficient absorption or degradation in the digestive system.

(364) (A) ISMP.

In general, sound-alike problems may be caused by confusion with brand-brand, generic-brand, or generic-generic drug names. Look-alike problems may occur because different drugs may look the same and one drug from different sources may look different. To avoid this, the FDA and the Institute for Safe Medication Practices (ISMP) recommend the use of tall man lettering for certain drug names.

(365) (D) LASA medications.

"Look-alike, sound-alike medications" (LASA) is the term used to identify pharmaceuticals that have similar spelling or pronunciation that could cause medication errors. Because of their phonetic and orthographic similarities, LASA drugs carry a risk of confusion during the dispensing, administering, and prescription procedures. These parallels may result in mistakes like choosing the wrong drug or giving the wrong dosage. The FDA and groups like the Institute for Safe Medication Practices (ISMP) support techniques like tall man letters to set apart similar drug names and lower the possibility of mistakes as a way to lessen this danger.

(366) (A) The fraction of the administered drug that reaches systemic circulation.

After administration, a drug has to be absorbed. The rate of absorption varies according to the administration route and various characteristics of the drug (dissolution rate, concentration, and other biochemical variables). An important factor to consider, especially when a drug is taken orally, is the bioavailability of the drug, which is the fraction of the administered drug that reaches systemic circulation. Bioavailability varies when drugs are taken orally due to inactivation by digestive enzymes, rate of gastrointestinal absorption, metabolism in the liver, etc.

(367) (B) Intravenous administration.

IV administration is the route of delivery that usually yields 100% bioavailability. A medication that is injected intravenously enters the circulation directly, avoiding any gastrointestinal system absorption barriers. This ensures that the whole dosage of the medication enters the bloodstream without being lost or changed. Conversely, different modes of delivery, such as topical or oral, can have a reduced bioavailability due to things like inadequate absorption, metabolism, or the liver's first-pass effect.

(368) (A) Kidneys.

The kidneys are the organ principally in charge of excreting the majority of medications. Through the production of urine, the kidneys are essential in filtering blood and getting rid of waste items, including medications. They help the body eliminate drugs by drawing them out of the bloodstream and concentrating them in the urine. It is important to remember, though, that the liver also aids in the removal of medications by breaking them down into more water-soluble substances that can be expelled in bile, which ultimately travels to the intestines for removal.

(369) (C) Macronutrients and micronutrients.

The two primary categories of nutrients are macronutrients and micronutrients. The body uses macronutrients—proteins, lipids, and carbs—as building blocks and energy when they are ingested in substantial amounts. Vitamins and electrolytes are examples of micronutrients, which are ingested in tiny amounts and assist a number of bodily processes. The preservation of general health and wellbeing depends heavily on these two categories.

(370) (D) Dietary fiber.

Carbohydrates include monosaccharides or simple sugars like glucose, disaccharides like sucrose or lactose, oligosaccharides, and polysaccharides like starch, all of which are important sources of energy. Dietary fiber is a type of carbohydrate that is not broken down into simple sugars but helps the digestion process instead.

(371) (C) Side or back labels.

Side or back labels include a list of ingredients in order of weight (the ingredient that weighs the most goes first and the ingredient that weighs the least goes last). Added sugars may appear with different names, such as honey, evaporated cane juice, or high fructose corn syrup, among others. These labels also contain shelf-life information (sell-by, best-by, use-by dates) and allergy information related to the presence (or potential presence) of milk, fish, tree nuts, peanuts, shellfish, wheat, eggs, and soybeans.

(372) (B) Warning labels.

Front-of-package labels are voluntary and food manufacturers frequently use them to display positive nutritional qualities of their foods. However, this selective display of information (when negative qualities are left out) may deceive the consumer. For this reason, public health advocates are recommending the use of warning labels as front-of-package labels to warn consumers about added sugars, high levels of saturated fats, and other potentially negative qualities of food.

(373) (A) Foods containing gluten.

Foods containing gluten should be avoided by those who have celiac disease. Grains like wheat, barley, rye, and triticale all contain gluten. Celiac disease sufferers should carefully read food labels and avoid anything that contains these gluten-containing cereals or their derivatives. This entails staying away from items that could include hidden sources of gluten, such as bread, pasta, cereal, baked goods, and many processed foods. For those who have celiac disease, naturally gluten-free meals and gluten-free substitutes are advised.

(374) (A) Carbohydrate.

A diet for people with kidney disease should include low-sodium foods. Packaged foods should be avoided, and fresh foods are recommended. The consumption of proteins, potassium (bananas, oranges, potatoes, nuts, dairy foods), and phosphorus (dark-colored sodas, bran cereals, nuts, and dairy foods) should be limited.

(375) (A) Binge-eating disorder.

Binge-eating disorder is a condition characterized by episodes of excessive or uncontrolled eating (binge-eating), which is not followed by purging or other compensatory behaviors. Patients are usually overweight or obese.

(376) (C) Bulimia nervosa.

Bulimia nervosa is a condition characterized by binge-eating episodes followed by excessive behaviors aimed at preventing weight gain (such as vomiting, excessive exercise or fasting, use of laxatives or diuretics, etc.). In contrast with patients with anorexia nervosa, those with bulimia nervosa may be overweight or have a normal weight.

(377) (D) Avoidant restrictive food intake disorder (ARFID).

Avoidant restrictive food intake disorder (ARFID) is a condition characterized by excessive selectivity with the amount and type of food consumed and low-calorie intake. ARFID usually starts during middle childhood and may impair the child's growth and development. It is not characterized by body image issues or fear of being overweight or obese.

(378) (A) Stage 1 (trust vs. mistrust).

The theory of psychosocial development was postulated by Erik Erikson and establishes eight sequential stages of development. Stage 1 (trust vs. mistrust) occurs from infancy to one year. When parents provide a safe environment for their child, the child learns to trust others.

(379) (B) Stage 6 (intimacy vs. isolation).

Stage 6 generally occurs between the ages of eighteen and forty. In this stage, young adults focus on forming intimate, loving relationships with people in their lives. If they are unable to form these connections, they may experience isolation, which includes feelings of loneliness and exclusion.

(380) (C) Depression.

A major depressive disorder is characterized by a persistent and deep feeling of sadness and lack of pleasure. Symptoms include persistent sadness, anhedonia (loss of interest and pleasure in activities that used to be enjoyable), unwanted weight loss or gain, changes in appetite, sleeping problems, fatigue, feelings of guilt, pain, and recurrent thoughts of death, harm, or suicide.

(381) (B) ADHD.

Attention Deficit Hyperactivity Disorder (ADHD) is a behavioral disorder characterized by disorganized, excessive, and impulsive activity. Symptoms include hyperactivity, difficulty with attention and following instructions, repetitive movements of hands and feet, and excessive talking and interruption.

(382) (A) Denial.

In the field of medicine, denial is a defensive tactic frequently used by patients who will not accept their illness. It entails denying the existence of the sickness or the severity of it, frequently out of fear, anxiety, or a need to avoid dealing with uncomfortable feelings. Adherence to medical advice, appropriate diagnosis, and treatment might be impeded by denial. Effective patient care and support require healthcare providers to identify and delicately handle denial.

(383) (C) Repression.

In medicine, repression is the term used to describe the unconscious hiding of upsetting or traumatic memories or events as a defensive strategy. Within the medical setting, people may suppress distressing experiences associated with their disease, such excruciating tests or diagnoses. The goal of repression is to shield the person from intense feelings of emotion or worry brought on by those memories. Repressed memories, however, can negatively affect mental health and impede the effectiveness of therapy. Healthcare professionals should be aware of the possible consequences of repression and provide the proper assistance and remedies.

(384) (D) Rationalization.

In the field of medicine, rationalization is a defensive tactic frequently seen in patients who try to provide coherent or acceptable justifications for their illness, symptoms, or results. This enables people to downplay feelings of shame or blame or to rationalize or make sense of their experiences in a way that maintains their sense of self. Patients who rationalize their sickness may do so by discounting warning indicators or attributing it to outside causes. To guarantee proper assessment and suitable treatment planning, healthcare providers should be aware of rationalization and take necessary action.

(385) (D) Assessing blood flow, cancer, and neurological conditions.

Positron emission tomography (PET) scan is a functional imaging technique that employs a tracer, which is a radioactive substance. It helps to visualize blood flow, cancer, and neurological conditions.

(386) A) To analyze tissue or cell samples.

Obtaining a tissue or cell sample from a particular part of the body for further study is the primary goal of a biopsy. To check for anomalies like cancer, infections, inflammatory disorders, or other diseases, the sample is taken, analyzed under a microscope, and subjected to additional laboratory testing. Biopsies are useful tools for medical decision-making because they aid in precise diagnosis, the formulation of suitable treatment regimens, the evaluation of disease development, and the provision of important data.

(387) (C) Excisional biopsy.

A surgical procedure called an excisional biopsy includes the total removal of a suspicious or abnormal tumor or tissue. Usually, either local or general anesthetic is used during the procedure. After that, the removed tissue is transported to a pathology lab for a thorough inspection and analysis. Excisional biopsies are frequently performed when a larger sample is required for diagnosis or when there is a possibility of malignancy. The process helps determine the best course of action for treatment by enabling a comprehensive assessment of the tissue.

(388) (A) Ultrasound.

The imaging method most frequently employed to direct a needle biopsy is ultrasound. The healthcare provider can precisely guide the biopsy needle to the intended region because of the ultrasound's real-time view of the target area. The thyroid gland, liver, breast, prostate, and lymph nodes are among the organs and tissues that are frequently subjected to ultrasound-guided needle biopsies because they are readily accessible and observable. By guaranteeing precise needle placement, this technique enhances the safety and precision of the biopsy process.

(389) (C) Colonoscopy.

Colonoscopy is an endoscopic procedure that is used to diagnose conditions that affect the large intestine. It can also be used to take biopsy samples. On the contrary a gastroscopy is an endoscopic procedure used to diagnose conditions that affect the gastric tissues. It can be used to take biopsy samples.

(390) (A) Pharmacological therapy.

The use of drugs to treat or manage a range of medical disorders is known as pharmacological therapy. It entails the use of particular pharmaceuticals or medications that are given orally, topically, intravenously, or through other means in order to treat the underlying disease or symptoms. The goals of pharmacological treatment are to cure the illness completely, relieve symptoms, stop the disease from getting worse, and restore normal physiological processes. Depending on the particular medical condition being treated, these medications may include antibiotics, painkillers, antihypertensives, antidiabetic agents, and many others.

(391) (C) Immunotherapy.

Immunotherapy is a type of treatment that uses biologics, a type of medication that modulates the body's immune response to help it destroy cancer cells. It is one of the cornerstones of cancer treatment.

(392) (D) Number of new-onset cases during a period of time.

The number of new cases of an illness within a defined population over a specified period of time is measured by incidence in epidemiology. This focuses on documenting the emergence of new instances in order to provide insights into the pace at which the disease progresses. A useful tool for studying acute diseases, incidence also aids in determining the risk and burden of a given disease within a population. It helps with trend identification, assessment of the need for interventions, and evaluation of preventive actions.

(393) (B) Increased risk of developing a specific condition.

In the field of epidemiology, risk factors refer to attributes or features that raise the possibility of contracting a certain illness or condition. These variables may be linked to other facets of a person's health or they may be demographic, genetic, behavioral, or environmental factors. Epidemiologists can learn more about the origins and mechanisms of diseases, evaluate a population's or an individual's susceptibility to a condition, create preventive measures, and guide public health activities by identifying and researching risk factors. Comprehending risk factors is essential for preventing diseases, identifying them early, and managing them effectively.

(394) (A) Increase in the incidence of a specific infectious disease within a specific facility.

An outbreak occurs when the prevalence of a specific infectious illness suddenly rises in a given facility, community, or geographic area. It describes a localized incidence of instances that is higher than anticipated for that demographic or region. Outbreaks can occur in a variety of contexts, including schools, hospitals, nursing homes, and even within a particular community. They are distinguished by the disease spreading quickly among people who are in close proximity to one another or within a specific demographic. A new pathogen's introduction, flaws in infection control procedures, or other environmental or behavioral factors are some of the causes of outbreaks.

(395) (C) Outbreak with a global threat to the health of the general population.

Within the discipline of epidemiology, a pandemic is an outbreak of a disease that has swept across large geographical regions, which transcends national borders and impacts a substantial segment of the world's populace. A pandemic provides a worldwide threat to public health, in contrast to an epidemic, which is confined to a particular area or population. A virus with high rates of disease and death spreading continuously from person to person defines a pandemic. These frequently cause widespread sickness, upend social and economic structures, and necessitate concerted worldwide efforts for treatment, mitigation, and control. The influenza pandemics of the previous century, such the COVID-19 pandemic and the H1N1 pandemic of 2009, are two notable instances of pandemics.

(396) (B) 12-20 respirations per minute.

Rate is the number of respirations per minute. The normal range in healthy adults is between twelve and twenty respirations per minute. Higher rates are known as tachypnea and lower rates as bradypnea.

(397) (C) Apnea.

The lack or cessation of breathing is referred to as apnea. This is a condition in which there is a brief, several-second-long stop in breathing. Sleep apnea is a type of apnea that happens while you are asleep. Other causes of apnea include neurological or respiratory issues. If left untreated, it frequently causes a reduction in blood oxygen levels and can cause irregular sleep patterns, excessive daytime sleepiness, and other health issues.

(398) (C) Wheezing.

The peculiar respiratory sound known as wheezing is typified by a high-pitched whistling or melodic noise made while breathing. It happens when the lungs' small airways are obstructed to airflow. Conditions like asthma, bronchitis, chronic obstructive pulmonary disease (COPD), and allergic responses are frequently linked to wheezing. It is brought on by inflammation, an overabundance of mucus, and airway constriction. Chest tightness, coughing, and shortness of breath can all occur with wheezing. For an accurate diagnosis and course of treatment, medical assessment is required.

(399) (C) Dyspnea.

Breathlessness or shortness of breath is referred to as dyspnea. Breathing difficulties are a subjective feeling that can be brought on by a number of situations, including heart problems, lung ailments, anxiety, and physical effort. The severity of dyspnea varies, and in order to choose the best course of action, its underlying cause should be thoroughly assessed.

(400) (A) When lying down.

Breathing becomes harder for those with orthopnea when they are in a lying position. Increased fluid buildup in the lungs, which is frequently observed in diseases including heart failure and chronic obstructive pulmonary disease (COPD), is the cause of this. The fluid redistributes when you lie flat, making breathing difficult. Sitting upright or elevating the upper body while sleeping with additional pillows are two ways to alleviate orthopnea.

(401) (D) There is no point in doing that.

The measurement of a patient's respiratory rate usually requires doing so without the patient noticing. Since respiration is automatic, the respiratory rate may be altered if the patient is actively thinking about breathing. A common technique involves measuring the patient's respiratory rate just after measuring their pulse: keep your fingers on the patient's wrist, as if you were still measuring their pulse, and start measuring their respiration.

(402) (B) Oxygen saturation.

Pulse oximetry is a simple and noninvasive method to measure oxygen saturation. These devices also display the patient's pulse rate. Oxygen saturation reflects the percentage of oxygenated hemoglobin in relation to total hemoglobin.

(403) (D) Throat.

A healthy individual should have a reading above 95% saturation. The measurement is usually performed on a finger, toe, or earlobe. Oxygen saturation below 90% can be due to a disease process that results in an oxygenation issue, such as a pulmonary infection, asthma, bronchitis, etc. Oxygen therapy and other treatment options may be required to enhance the patient's oxygenation during such scenario.

(404) (D) Numeric pain scale.

Pain scales are tools to help patients and health care providers describe pain in a relatively standardized manner. The most common way to measure pain is with a numerical scale from zero to ten where zero is the absence of pain and ten is the worst pain of your life. The visual analog scale presents the patient with a horizontal line where the farthest left is no pain at all and the farthest right is the worst pain, and the patient draws a line at the point they feel describes their pain. Many other variables of the pain scales exist, and their usage may vary between institutions and age groups.

(405) (B) Menarche.

After their first menstruation (also known as menarche), which usually occurs after puberty and between the ages of nine and seventeen, female patients initiate their menstrual and ovarian cycles. These cycles last approximately one month, and they are characterized by hormonal changes that promote the proliferation of the endometrium and maturation of ovarian follicles for ovulation in preparation for fecundation and pregnancy.

(406) (A) Last Menstrual Period.

The last menstrual period (LMP) is the first day of the patient's last menstrual period. It is most commonly used to determine the beginning of a pregnancy and calculate the estimated date of delivery. In the absence of fecundation and/or pregnancy, the menstrual phase begins in the form of the discharge of endometrial tissue in a process known as menstruation (also known as periods), which can last up to seven days.

(407) (A) Diaper and a shirt.

It is advised that small children wear a shirt and diapers when having their height measured. Without any extra clothing interfering with the measurement procedure, this minimum attire enables accurate measurement. It makes it simple to get at the child's body and guarantees that the measurement is made from the child's true height without the presence of other layers or fabric that could skew the results.

(408) (B) Place the tape measure just above the ears and eyebrows.

When measuring a baby's head circumference, the tape measure should be placed just above the ears and eyebrows to ensure accuracy. This method provides a consistent point of reference and helps monitor the baby's growth and development.

(409) (B) Two people.

To maximize the accuracy of height measurement in children, two people should participate in the measurement (an assistant helping to hold and position the child and a measurer).

(410) (A) Contamination.

Contamination is the stage of wound infection when pathogens are present but there is no host response or multiplication. In this phase, bacteria are present in the wound, but the host's immune system is not actively growing or reacting to them. It indicates that germs have been introduced to the site for the first time, necessitating cleansing and preventive steps to stop the infection from spreading.

(411) (A) Limited proliferation without host reaction.

Microorganisms only slightly proliferate during the colonization stage of wound infection, and there is little to no host response. In this stage, the incision becomes more infected with bacteria, but there is no visible inflammation or infection. In the event that the balance between the host and microorganisms is upset, colonization—the development of microorganisms in the wound—sets the foundation for possible local infection progression. To stop additional problems, wounds must be properly managed and monitored.

(412) (C) Hypergranulation, exudate, bleeding, and delayed healing.

In covert cases of local wound infection, there is hypergranulation, exudate, bleeding, and delayed healing. In overt cases, there are signs of inflammation alongside a purulent exudate.

(413) (C) Inflammation extension and wound dehiscence.

The extension of inflammation and possible consequences are characteristics of the spreading infection stage of wound infection. In this phase, the infection spreads beyond the original site of the lesion and symptoms including warmth, redness, and swelling may appear in adjacent tissues. Additionally, possible outcomes include lymphangitis, or inflammation of the lymphatic vessels, and wound dehiscence, or the partial or whole separation of the wound borders. This requires immediate medical attention and action to stop additional tissue damage and systemic problems.

(414) (D) Malaise, fever, and sepsis.

A systemic infection creates systemic symptoms like malaise, fever, and asthenia. The infection may complicate even further, which can result in sepsis, septic shock, and death.

(415) (B) To take a sample of breast tissue for study under a microscope.

Breast biopsy is a diagnostic test that consists of taking a sample of breast tissue or cells to study the morphology under a microscope. It is commonly performed to rule out malignancy in patients with signs or symptoms of breast cancer or neoplasms.

(416) (C) Replacing the clouded lens of the eye with an artificial lens.

Cataract surgery is a surgical procedure that consists of removing cataracts, which occur when the lens of the eye becomes cloudy, and replacing it with a new and clear artificial lens.

(417) (D) When the gallbladder becomes infected or in the treatment of gallbladder cancer.

Cholecystectomy is the surgical removal of the gallbladder, which may be required when a person presents gallstones and the gallbladder becomes infected (cholecystitis). It may also be required during the treatment of cancer that affects the gallbladder.

(418) (A) To remove the uterus.

Hysterectomy is a surgery that consists of removing the uterus, which may be required when patients present excessively heavy periods or pain, or when a patient has cancer that affects the uterus.

(419) (D) To remove infected and nonviable tissue from wounds.

The debridement procedure is frequently part of wound care plans. It consists of removing infected and nonviable tissue from wounds, which allows the tissue to heal effectively.

(420) (A) An urgency requires immediate examination and/or treatment within twenty-four hours, while an emergency requires immediate examination and/or treatment in the emergency department.

The terms "urgency" and "emergency" are frequently used interchangeably, even by health care workers. Although these terms are closely related, they refer to different things. Urgency is an injury or medical condition that requires immediate examination and/or treatment by a health care provider, usually within twenty-four hours in an outpatient setting. An emergency is a severe or life-threatening injury or medical condition that requires immediate examination and/or treatment in the emergency department of a hospital.

(421) (D) Make sure somebody holds the hands and legs of the patient.

The use of an AED is especially important in patients who have collapsed. In patients with probable asphyxia, high-quality CPR is the priority. Before using the AED, make sure there is no water in the area, remove the patient's clothing, dry their chest, and finally announce that you are going to use the defibrillator and make sure no one is touching the patient.

(422) (C) 100-120 compressions per minute.

Adult CPR compressions should be performed at a pace of between 100 and 120 per minute. This raises the likelihood of successful resuscitation and guarantees proper blood flow to essential organs. For adult patients undergoing cardiac arrest, maintaining a steady and proper compression rate is essential to the overall success of CPR in supporting the heart and oxygenation.

(423) (B) Two inches.

High-quality CPR is characterized by fast compressions that push the chest down (two inches or five centimeters) and allow complete recoil of the chest. The airway can be opened by tilting the chin up.

(424) (A) Call for help and activate the emergency response system.

The first step for providing Basic Life Support is to call for help and activate the emergency response system. This ensures that additional medical assistance is on the way while you begin to assess and provide initial care to the patient.

(425) (C) Birth year of the patient.

Medication logs are simple tools to document the administration of medication and keep track of the inventory. These logs consist of the name of the drug, strength, amount administered, date, time, patient name, prescriber name, and who administered the medication (e.g., in the case of injectables). Medication logs can be kept on paper or electronically.

(426) (A) Specialty drugs.

Specialty pharmacies are pharmacies that handle specialty drugs and services, which are usually employed in the management of rare or complex medical conditions. These are drugs that a small portion of the total population needs and, therefore, a typical pharmacy does not keep them in stock.

(427) (C) Patients with asthma.

Patients who may at some point need services from a specialty pharmacy include those with multiple sclerosis, rheumatoid arthritis, hemophilia, cancer, HIV, and Crohn's disease.

(428) (D) Every time the patient is evaluated.

The progress notes contain essential information about the clinical evolution of the patient's condition, which should be updated every time the patient is evaluated. This includes information about the progress of signs and symptoms, application and response to treatments or procedures, and consideration of laboratory and imaging results. The documentation process should not include a future action or procedure—this promotes accuracy and reduces the presence of mistakes. However, if a mistake is made for any reason, it is important to correct it in a clear manner, which includes strikethrough the entry with the mistake (in paper), write a new entry specifying there was a mistake and proceed with the correction, and date and sign the correction.

(429) (A) To replace traditional in-person care.

Telehealth care provides health care providers with different ways to deliver care like remote monitoring or chat-based care, as well as extending many benefits of traditional care visits to e-visits, which contributes to the continuum of care (usually as an on-demand service). For this reason, telehealth should not be seen as a simple replacement or alternative for traditional care, but as a different approach that can be used alongside traditional care.

(430) (C) Stay on line with the patient and call the emergency medical service.

Some patients with a life-threatening condition may contact the medical office and ask for telehealth care. In this situation, a professional medical assistant must be able to recognize the problem, stay on line with the patient and call the emergency medical service.

(431) (C) Electronic prescribing.

Electronic prescribing (or e-prescribing) is the electronic generation, transmission, and filling of medical prescriptions with the help of computer-based applications. These applications facilitate the electronic transmission of new or renewed prescriptions. These prescriptions are easier to read, which reduces medication errors. Pharmacies can also request refills directly via the electronic prescription software, which must be approved or declined by the original prescriber (or someone authorized by them). Examples of electronic prescribing software include RXNT, Kareo Clinical, Benchmark Systems, CharmHealth, ScriptSure, AthenaOne, and Elation Health, among others.

(432) (C) Anaphylactic shock.

Anaphylaxis can cause a serious and sometimes fatal condition known as anaphylactic shock. It is typified by an extremely quick and severe systemic reaction to an allergen, which causes a sharp decrease in blood pressure and insufficient blood supply to essential organs. Breathing problems, a fast heartbeat, lightheadedness, disorientation, unconsciousness, and pale or bluish skin are among the symptoms. Anaphylactic shock requires immediate medical attention, which includes giving epinephrine and performing emergency resuscitation techniques.

(433) (D) Fever.

Fever is not seen as a typical anaphylactic sign. The main clinical manifestation of anaphylaxis is an acute allergic reaction, which includes a range of systemic symptoms such breathing difficulties, swelling, hives, low blood pressure, and gastrointestinal problems. Rather than being related to anaphylaxis, fever is more frequently linked to infectious or inflammatory diseases. Individual responses may differ, though, and in certain instances, fever can happen as a secondary reaction to anaphylaxis because of comorbidities or infections. It is advisable to get medical help for a comprehensive evaluation and diagnosis if you think you may be having an allergic response.

(434) (C) Sharps containers.

Sharps containers should be used to dispose of needles and other sharp objects. Sharps containers are made expressly to hold and gather used lancets, syringes, needles, and other sharp medical supplies in a secure manner. These containers are marked with biohazard symbols for accurate identification and are puncture-resistant to minimize unintentional needlestick injuries. By ensuring the proper handling and disposal of potentially infectious materials, the use of sharps containers helps prevent needle-related injuries and the spread of bloodborne diseases, which serves to safeguard both the public and healthcare professionals.

(435) (A) Contaminated gloves.

Reg bags are used for medical/biohazardous waste, which includes tissues and other organic waste, blood, items with blood (gowns, gauzes, gloves, vials, tubes, etc.), body fluids, and sharps containers.

(436) (B) In yellow biohazard bags.

Soiled dressings and bandages should be disposed of in yellow biohazard bags. These bags are designed to safely contain medical waste that may be contaminated with blood or other potentially infectious materials.

(437) (A) Review the product's safety data sheet.

Reading the safety data sheet for any chemical product should be your first step before using it. This paper gives you all the information you need to handle the chemical safely and effectively by outlining the product's risks, handling guidelines, and required safety measures.

(438) (B) Keep the chemical products stored in a tight container.

All of the following cautions should be taken in relation to the use of chemicals: review the product's safety data sheet, use chemical products in accordance with your training and duties, do not use a chemical product if you do not know how to handle it, use protective equipment when handling potentially dangerous chemical products, verify that the product inside the container is the correct one, as stated by the label, perform hand washing after handling chemical products, do not consume foods or drinks when handling chemical products, do not handle contact lenses and other personal objects when handling chemical products, follow the facility's plan in case of an accident or injury and keep the chemical products stored in a ventilated and dry area.

(439) (B) To provide an environment for the microorganism to multiply.

The source, also known as the reservoir, serves as a place where the pathogen may multiply and propagate across the chain of infection. The disease can multiply and proliferate by using the source or reservoir as a breeding environment. The pathogen's amplification raises the possibility that it will be transmitted to vulnerable hosts, which aids in the infectious condition's dissemination among a population or community.

(440) (D) Fever.

The clinical findings associated with an infectious disease can be caused by the direct effect of the pathogen's actions. However, the host's immune response against the pathogen also produces a wide variety of responses that can be more detrimental than the pathologic action of the infectious agent. Some of the most common signs and symptoms associated with an infectious disease include: fever (most common, sometimes present in isolation), asthenia, cough, nausea, vomiting, sore throat, inflammation or exudate in wounds, diarrhea, shortness of breath, chills, burning sensation during urination, swollen lymph nodes, headache, pain and neck stiffness.

(441) (A) Vaccines and immunizations.

One of the most important tools for the prevention and response to epidemics and pandemics is the use of vaccines and immunizations. This is important for both the general population and health care workers.

(442) (D) Adults.

Some infectious diseases can spread rapidly and pose a risk to the health of the general population, especially vulnerable people like the elderly, pregnant women, and children. To prevent the deleterious effects of outbreaks, epidemics, and pandemics, various research groups and federal agencies study these phenomena and work on the development of response plans.

(443) (A) Individuals with no underlying health conditions.

A susceptible host is a person that is at risk of becoming infected with the infectious microorganism due to other health conditions, age, nutrition, medication use, immunodeficiency, etc.

(444) (A) pH below 5.5.

Bacterial growth can be influenced by various factors, both environmental and nutritional. In relation to pH, bacteria can be acidophilic (prefer a pH below 5.5), alkaliphilic (prefer a pH above 8.5), or neutrophilic (prefer a pH from 5 to 8). An important factor that is commonly considered is temperature: bacteria can withstand various ranges of temperature, although pathogen bacteria and bacteria from the human flora live between 25°C and 45°C (mesophiles).

(445) (C) Measure hearing threshold.

An audiometer measures sound intensity (decibels) and tone (hertz or cycles per second). The procedure simply requires the patient to raise their hand if they hear a tone produced by the device to measure the hearing threshold of the patient.

(446) (D) Rinne test.

A tuning fork can be used to administer the clinical Weber and Rinne tests. A tuning fork is put on the patient's forehead or head during the Weber test to determine whether there is a difference in hearing capacity between the ears. By positioning the tuning fork on the mastoid bone, close to the ear canal, the Rinne test contrasts air conduction versus bone conduction of sound. These tests aid in the assessment of auditory function, the detection of any anomalies in hearing, and the distinction between sensorineural and conductive hearing loss.

(447) (D) Flow rate during forced expiration after deep inspiration.

Peak flow rate is a very simple test that measures the flow rate during a forced expiration after a deep inspiration. The patient only needs a reusable and small hand-held device with a mouthpiece, a cylinder, and an indicator (red zone or 50%, yellow zone or 50-80%, and green zone or 80-100%). A peak flow rate can be used by patients with respiratory conditions to adapt their treatment (i.e., an increased dose of inhaled corticosteroids) or identify the need for acute care.

(448) (C) Measure lung function.

Spirometry is used in respiratory testing to monitor and evaluate lung function. It provides useful data on a number of respiratory parameters, which include tidal volume, forced vital capacity (FVC), and forced expiratory volume in one second (FEV1). Respiratory disorders such as pulmonary fibrosis, asthma, and chronic obstructive pulmonary disease (COPD) can be diagnosed with the use of spirometry. It helps in assessing lung disease severity, tracking the course of the illness, and figuring out how well treatment plans are working.

(449) (B) Asthma.

Spirometry is a pulmonary function test that measures general lung function (not only expiratory flow rate). It requires a spirometer and can be used to determine various respiratory parameters (forced expiratory volume in one second, forced vital capacity, tidal volume, etc.). Spirometry is employed during the diagnosis of various respiratory conditions like asthma, chronic obstructive pulmonary disease, and pulmonary fibrosis.

(450) (B) Snellen charts.

testing visual acuity in a clinical setting consists of employing eye charts like the Snellen chart or the logMAR chart. Refractor devices are specialized vision testing devices mostly used by ophthalmologists and other eye care professionals.

(451) (A) Ishihara charts.

The Ishihara charts are used to study color vision/blindness, which may affect various groups of colors, such as red-green color blindness (deuteranopia and protanopia) and blue-yellow color blindness (tritanopia).

(452) (B) The patient stands twenty feet away from the chart.

The Snellen chart should be viewed at a distance of twenty feet when evaluating visual acuity. Accurate measurement and comparison of visual acuity are ensured by this standard distance. Every line on the Snellen chart denotes a distinct visual acuity level. Normal vision (20/20) is represented by line eight. The person can read the lines by standing at the designated distance, and to determine their visual acuity, they can identify which is the lowest line that they can read with accuracy.

(453) (C) Collection errors.

The preanalytical stage consists of variables related to specimen ordering, collection, storage, transport, and preanalytical processing (for example, centrifugation). Errors in this stage include: ordering errors (no order, deficient patient preparation, wrong test ordered, incomplete order), collection errors (incorrect technique, wrong container, lost specimen, sample contamination), storage errors (wrong temperature, wrong light conditions, contamination, specimen lost), transportation errors (specimen lost, contamination, damage) and processing errors (wrong timing, wrong temperature, wrong technique).

(454) (C) Calibration errors.

The analytical stage consists of variables related to the analysis of the specimen. Errors in this stage include calibration errors (lack of quality control, handling error, wrong technique), reagent errors (lack of quality control, handling error, wrong technique), and machine errors (lack of quality control, handling error, computer or technical error, power failure, wrong technique).

(455) (C) Postanalytical stage.

The postanalytical stage consists of variables related to the reporting and delivery of the results, as well as the disposal of the specimen. Errors in this stage include disposal errors (wrong technique), reporting errors (delay, wrong patient, incorrect result, and documentation error), delivery errors (delay, wrong patient, incorrect results) and interpretation error (wrong diagnosis).

(456) (C) Interpretation error.

One mistake connected to the postanalytical phase of quality assurance is interpretation error. This error pertains to misinterpretations or errors in the test results. Misdiagnosis or inaccurate evaluation of the patient's condition based on test results may be involved. Errors in interpretation can have a big impact on patient care by resulting in misdiagnoses or ineffective treatments. In order to properly interpret test results and make therapeutic decisions based on them, healthcare practitioners must possess the requisite knowledge, skills, and training.

(457) (A) Preanalytical stage.

Variables connected to the many procedures that take place prior to the actual examination of the specimen are included in the preanalytical stage of quality assurance. Ordering, collecting, preserving, delivery, and preanalytical processing of specimens are all included in this.

(458) (B) 14-18 g/dL.

Red blood cells contain a protein called hemoglobin, which transports oxygen throughout the body. An adult male in a healthy state usually has hemoglobin concentrations in the range of 14–18 g/dL, which guarantees adequate oxygen-carrying capacity.

(459) (D) 46%-55%

The normal reference range for hematocrit (Hct) in a healthy adult man is 46%-55%. Hematocrit measures the proportion of red blood cells in the blood, which is important for assessing conditions like anemia or polycythemia.

(460) (D) 80-100 fL/cell.

Red blood cell average size is measured by MCV. The normal range of red blood cells in a healthy individual is 80–100 fL/cell, which helps to determine the underlying causes of anemia and assess its different types.

(461) (A) 4.5-11.0 x 10^3 cells/mm^3.

The term "WBC count" refers to the quantity of white blood cells in a given blood volume. The standard range of white blood cell counts in a healthy individual is 4.5-11.0 x 10^} cells/mm^3. This range helps with immune function evaluation and helps to identify infections or other abnormalities.

(462) (B) 150,000-350,000 cells/mm^3.

The amount of platelets in a specific volume of blood is measured by the platelet count. A healthy person's blood usually has between 150,000 and 350,000 cells/mm^3 of platelets, which are essential for blood clotting and controlling excessive bleeding.

(463) (A) 0.9-1.1.

INR is a standardized blood clotting time measurement that is mainly used to track how well anticoagulant medication is working. For the majority of people, the range of 0.9–1.1 is the ideal therapeutic range since it promotes proper blood clotting and reduces the risk of bleeding or clotting disorders.

(464) (B) 10-13 seconds.

The duration needed for blood to clot is measured by PT. The normal clotting time in a healthy individual is within the range of 10–13 seconds. This can be used to assess the success of anticoagulant therapy and provide important information about the integrity of the coagulation system.

(465) (A) CBC.

CBC (Complete Blood Count) assesses the red, white, and platelet components of blood among other things. There are no light-sensitive materials or analytes involved that need to be shielded from light. However, during testing, riboflavin, vitamin E, and bilirubin must be shielded from light because they are all light-sensitive chemicals.

(466) (B) 4-8°C without freezing.

The suggested storage temperature range for most whole blood samples is 4°C to 8°C (refrigerated storage) without freezing. This temperature range helps to ensure reliable test findings by preventing sample degradation or change and maintaining the stability of the blood components. Sample integrity may be compromised and cellular damage may result from freezing whole blood.

(467) (A) Wrapped with aluminum foil.

Blood samples that need to be kept out of the sun, particularly those used for bilirubin analysis or other tests involving light-sensitive compounds like vitamin E or riboflavin, should be wrapped in aluminum foil or another appropriate light-blocking material. Exposure to light can cause the compounds of interest in the sample to deteriorate or change, which could result in unreliable test findings. Sample integrity is maintained and light exposure is reduced when the sample is wrapped.

(468) (C) Incineration.

The majority of the time, remaining blood samples are incinerated. High-temperature burning through incineration guarantees the total annihilation of biological components, including blood samples. By guaranteeing correct treatment and reducing the chance of contamination or pathogen exposure, this disposal technique helps to avoid any potential biohazards or risks connected with the blood samples.

(469) (C) 15-degree angle.

A precise angle must be maintained when inserting the needle into the vein during venipuncture in order to guarantee correct insertion and lower the possibility of problems. Generally speaking, an angle of about fifteen degrees is advised while inserting needles. This angle facilitates a smooth entrance into the vein without subjecting the surrounding tissues to undue stress or injury. A shallow angle of insertion of the needle reduces patient discomfort and improves the chances of a successful blood collection.

(470) (A) 3.5-5 g/dL.

Blood contains a protein called albumin, which is essential for transferring different chemicals including hormones and prescription drugs and for preserving the ideal fluid balance. Adults' normal albumin levels normally fall between 3.5-5 g/dL. Enough protein is present in this range to support regular body processes. Deviations from this range could be a sign of inflammation, malnourishment, liver or kidney problems, or other illnesses.

(471) (A) 8-23 mg/dL.

When proteins are broken down in the liver, a waste product known as blood urea nitrogen (BUN) is created and then eliminated by the kidneys. It is frequently employed as a kidney function indicator. Adults' normal BUN ranges normally fall between 8-23 mg/dL. Elevated levels could signify compromised kidney function, dehydration, blockage of the urinary system, or further ailments that impact the kidneys' capacity to efficiently filter waste materials.

(472) (C) 8.2-10.2 mg/dL.

Calcium is a vital mineral that is involved in many body processes, which include nerve signaling, muscular contraction, and bone health. Total serum calcium, which measures all of the calcium in the blood—both bound and ionized—normally ranges from 8.2-10.2 mg/dL. Deviations from this range may point to anomalous metabolism of calcium, such as hypo- or hypercalcemia (low or high calcium levels), which can be brought on by problems with the kidneys, hormonal imbalances, or other underlying illnesses.

(473) (B) 0.3-1.2 mg/dL.

The yellow pigment known as bilirubin is created when red blood cells degrade. The liver breaks it down and excretes it as bile. The combined amount of conjugated and unconjugated bilirubin is known as total bilirubin. Total bilirubin usually has a normal range of 0.3-1.2 mg/dL. Increased levels could be a sign of bilirubin metabolism-affecting disorders, liver disease, or obstruction of the bile duct. The underlying cause of aberrant bilirubin levels can be ascertained by evaluating the direct and indirect bilirubin levels independently.

(474) (D) Light green.

Lithium heparin and gel for plasma separation are contained in the light green tube. The gel helps separate plasma from the blood's cellular components during centrifugation, while the lithium heparin functions as an anticoagulant to stop blood from clotting. This tube makes it possible to measure plasma levels in chemical tests with accuracy.

(475) (B) Pull the plunger with the non-dominant hand.

Blood is flowing into the syringe and the needle has successfully reached the vein when blood is visible inside the syringe's hub. The healthcare provider should move the plunger backward with their non-dominant hand to fill the syringe barrel with the required amount of blood. By doing this, the syringe creates a vacuum, which forces the blood into the barrel. This stage guarantees that a sufficient sample is obtained for examination or additional steps.

(476) (B) 70-110 mg/dL.

The amount of glucose (sugar) in the blood is measured by serum glucose, which has a normal range of 70-110 mg/dL. The body uses glucose as its main energy source for cells, so it is important to keep blood glucose levels within this range for normal physiological processes. Atypical glucose metabolism, characterized by hypo- or hypoglycemia (low blood sugar) or hyperglycemia (high blood sugar), may be indicated by values outside of this range and linked to a number of illnesses, including diabetes.

(477) (C) 3.5-5.0 mEq/L.

Potassium, a vital electrolyte in the body, usually ranges from 3.5-5.0 milliequivalents per liter (mEq/L). Potassium is essential for sustaining healthy neuron and muscle function, as well as cellular function. Disturbances from this spectrum may result in health problems.

(478) (A) 4%-7%.

A blood test called hemoglobin A1C (HbA1C) measures the average blood glucose levels over the previous two to three months. It is mostly used to track how well people with diabetes are managing their blood sugar over the long term. The conventional consensus is that the normal range for hemoglobin A1C is 4%-7%.

(479) (B) 136-142 mEq/L.

Sodium, a vital electrolyte involved in preserving fluid balance and neuronal function, has a normal range of 136-142 mEq/L. The unit of measurement for blood sodium levels is milliequivalents per liter, or mEq/L.

(480) (A) 4-8 mg/dL.

One waste product produced by the body's breakdown of purines is uric acid. Uric acid usually ranges between 4-8 mg/dL (milligrams per deciliter). A kind of arthritis called gout can be brought on by the accumulation of urate crystals in tissues and joints as a result of high uric acid levels. It is critical to track uric acid levels when treating gout and other disorders involving improper purine metabolism.

(481) (C) Fifth intercostal space (left mid-clavicular line).

Using the left mid-clavicular line as a guide, position the precordial electrode V4 in the fifth intercostal gap. This entails finding the area on the left side of the chest between the fifth and sixth ribs and aligning the electrode in a vertical line with the clavicle's (collarbone) midway. For an EKG to yield appropriate readings from the chest leads, V4 must be positioned correctly.

(482) (A) White.

White is the proper lead wire color code for the electrode on the right arm. Lead wires in conventional EKG lead systems are color-coded in accordance with a particular standard. The color white designates the lead wire for the electrode on the right arm. Accurate signal capture and interpretation during the EKG procedure are ensured by correctly attaching the lead wires to their corresponding electrodes.

(483) (D) Red.

Red is the proper lead wire color coding for the electrode in the left leg. In the EKG system, every lead wire has a unique color assigned to it for convenience and correct connection. Usually, the lead wire for the electrode on the left leg is colored red. Maintaining consistency and accuracy in the EKG recording is facilitated by making sure the lead wires are attached using the appropriate color coding.

(484) (B) Fourth intercostal space (left parasternal line).

The fourth intercostal gap along the left parasternal line is where the precordial electrode V2 should be positioned. This entails finding the area on the left side of the chest between the fourth and fifth ribs and aligning the electrode with the line parallel to the sternum. For the EKG to record electrical activity from the particular area of the heart, V2 must be positioned correctly.

(485) (D) Purple.

Purple is the proper color coding for the precordial electrode V6 lead wire. Every precordial electrode, including V6, has a corresponding lead wire that is color-coded. V6 is usually attached to a lead wire with a purple color code in conventional EKG devices. Accurate connection and reliable EKG readings from the matching precordial leads are guaranteed when the specified color coding is followed.

(486) (D) Fifth intercostal space (left mid-axillary line).

Precordial electrode V6 should be positioned correctly in the fifth intercostal space on the left mid-axillary line. This entails finding the area on the left side of the chest between the fifth and sixth ribs and aligning the electrode in a vertical line with the side of the body's middle (axillary line). For an EKG to accurately record electrical activity from the particular area of the heart, V6 positioning is important.

(487) (D) Well above the site of amputation.

When performing an ECG on a patient with an amputated limb, electrodes should be placed well above the site of amputation to ensure proper attachment and accurate readings. This placement avoids any complications or interference that may arise from placing electrodes too close to the amputation site.

(488) (B) Place them on the right side of the chest.

In these cases, the limb electrodes are placed in the same manner, but the precordial electrodes should be placed on the right side of the chest, in a manner which will mirror the usual position on the left side.

(489) (B) Close to the injury or incision.

Do not place an electrode on an injury or incision. It can be placed close to the site. The modification should be documented. Directly applying an electrode to such regions may exacerbate the damage, slow down the healing process, or make the patient more uncomfortable.

(490) (B) Move V3 to the right side of the chest.

The placement of electrodes is the same, but considering the smaller size of the chest, the third precordial lead (V3) can be moved to the right side of the chest to reduce clutter. This lead change is known as V3 right or V3R and should be documented.

(491) (C) Atrial flutter.

Atrial flutter can be identified as an extremely fast heartbeat (>200 beats per minute) and a sawtooth pattern (a string of multiple P waves that resembles a sawtooth) followed by a QRS complex.

(492) (A) Increased heart rate with irregular and wide QRS complexes.

Ventricular arrhythmias can occur due to ectopic foci or altered conduction in the ventricles. The most common examples are ventricular tachycardia and ventricular fibrillation. Ventricular tachycardia is characterized by an increased heart rate with irregular and wide QRS complexes. Ventricular fibrillation is a life-threatening condition in which the ventricles contract erratically—no waves are identifiable.

(493) (D) Valvular disorders.

Metabolic arrhythmias are caused by metabolic derangements. They include increased or decreased potassium, as well as toxicity due to treatment with digitalis (for example, patients who use digoxin).

(494) (C) 25 mm per second.

Electrocardiographs are calibrated according to international guidelines to present a standardized sensitivity that can be interpreted in the same manner anywhere in the world. This international sensitivity standard dictates that 1 mV of electricity translates to a 10 mm vertical movement (x-axis). This is known as 1 STD (one standard), which is the standard mode of an EKG. This can be altered to double standard (1 mV = 20 mm) or one-half standard (1 mV = 5 mm). This can be seen at the start of the tracing (as a short 10 mm trace at 1 STD) or written down on the paper. At the same time, the standard speed is 25 mm per second. This can be altered as well: a faster speed (usually 50 mm per second) is useful to inspect faster heart rates or waves that are too close together.

(495) (B) Referral coordinator.

A referral is a document provided by a primary care provider when a patient needs to see a specialist due to a specific medical condition. A referral coordinator from the medical office manages the referral process by scheduling the visit with the required specialist, which involves a referral form alongside the patient's relevant information.

(496) (C) The specialist cannot ask for extra information besides the one mentioned on the referral paper.

The specialist may ask for extra information (in some cases, they may provide their own referral form to include the specific information they need). The exchange of information is very important to avoid delays and duplication of imaging or tests.

(497) (C) Unapproved acronyms.

An efficient referral process requires organization, and the first step is a standardized form, which may be filled out on paper or electronically. Referral forms may include: date of the appointment, name of the primary care provider, current diagnosis, urgency (from immediate to routine), type of specialist required and motive of referral and required service (consultation, diagnosis, follow-up, etc.).

(498) (B) There is ample evidence that supports a ketogenic diet.

Patients should learn that nutrition goes beyond losing weight. It helps to lower the risk of various conditions (cancer, cardiovascular disease, diabetes) and promotes better health and quality of life. There are multiple types of diets (Mediterranean diet, DASH diet, low-fat diet, plant-based diet), and patients may benefit from one over the other due to personal preferences, nutritional needs, cultural or religious background, cost, etc. Diets with limited evidence include a low-carbohydrate diet, ketogenic diet, gluten-free diet, and organic diet.

(499) (B) Fiber.

In general, the most important components of a healthy diet are: whole grains, fruits, vegetables, fiber, healthy fats (monounsaturated and polyunsaturated fats) and proteins. It is also important to avoid added sugars, processed foods and meats, red meats, alcohol, and unhealthy fats (saturated and trans fats).

(500) (B) Receptionist.

In addition to handling calls, emails, and appointments, the receptionist is responsible for patient registration and information verification. When a patient calls or visits the medical office, the receptionist is their first point of contact. They are essential to the efficient completion of administrative duties. In addition to scheduling appointments, taking phone calls, responding to emails, and gathering and confirming patient information, receptionists often handle a variety of administrative tasks.

(501) (C) Office manager.

Coordinating the office workflow in a patient-centered medical home is the responsibility of the office manager. In charge of the medical office's administrative activities, the office manager is essential. They are in charge of assuring that procedures are effective and well-organized, scheduling employees, taking care of money, scheduling patient visits, managing administrative personnel, and making sure that rules and policies are followed.

(502) (B) NSAIDs.

NSAIDs (non-steroidal anti-inflammatory drugs) increase the risk of stomach bleeding and hepatic (liver) damage when used with alcohol. Drinking alcohol can amplify the negative effects of NSAIDs on the liver and digestive tract, which increases the risk of concerns.

(503) (D) Ciprofloxacin.

Antibiotics — Milk consumption may reduce the absorption of certain antibiotics (e.g., ciprofloxacin and tetracycline). Food reduces the absorption of azithromycin. When taken with milk, the antibiotic ciprofloxacin is less well absorbed. Calcium present in milk and dairy products has the ability to bind to ciprofloxacin and prevent its absorption.

(504) (A) Medical consultation for patients.

Mobile healthcare apps provide various services. Apps like Teladoc, MDLIVE, and Amwell provide medical consultation for patients. Apps like Lecturio and Osmosis Med provide education to health care students. And apps like Epocrates, UpToDate, and Drugs.com provide clinical and drug information for health care providers.

(505) (B) It is possible to perform a throughout physical exam during a virtual visit.

There are multiple barriers to access for virtual visits which includes some patients or healthcare providers who may not have the knowledge required to manage telehealth software and apps. Additionally, it is not possible to perform a throughout physical exam during a virtual visit. Examinations can only employ visual examination and remote monitoring, when available. Finally, the patient and the health care provider may not speak the same language and technical issues like incompatibility, software bugs, and poor internet connection might arise.

(506) (A) COVID-19 pandemic.

Although telehealth started with remote consultations via telephone or radio, this practice has become truly prevalent now in the digital era, especially after the COVID-19 pandemic in 2020. Virtual visits, remote patient monitoring, remote surgery, telepharmacy, patient portals, and other health care services can be provided through telehealth.

(507) (D) Zoom.

Video communication software (Zoom, Google Meets, Microsoft Teams, and other platforms) programs usually allow users to communicate via video, audio, and text. The majority of these programs are also available for various devices and operating systems.

(508) (C) Sterilization equipment.

The required inspection schedule may vary between devices due to their function, usage, and safety profile. For example, stethoscopes or wheelchairs do not need frequent inspections, especially when compared with sterilization equipment. The main regulatory bodies in relation to equipment inspection and maintenance of equipment in health care facilities are the U.S. Food and Drug Administration (FDA) and the Occupational Safety and Health Administration (OSHA), and the CMS (2013) provides thorough guidance in "Hospital Equipment Maintenance Requirements ".

(509) (B) To standardize and simplify the reporting of medical services for billing purposes.

The main purpose of medical coding is to standardize and simplify the reporting of medical services, procedures, and diagnoses for billing and reimbursement purposes. Medical codes, such as ICD and CPT codes, ensure consistency and accuracy in healthcare documentation.

(510) (B) ICD-10-CM.

The International Classification of Diseases (ICD) is a commonly used classification system in the United States. The most recent revision (ICD-11) became available globally as of January 01, 2022. However, the United States employs the ICD-10-CM (for diagnostic codes) and ICD-10-PCS (for procedure codes in inpatient settings).

(511) (B) To standardize procedure codes for outpatient settings.

The American Medical Association (AMA) publishes a classification system called Current Procedural Terminology (CPT). Its objective is to create uniform procedure codes for outpatient settings. Specific medical procedures, services, and treatments provided by doctors or other healthcare professionals in outpatient settings are denoted by five-digit CPT codes.

(512) (B) Superbill.

A superbill is a detailed itemized bill that lists all the services and procedures performed during a patient visit. It includes codes and descriptions for the procedures, diagnoses, and any other relevant information needed for billing purposes. This document is used by healthcare providers to submit claims to insurance companies for reimbursement.

(513) (A) Level I, Level II, Level III.

Medicare beneficiaries' medical services are reported using the three tiers of HCPCS codes. Level I codes (repeats CPT codes), level II codes (eighteen sections with new codes, not listed in CPT), and level III codes (local codes used only by insurance companies in their specific region).

(514) (B) To ensure patient confidentiality and privacy.

Data entry is an integral part of the recording, coding, and billing processes that MAs perform. The management of patient and insurance data demands accuracy and the adequate use of standardized terminology (diagnostic and procedural codes), as well as agility during the data entry process to avoid unnecessarily slowing down the delivery of medical care. Data management in medical offices and other health care settings also implies the use of private and confidential patient information. As a result, MAs must be compliant with HIPAA regulations when handling private information.

(515) (B) To ensure patient safety.

To guarantee patient safety, certain medical equipment needs to be inspected more frequently than others. Frequent inspections assist in locating any possible flaws, problems, or malfunctions with the apparatus that can jeopardize patient safety or treatment. Healthcare facilities can proactively address issues, carry out required maintenance or repairs, and make sure the equipment is operating as intended by regularly inspecting the facility.

(516) (C) Monitoring carbohydrate intake.

For diabetic patients, monitoring carbohydrate intake is necessary to manage blood sugar levels. Carbohydrates have the most significant impact on blood glucose, so balancing carbohydrate consumption with medication, physical activity, and blood sugar monitoring helps to maintain target blood glucose levels.

(517) (B) Treat everyone with attention and respect.

MAs may handle various types of calls as part of their work activities. Calls from patients (for scheduling new and recurring patients, or answering questions from patients) are very common, but MAs will also interact with laboratories, insurance companies, other medical offices, and salespeople. Regardless of who is calling, everyone should be treated with attention and respect.

(518) (B) Greet the caller and introduce themselves.

When handling calls, remember to greet the person calling and introduce yourself. The scheduling process requires you to ask for certain information. For new patients, do not forget to ask about insurance details and the name of the referring physician when applicable. For recurring patients, ask for the patient's name, reason for visiting, and if any insurance information has changed.

(519) (C) To enhance patient development for the future.

Coaching is developmental and aims toward the future. It can be used to enhance the patient's development through active listening and guidance. This approach is mainly useful to help the patient understand their medical condition and treatment options, which increases patient compliance and capacity for self-care. It also allows the patient to participate meaningfully in their care.

(520) (A) To reflect on past actions.

MAs can use feedback and coaching as communication tools to the benefit of patients in various ways. Feedback is mainly retrospective and can be used to reflect on past actions or events. For example, it can be used to highlight positive behaviors and encourage the patient. Feedback can also be constructive, which helps the patient to identify a problem and improve.

(521) (C) For non-urgent communication.

Emails are frequently used for correspondence that is not urgent. They provide a practical and effective means for individuals or groups to communicate, share documents, and exchange information. Emails, in contrast to urgent matters that demand immediate attention, allow for asynchronous communication in which the recipient can reply whenever it is most convenient for them.

(522) (A) A concise description of the email contents.

An email with proper structure should have a subject line that sums up what is inside in clear and concise terms. The email's subject line acts as a synopsis or sneak peek at its contents, giving the recipient a quick overview of the message's goal or subject. The recipient can more efficiently prioritize and arrange their emails when the subject line is clear and succinct.

(523) (D) Start with a salutation, end with a closing and contact information.

An email should always begin with a salutation, such as "Dear...," to greet the recipient and uphold proper email etiquette. This sets a tone of civility and professionalism. After a closing like "Best regards," the sender's name and contact details should be included in the email. Giving the sender's contact information makes it simple for the recipient to reply or get in touch if necessary. Appropriate salutations and closings at the beginning and end of an email contribute to a courteous and professional communication tone.

(524) (A) To assess the quality of care provided.

Patient satisfaction surveys are used to assess the quality of care provided in a healthcare facility. These surveys can be varied, and they can be created by the facility or commissioned to a third party.

(525) (B) Hospital Consumer Assessment of Healthcare Providers and Systems Survey (HCAHPS).

Most hospitals use the Hospital Consumer Assessment of Healthcare Providers and Systems Survey (HCAHPS), which was created by the CMS alongside the AHRQ to facilitate the evaluation and comparison of care quality between hospitals. The HCAHPS is a standardized survey with twenty-seven questions.

(526) (A) Assessment, Communication, Tactics.

The Dix and Page model is a de-escalation model based on three components: assessment, communication, and tactics (ACT). Assessment refers to the recognition of aggressive behavior. Communication refers to verbal and nonverbal communication strategies used during de-escalation (therapeutic communication, active listening, avoiding physical contact, avoiding medical terminology, and being sincere). Finally, tactics refer to context-specific actions which are used to invalidate the patient's need for aggression.

(527) (B) Providing solutions and gaining the patient's trust.

Some strategies to de-escalate aggressive behavior may include: early recognition of aggression, active listening, non-threatening body language, gain the trust of the patient by answering to their problem and acknowledging their feelings, provide solutions and practice de-escalation with all the staff.

(528) (A) Concern-Uncomfortable-Safety Issue.

"Concern-Uncomfortable-Safety Issue" is the acronym for the CUS process, which is used in healthcare settings to escalate troublesome circumstances. The Agency for Healthcare Research and Quality (AHRQ) created this technique to motivate medical personnel to voice their concerns and elevate them as needed.

(529) (C) If the concern remains unresolved.

The AHRQ developed the CUS ("Concern-Uncomfortable-Safety Issue") method to encourage health care professionals to speak up and escalate when necessary by stating they are concerned and why. If unresolved, the health care professional states "I am uncomfortable" and if the concern remains, the health care professional declares that there is a safety issue in place. At this point, if the issue persists unresolved, the health care professional may escalate the concern to a defined contact in the office or department.

(530) (A) To document and report unwanted or unexpected events.

Any unwanted or unexpected event, incidental or accidental, that may potentially result in harm to the staff, patients, or visitors must be documented and reported to a superior and/or someone in charge of risk management in the facility. The tool utilized for reporting these issues is an Unusual Occurrence Report (also known as an Incident Report or Event Report).

(531) (B) It results in jealousy among coworkers.

A professional presence is necessary to establish a positive relationship with patients and colleagues. It inspires and transmits respect, integrity, responsibility, and confidence.

(532) (C) Acting in self-interest.

Being a professional means having traits like respect, accountability, and honesty. Self-serving behavior is contrary to these values and is not regarded as professional presence.

(533) (D) It will attract more clients than your colleagues.

Patients prefer when health care providers dress formally or wear scrubs. Hygiene and grooming are also very important. Although projecting a professional image is important, gaining clients over colleagues is not the main goal of appearance.

(534) (C) Nonfeasance.

The act of not carrying out a required act or duty is referred to as nonfeasance. In this case, a health care worker's failure to contact a doctor in an emergency is considered nonfeasance because the provider did not carry out their duty to take the required action.

(535) (B) Malfeasance.

Malfeasance is the act of committing an unlawful crime. Since it is outside of their scope of practice, it is illegal for a medical assistant to provide drugs in this situation. Licensed medical practitioners, such as physicians or nurse practitioners, are usually the only ones authorized to prescribe drugs.

(536) (A) Misfeasance.

Misfeasance is the improper performance of a lawful act. In this instance, misfeasance is defined as the wrong or inappropriate performance of a legal action, such as when a non-sterile instrument is used during a sterile treatment. The act may be lawful in and of itself, but the way it was carried out was improper and could endanger the patient.

(537) (D) Women.

The reporting of mistreatment and abuse is a legal duty for workers (like health care providers) who are frequently in contact with vulnerable populations. The exact populations protected may vary from state to state, but it generally includes children, people with disabilities, and the elderly. In the particular case of health care professionals, reporting laws also include certain infectious diseases. The National Notifiable Conditions is published annually by the CDC.

(538) (A) Whenever the healthcare professional wishes to.

The legal guardian or parents of a minor are generally allowed access to the information of the minor, except in situations in which the minor is able to consent, care is authorized by a court, or whenever the minor, provider, and parents agree that the minor and the provider can have a confidential relationship.

(539) (D) Being young.

Medical malpractice stems from negligence or substandard care due to a lack of knowledge or experience of a healthcare professional during a professional act that results in harm to the patient. To avoid malpractice claims, it is important to follow professional guidelines and learn to communicate effectively with patients.

(540) (A) Shredding.

When destroying paper records, they should be rendered forever unintelligible. Shredding is a popular technique for accomplishing this because it breaks the paper into tiny, unreadable fragments.

Test 4

(541) Healthcare professionals who assist physicians in outpatient and inpatient settings are known as:

(A) Physician associates.

(B) Medical assistants.

(C) Physician helpers.

(D) Healthcare aides.

(542) Which of the following tasks might medical assistants (MAs) be involved in?

(A) Arrange hospital admissions.

(B) Perform complex surgical procedures.

(C) Analyze complex diagnostic test results.

(D) Conduct research studies.

(543) Which healthcare professional practices medicine and includes medical doctors (M.D.) and doctors of osteopathic medicine (D.O.)?

(A) Physician.

(B) Nurse Practitioner (NP).

(C) Physician Assistant (PA).

(D) Licensed Practical Nurse (LPN).

(544) Which health care professional provides patient care under the supervision of a physician and may prescribe medication?

(A) Physician.

(B) Nurse Practitioner (NP).

(C) Physician Assistant (PA).

(D) Registered Nurse (RN).

(545) What is the role of a Physician Assistant (PA) in the healthcare system?

(A) Prescribe medication independently.

(B) Work as a primary care provider.

(C) Provide patient care under physician supervision.

(D) Perform specialized surgeries.

(546) Which healthcare professional must complete a nursing program and a state board examination to practice?

(A) Physician.

(B) Nurse Practitioner (NP).

(C) Physician Assistant (PA).

(D) Registered Nurse (RN).

(547) What is a key characteristic of the ketogenic (keto) diet?

(A) High carbohydrate, low fat.

(B) High protein, high carbohydrate.

(C) Low carbohydrate, high fat.

(D) Low protein, high carbohydrate.

(548) How often must the CCMA credential be recertified for medical assistants?

(A) Every year.

(B) Every two years.

(C) Every five years.

(D) Every ten years.

(549) Which organization awards the CCMA certification for medical assistants?

(A) National Healthcareer Association.

(B) Certifying Board of the American Association of Medical Assistants.

(C) American Medical Technologists.

(D) National Center for Competency Testing.

(550) Which type of care is mainly concerned with end-of-life care?

(A) Outpatient care.

(B) Hospice care.

(C) Home health care.

(D) Community health clinics.

(551) What is the main characteristic of concierge medicine?

(A) Affordable health care services for everyone.

(B) 24/7 access to primary care.

(C) Monthly or annual fee for access to a physician.

(D) Customizable mobile health unit.

(552) What is a managed care organization's primary goal?

(A) Provide lower costs without compromising quality.

(B) Provide specialized care for rare medical conditions.

(C) Provide free healthcare services to the community.

(D) Provide 24/7 access to primary care.

(553) What is the main focus of primary care?

(A) Provide specialized care for complex conditions.

(B) Provide supplementary services.

(C) Be the first line of defense in the healthcare system.

(D) Conduct genetic testing.

(554) What does the abbreviation "BID" or "bid" stand for?

(A) Two times a day.

(B) Before meals.

(C) Body mass index.

(D) Blood pressure.

(555) When a prescription is written as "OD," what does it indicate?

(A) Once a day.

(B) Outpatient.

(C) Operating room.

(D) Over the counter.

(556) What is the meaning of the abbreviation "postop" in healthcare terminology?

(A) Preoperative.

(B) Papanicolaou smear.

(C) Peripheral nervous system.

(D) Postoperative.

(557) Which abbreviation represents "suppository?"

(A) SQ, SubQ.

(B) Supp., suppos.

(C) Sx.

(D) Tx.

(558) Which suffix refers to a tumor in medical terminology?

(A) –auto.

(B) –oma.

(C) –iasis.

(D) –rrhea.

(559) What does the prefix "dys-" signify in medical terms?

(A) Painful, difficult, bad.

(B) Condition.

(C) Development.

(D) Inflammation.

(560) Which suffix refers to a surgical aperture?

(A) –penia.

(B) –stasis.

(C) –stomy.

(D) –tomy.

(561) What does the term “pruritus” refer to?
(A) Itching, scratchy.
(B) Weakness, lack of strength.
(C) Puffiness, swelling.
(D) High sugar, too much sugar, diabetes.

(562) What does the term “vertigo” refer to in the field of medicine?
(A) Earache, pain in the ear.
(B) Shortness of breath, difficulty breathing.
(C) Cold, stuffy nose, runny nose.
(D) Dizziness, lightheadedness.

(563) What is the description of “emesis” in simpler terms?
(A) Cold, stuffy nose, runny nose.
(B) Loose or watery poo.
(C) Throwing up, vomiting.
(D) Earache, pain in the ear.

(564) Which term refers to the frontal part of the body?
(A) Anterior/ventral.
(B) Posterior/dorsal.
(C) Deep.
(D) Superficial.

(565) What does the term “inferior/caudal” mean in anatomical terms?
(A) Toward the head, away from the feet.
(B) Toward the feet, away from the head.
(C) Toward the midline of the body.
(D) Away from the midline of the body.

(566) Which category of drugs is mainly used to diagnose a condition?

(A) Therapeutic.

(B) Diagnostic.

(C) Palliative.

(D) Preventive.

(567) Which drug category is commonly used to treat constipation?

(A) Hormones.

(B) Hypnotics.

(C) Laxatives.

(D) Muscle relaxants.

(568) What is the primary function of immunosuppressive drugs?

(A) To induce and prolong sleep.

(B) To increase immune response.

(C) To reduce blood glucose levels.

(D) To decrease immune response.

(569) What are thrombolytic drugs mainly used for?

(A) To induce and prolong sleep.

(B) To treat constipation.

(C) To reduce blood glucose levels.

(D) To dissolve clots.

(570) What is the function of the OTC medication guaifenesin?

(A) Analgesic.

(B) Antipyretic.

(C) Cough medicine.

(D) Sleep aid.

(571) What is the primary characteristic of the parenteral route of administration?

(A) The drug dissolves under the tongue.

(B) The drug is placed in the mouth and not swallowed.

(C) It bypasses the gastrointestinal tract.

(D) The drug is instilled into the affected ear.

(572) What is the purpose of the otic route of administration?

(A) To bypass the gastrointestinal tract.

(B) To instill the drug into the affected ear.

(C) To dissolve the drug under the tongue.

(D) To apply the drug onto the skin.

(573) In which route of administration is the drug administered into a bone?

(A) Nasal route.

(B) Intraarterial route.

(C) Intraosseous route.

(D) Urethral route.

(574) Individuals with celiac disease should avoid all of the following in their diet except:

(A) Gluten.

(B) Wheat.

(C) Barley.

(D) Saturated fat.

(575) What dietary component should individuals with inflammatory bowel disease increase in their diet?

(A) Dietary fiber.

(B) Gluten.

(C) FODMAPs.

(D) Saturated fats.

(576) What disorder is characterized by delayed responses to a traumatic situation, with symptoms like vivid flashbacks, intense fear, and difficulty concentrating?

(A) Generalized anxiety.

(B) Panic attacks.

(C) Depression.

(D) PTSD.

(577) Which mental health condition is characterized by persistent excessive worry that is difficult to control, along with symptoms such as restlessness, irritability, and muscle tension?

(A) PTSD.

(B) ADHD.

(C) Autism spectrum disorder.

(D) Generalized anxiety.

(578) What disorder involves recurrent and unpredictable attacks of severe anxiety, with symptoms like chest pain, feeling of suffocation, and fear of losing control or dying?

(A) Generalized anxiety.

(B) Panic attacks.

(C) Depression.

(D) ADHD.

(579) What are the building blocks of proteins?

(A) Monosaccharides.

(B) Fatty acids.

(C) Amino acids.

(D) Electrolytes.

(580) Which type of vitamin is water-soluble?

(A) Vitamin A.

(B) Vitamin D.

(C) Vitamin E.

(D) Vitamin C.

(581) What is the main function of mitochondria?

(A) Provide energy in the form of ATP.

(B) Synthesize proteins.

(C) Store newly synthesized proteins.

(D) Digest molecules.

(582) Which organelle is a cylindrical structure of microtubules that is required during cell division?

(A) Ribosomes.

(B) Mitochondria.

(C) Endoplasmic reticulum.

(D) Centriole.

(583) What is the main function of lysosomes?

(A) Protein synthesis.

(B) Energy production.

(C) Digestion of molecules.

(D) Cell division.

(584) Which tissue type protects and regulates the flow of substances in the body?

(A) Epithelial.

(B) Connective.

(C) Muscle.

(D) Nervous.

(585) Which system is responsible for the exchange of oxygen and carbon dioxide?

(A) Respiratory.

(B) Musculoskeletal.

(C) Nervous.

(D) Endocrine.

(586) What is the main function of the urinary system?

(A) Exchange of oxygen and carbon dioxide.

(B) Motion and posture.

(C) Filtration of blood and waste removal.

(D) Regulation of other body systems.

(587) Which condition is characterized by acute inflammation of the gallbladder?

(A) Acute cholecystitis.

(B) Acute pancreatitis.

(C) Allergic rhinitis.

(D) Acute appendicitis.

(588) What clinical finding is associated with acute appendicitis?

(A) Mild abdominal pain worsened by eating fatty foods.

(B) Fever, pain in the lower right flank, nausea and vomiting.

(C) Sneezing and rhinorrhea.

(D) Progressive cognitive decline.

(589) What is the characteristic clinical finding of cellulitis?

(A) Chest pain and palpitations.

(B) Vaginal discharge with a strong odor.

(C) Redness, pain, and inflammation of the skin.

(D) Cough, sneezing, and rhinorrhea.

(590) Febrile seizures are commonly seen in which age group?

(A) Adults.

(B) Elderly individuals.

(C) Children.

(D) Individuals with epilepsy.

(591) Which blood test investigates various substances in the blood, such as glucose, electrolytes, proteins, and bilirubin?

(A) Complete blood count (CBC).

(B) Blood chemistry.

(C) Urinalysis.

(D) Stool analysis.

(592) What does prevalence measure in epidemiology?

(A) Number of new-onset cases.

(B) Number of acute conditions.

(C) Number of cases during a period of time.

(D) Number of risk factors.

(593) Which term describes an increase in the incidence of a particular infectious disease within a specific facility or institution?

(A) Outbreak.

(B) Epidemic.

(C) Pandemic.

(D) Incidence.

(594) What is the purpose of chemotherapy?

(A) To employ medication to treat or manage a medical condition.

(B) To destroy fast-growing cells, including cancer cells.

(C) To use X-rays or radiation to treat cancer.

(D) To modulate the body's immune response.

(595) Which of the following parameters cannot be used as a patient identifier?

(A) Street address.

(B) Telephone number.

(C) Room number.

(D) Social security number.

(596) All of the following criteria are used for lung cancer screening except:

(A) History of 30 pack-years (at least).

(B) Age between 55 and 74 years.

(C) Recent smoking cessation within the last 15 years.

(D) Female sex.

(597) What medical condition is neonatal thyroid-stimulating hormone (TSH) testing used to screen?

(A) Congenital hypothyroidism.

(B) Hypopituitarism.

(C) Prolactinoma.

(D) Heart disease.

(598) Which of the following is not recommended before measuring vital signs in a patient who has engaged in physical activity?

(A) Ask the patient to relax.

(B) Ask the patient to sit down for a few minutes.

(C) Allow time for the patient's vital signs to return to baseline levels.

(D) Allow the patient to have a cup of coffee.

(599) Blood pressure is normally measured with what?

(A) Sphygmomanometer and stethoscope.

(B) Stethoscope only.

(C) Thermometer.

(D) Penlight.

(600) All of the following clinical findings are suggestive of hypotension except which?

(A) Dizziness.

(B) Vertigo.

(C) Lightheadedness.

(D) High blood pressure.

(601) Which one of the following thermometers should be avoided if the patient complains of pain or has bilateral otitis externa?

(A) Tympanic thermometer.

(B) Digital thermometer.

(C) Temporal artery scanner.

(D) Oral thermometer.

(602) Which one of the following thermometers should be avoided if the patient has recently consumed cold or hot foods or fluids, smoked, or exercised?

(A) Tympanic thermometer.

(B) Rectal thermometer.

(C) Temporal artery scanner.

(D) Oral digital thermometer.

(603) Which of the following is not a characteristic used to describe a pulse?

(A) Rate.

(B) Rhythm.

(C) Amplitude.

(D) Depth.

(604) What is the medical term for an abnormally fast heart rate?

(A) Tachycardia.

(B) Bradycardia.

(C) Feeble pulse.

(D) Hypothermia.

(605) What is the medical term for an abnormally slow respiratory rate?

(A) Tachypnea.

(B) Bradypnea.

(C) Dyspnea.

(D) Hypopnea.

(606) All of the following are characteristics used to describe normal breathing except which?

(A) Amplitude.

(B) Rhythm.

(C) Depth.

(D) Rate.

(607) What is the range of numbers in the numerical scale used to measure pain?

(A) 0 to 1.

(B) 0 to 10.

(C) 0 to 20.

(D) 0 to 50.

(608) Which of the following is not part of the menstrual phase?

(A) Discharge of endometrial tissue.

(B) Preparation for fecundation and pregnancy.

(C) Maturation of ovarian follicles.

(D) Preparation for lactation.

(609) How long does a normal menstruation in humans last?

(A) Up to 7 days.

(B) Up to 14 days.

(C) Up to 21 days.

(D) Up to 28 days.

(610) What is the approximate frequency of a normal menstrual cycle?

(A) Every 14 days.

(B) Every 28 days.

(C) Every 2 months.

(D) Every 3 months.

(611) What should a patient do if they experience severe pain, fever, or rectal bleeding after a colonoscopy?

(A) Contact their healthcare provider immediately.

(B) Drink a lot of water.

(C) Take metronidazole.

(D) Nothing, as it is normally expected after a colonoscopy.

(612) What is rubella commonly known as?

(A) Measles.

(B) Chickenpox.

(C) German measles.

(D) Mumps.

(613) How many doses of the varicella vaccine are recommended for adults without evidence of immunity?

(A) 1 dose.

(B) 2 doses.

(C) 3 doses.

(D) 4 doses.

(614) What is the recommended age group for the human papillomavirus (HPV) vaccine series?

(A) Up to 8 years old.

(B) Up to 13 years old.

(C) Up to 26 years old.

(D) Up to 50 years old.

(615) What is a life-threatening allergic shock that can occur in response to allergens?

(A) Hay fever.

(B) Allergic asthma.

(C) Anaphylaxis.

(D) Contact allergy.

(616) Which allergy test is performed when the reaction is expected to occur after a couple of days?

(A) Skin prick test (or scratch test).

(B) Patch test.

(C) Intradermal allergy test.

(D) Provocation test.

(617) Which allergy test involves injecting individual allergens through intradermal injection?

(A) Skin prick test (or scratch test).

(B) Patch test.

(C) Intradermal allergy test.

(D) Provocation test.

(618) Which allergy test involves exposing the patient's nose to potential allergens to evaluate the response?

(A) Skin prick test (or scratch test).

(B) Patch test.

(C) Intradermal allergy test.

(D) Provocation test.

(619) What is the recommended timing for administering intramuscular epinephrine in the treatment of anaphylaxis?

(A) Within the first 20 minutes.

(B) Within the first 30 minutes.

(C) Within the first 45 minutes.

(D) Within the first 60 minutes.

(620) Which of the following medications generally requires refrigeration for storage?

(A) Insulin.

(B) Diphenhydramine.

(C) Ketorolac.

(D) Methotrexate.

(621) In what format are expiration dates usually printed on medication labels?

(A) DD/MM.

(B) MM/YY.

(C) YYYY/MM.

(D) MM/DD.

(622) What is the purpose of pinching the skin before inserting a subcutaneous injection?

(A) To create an accessible skinfold.

(B) To reduce pain during the injection.

(C) To minimize the risk of infection.

(D) To ensure accurate dosage delivery.

(623) All of the following are recommended actions for fractures except:

(A) Immobilize the affected bone.

(B) Apply ice.

(C) Transfer the patient for emergency care.

(D) Apply warm compresses.

(624) Which surgical intervention is commonly performed to remove hemorrhoids?

(A) Appendectomy.

(B) Debridement.

(C) Hysterectomy.

(D) Hemorrhoidectomy.

(625) Which of the following is not a common indication to perform hysterectomy?

(A) Excessively heavy periods.

(B) Painful periods.

(C) Pregnancy.

(D) Cancer affecting the uterus.

(626) Which of the following is an example of a common emergency that requires immediate examination or treatment in the emergency department?

(A) Fever.

(B) Choking.

(C) Sprains.

(D) Contusions.

(627) Which of the following is considered a common urgency?

(A) Cough.

(B) Stroke.

(C) Seizure.

(D) Shock.

(628) What is the normal timeframe for examination or treatment of an emergency?

(A) Immediate examination and treatment in the emergency department.

(B) Within 24 hours in an outpatient setting.

(C) Within a week in an outpatient setting.

(D) Within minutes in an outpatient setting.

(629) What is a key characteristic of high-quality CPR?

(A) Slow compressions to avoid chest recoil.

(B) Compressions of one inch or three centimeters.

(C) Fast compressions that push the chest down and allow complete recoil.

(D) Tilt the chin down to open the airway.

(630) How often should a rescuer change during CPR in basic life support if possible?

(A) Every 30 seconds.

(B) Every minute.

(C) Every two minutes.

(D) Every five minutes.

(631) What is the correct definition of a microorganism?

(A) A macroscopic living being visible to the naked human eye.

(B) Any living being that is not visible to the naked human eye.

(C) A single-cell organism such as a bacterium or protozoan.

(D) A multicellular organism such as a fungus or algae.

(632) Which of the following is not a benefit provided by the normal flora of the body?

(A) Production of beneficial substances.

(B) Protection against potentially pathogenic microorganisms.

(C) Pathogenesis of disease.

(D) Digestion of various substances.

(633) What is the term used to describe microorganisms that cause diseases?

(A) Nonpathogens.

(B) Symbionts.

(C) Opportunistic infections.

(D) Pathogens.

(634) What disease is caused by the protozoan Plasmodium?

(A) Giardiasis.

(B) Malaria.

(C) Amoebiasis.

(D) Trichomoniasis.

(635) Which protozoan is associated with the cause of amoebiasis?

(A) Entamoeba duodenalis.

(B) Entamoeba plasmodium.

(C) Entamoeba histolytica.

(D) Entamoeba vaginalis.

(636) What disease is caused by the varicella virus?

(A) Influenza.

(B) Cold sores.

(C) Measles.

(D) Chickenpox.

(637) Which bacterium is responsible for causing cholera?

(A) Borrelia burgdorferi.

(B) Bacillus anthracis.

(C) Vibrio cholerae.

(D) Pseudomonas aeruginosa.

(638) Which element of the chain of infection represents the environment where microorganisms can multiply?

(A) Environment.

(B) Source or reservoir.

(C) Portal of exit.

(D) Modes of transport.

(639) Which element of the chain of infection represents the person at risk of becoming infected?

(A) Susceptible host.

(B) Source or reservoir.

(C) Portal of exit.

(D) Modes of transport.

(640) Which pH range do alkaliphilic bacteria prefer for growth?

(A) Below 5.5.

(B) Above 8.5.

(C) Between 5 and 8.

(D) Above 11.

(641) What should be done with used needles?

(A) Dispose of them in sharps containers.

(B) Recycle them.

(C) Sterilize them for reuse.

(D) Recap and use them again.

(642) When is surgical asepsis needed?

(A) During non-invasive procedures.

(B) During medical research.

(C) During outbreaks, epidemics, and pandemics.

(D) During invasive procedures like surgeries.

(643) Which of the following are considered vulnerable populations during outbreaks, epidemics, and pandemics?

(A) Federal agents.

(B) Pregnant women.

(C) Adults.

(D) Construction workers.

(644) What is a common use of hydrogen peroxide in a medical setting?

(A) Treating chronic diseases.

(B) Disinfecting wounds.

(C) Treating dehydration.

(D) Diagnosing infections.

(645) What should medical assistants do when a specimen must be collected by the patient?

(A) Provide clear instructions.

(B) Collect the specimens themselves.

(C) Use specialized collection techniques.

(D) Avoid providing any guidance.

(646) Why is the quality of the specimen important for accurate test results?

(A) It determines the type of collection technique.

(B) It impacts the potential accuracy of the results.

(C) It affects the patient's ability to collect the sample.

(D) It does not affect the provisional diagnosis.

(647) All of the following specimens are commonly collected by medical assistants except:

(A) Blood.

(B) Urine.

(C) Renal biopsy.

(D) Swabs.

(648) Why is a clean-catch midstream urine specimen usually collected?

(A) To assess proteins like Bence Jones proteins.

(B) To diagnose urinary tract infections.

(C) To measure clearance rates with creatinine levels.

(D) To assess the presence of pregnancy hormones.

(649) Which urine collection technique is commonly used for most clinical purposes and requires at least 12 mL of urine?

(A) Random specimen.

(B) Early morning specimen.

(C) Clean-catch midstream specimen.

(D) Catheterization.

(650) When is an early-morning or first-morning urine specimen collected?

(A) Early in the morning after the patient wakes up.

(B) During the day after the patient has eaten.

(C) In the evening before going to bed.

(D) After physical activity or exercise.

(651) When is a sputum specimen usually collected?

(A) After a meal.

(B) Early in the morning.

(C) Before going to bed.

(D) During physical activity.

(652) All of the following should be performed by a patient before collecting a sputum specimen except which action?

(A) Perform mouth washing.

(B) Take cough medication.

(C) Perform chest clearance exercises.

(D) Perform hand washing.

(653) What is the correct way for a patient to cough when collecting a sputum specimen?

(A) Into a clean container.

(B) On the floor.

(C) Into a tissue.

(D) Into their hand.

(654) In the case of tuberculosis assessment, how many sputum samples may be requested across three consecutive days?

(A) One.

(B) Two.

(C) Three.

(D) Six.

(655) What type of results do the positive control solution show in the quality control process of urine specimens?

(A) Abnormal results.

(B) Normal results.

(C) Inconclusive results.

(D) No results are shown.

(656) What is the normal range for white blood cells in urinalysis?

(A) 0 to 2 cells per high-power field.

(B) 0 to 5 cells per high-power field.

(C) 0 to 8 cells per high-power field.

(D) 0 to 10 cells per high-power field.

(657) Which parameter is used to assess the presence of bacteria in urinalysis?

(A) Blood.

(B) Glucose.

(C) Nitrite.

(D) Protein.

(658) Which parameter is used to assess the presence of liver dysfunction in urinalysis?

(A) Bilirubin.

(B) Ketones.

(C) Crystals.

(D) Casts.

(659) What does tidal volume measure in respiratory physiology?

(A) The total lung capacity.

(B) The volume of air inhaled and exhaled during a normal breath.

(C) The maximum amount of air exhaled after a deep breath.

(D) The amount of air remaining in the lungs after exhalation.

(660) What is the forced expiratory volume in 1 second (FEV1) for a 40-year-old male patient?

(A) 2.8 L.

(B) 4.0 L.

(C) 3.4 L.

(D) 5.0 L.

(661) Which type of blood cells can be divided into granulocytes and agranulocytes?

(A) Red blood cells.

(B) White blood cells.

(C) Platelets.

(D) Reticulocytes.

(662) Hepatitis C virus (HCV) can transmitted through all of the following ways except:

(A) Blood transfusions.

(B) Sharing needles/syringes.

(C) Inhalation of respiratory droplets.

(D) Contact with infected body fluid.

(663) What is the normal reference range for the mean corpuscular hemoglobin concentration (MCHC)?

(A) 33-37 g/dL.

(B) 40-45 g/dL.

(C) 25-30 g/dL.

(D) 50-55 g/dL.

(664) What is the normal reference range for the partial thromboplastin time (PTT)?

(A) 10-20 seconds.

(B) 25-40 seconds.

(C) 45-60 seconds.

(D) 5-10 seconds.

(665) What is the normal reference range for the red blood cell count (RBC) in men?

(A) 2.0-3.5 million cells/mm^3.

(B) 3.0-4.5 million cells/mm^3.

(C) 6.0-7.5 million cells/mm^3.

(D) 4.5-5.9 million cells/mm^3.

(666) Which of the following are normal reference ranges for reticulocyte levels?

(A) 0.5%-1.5%.

(B) 2%-4%.

(C) 10%-15%.

(D) 20%-25%.

(667) Which blood gas parameter is normally higher in venous blood compared to arterial blood?

(A) Partial pressure of carbon dioxide (PCO_2).

(B) Partial pressure of oxygen (Po_2).

(C) Oxygen saturation (SaO_2).

(D) Serum bicarbonate (HCO_3).

(668) What is the normal range for arterial pH?

(A) 7.35-7.45.

(B) 7.31-7.41.

(C) 1.35-3.45.

(D) 4.35-6.45.

(669) What machine is used to separate the plasma from the cells of whole blood?

(A) Separator.

(B) Centrifuge.

(C) Sterilizer.

(D) Refrigerator.

(670) What is the normal range for C-reactive protein (CRP)?

(A) 0.08-3.1 mg/L.

(B) 0.80-7.4 mg/L.

(C) 0.11-13.8 mg/L.

(D) 0.08-0.1mg/L.

(671) What is the main purpose of lead wires in EKG testing?

(A) To carry the recorded electrical activity to the electrocardiograph.

(B) To measure voltage.

(C) To assess arrhythmias.

(D) To diagnose myocardial infarction.

(672) What is represented on the x-axis of electrocardiograph paper?

(A) Voltage.

(B) Current.

(C) Time.

(D) Electrode number.

(673) What does the isoelectric line represent in an EKG?

(A) Depolarization of the ventricles.

(B) Repolarization of the atria.

(C) Relaxation of the ventricles.

(D) Baseline of the EKG.

(674) When would a faster speed setting on an EKG machine, such as 50 mm per second, be beneficial?

(A) To inspect slower heart rates.

(B) To inspect waves that are far apart.

(C) To inspect faster heart rates.

(D) To inspect waves that are spaced out.

(675) What is the standard sensitivity setting for an EKG machine according to international guidelines?

(A) 1 mV = 10 mm.

(B) 1 mV = 20 mm.

(C) 1 mV = 5 mm.

(D) 1 mV = 15 mm.

(676) How is the sensitivity of an EKG machine altered to double standard?

(A) 1 mV = 10 mm.

(B) 1 mV = 20 mm.

(C) 1 mV = 5 mm.

(D) 1 mV = 15 mm.

(677) Which arrhythmia is characterized by an irregular electrical discharge in the atria due to abnormal impulse formation in ectopic foci?

(A) Sinus arrhythmias.

(B) Atrial arrhythmias.

(C) Ventricular arrhythmias.

(D) Bradycardia.

(678) What is the defining feature of atrial fibrillation on an EKG?

(A) Regular P waves.

(B) Absence of P waves.

(C) Wide QRS complexes.

(D) Bradycardia.

(679) What is the correct placement for the precordial electrode V1?

(A) 2nd intercostal space (right parasternal line).

(B) 4th intercostal space (right parasternal line).

(C) 5th intercostal space (left mid-clavicular line).

(D) 6th intercostal space (right mid-axillary line).

(680) What is the correct placement for the precordial electrode V5?

(A) 2nd intercostal space (right parasternal line).

(B) 4th intercostal space (right parasternal line).

(C) 5th intercostal space (left anterior axillary line).

(D) 6th intercostal space (right mid-axillary line).

(681) What is the primary purpose of performing an ECG (electrocardiogram) test?

(A) To measure blood pressure.

(B) To assess lung function.

(C) To evaluate the electrical activity of the heart.

(D) To determine blood glucose levels.

(682) What is the correct lead wire color coding for the right leg?

(A) White.

(B) Black.

(C) Green.

(D) Red.

(683) Why is it important for the patient to not apply any skin substances prior to an ECG test?

(A) To ensure proper electrode attachment.

(B) To reduce skin irritation.

(C) To make the test more comfortable for the patient.

(D) To speed up the test process.

(684) What is the primary reason to position the patient in the supine position during an ECG test?

(A) To make it easier for the patient to breathe.

(B) To prevent interference from other electrical devices.

(C) To ensure proper electrode placement.

(D) To measure the patient's vital signs accurately.

(685) What should be done before placing the electrodes for an ECG test?

(A) Clean and dry the skin.

(B) Apply lotion to moisturize the skin.

(C) Rub alcohol on the skin.

(D) Use a rough scrub to exfoliate the skin.

(686) Why is it important to consider risk factors in medical condition screenings?

(A) Risk factors have no impact on disease development.

(B) Risk factors can help identify individuals who may benefit from early detection.

(C) Risk factors are irrelevant in preventive medicine.

(D) Risk factors only apply to certain age groups.

(687) Which of the following is an example of universal screening in preventive medicine?

(A) Screen patients with a history of smoking for lung cancer.

(B) Screen only overweight or obese individuals for heart disease.

(C) Screen all individuals over 45 years old for diabetes and prediabetes.

(D) Avoid screenings for communicable diseases.

(688) What is the primary goal of preventive medicine?

(A) To increase the prevalence of disease.

(B) To encourage unhealthy lifestyle choices.

(C) To promote the spread of communicable diseases.

(D) To reduce the prevalence of disease and its consequences.

(689) What factors should be considered when assessing a patient's educational needs in patient education?

(A) Age, language, level of education, and cultural background.

(B) Medical history, insurance coverage, and occupation.

(C) Favorite color, favorite food, and favorite TV show.

(D) Blood type, shoe size, and hair color.

(690) Why is it important for pregnant patients or those planning to get pregnant to receive folic acid supplementation daily?

(A) To enhance nutrient delivery to the fetus.

(B) To prevent neural tube defects in the developing fetus.

(C) To decrease the risk of APH during pregnancy.

(D) To promote weight loss in pregnant individuals.

(691) What is the effect of milk consumption on the absorption of certain antibiotics like ciprofloxacin and tetracycline?

(A) Increases absorption.

(B) Decreases absorption.

(C) Has no impact on absorption.

(D) Enhances antibiotic effectiveness.

(692) What potential risks are associated with consuming alcohol while taking NSAIDs?

(A) Increased risk of thromboembolism.

(B) Increased risk of gastric bleeding and hepatic damage.

(C) Decreased effectiveness of the medication.

(D) Reduced absorption of the drug.

(693) What steps should the medical office take if a patient misses their specialist appointment or the letter from the specialist does not arrive?

(A) Ignore the missed appointment.

(B) Reschedule the appointment without notification.

(C) Discharge the patient from further care.

(D) Call the patient or specialist's office to inquire.

(694) How can the exchange of information between the primary care provider, specialist, and referral coordinator help in the referral process?

(A) Avoid delays and duplication of imaging or tests.

(B) Increase administrative burden.

(C) Decrease patient satisfaction.

(D) Delay treatment initiation.

(695) In cases where the electronic health record is unavailable, what alternative method can the referral coordinator use to track the referral process?

(A) Create a referral tracking spreadsheet.

(B) Assume that the referral was successful.

(C) Discontinue monitoring the referral.

(D) Request additional referrals from the primary care provider.

(696) In which of the following circumstances are specialty visits not usually scheduled?

(A) With a referral by a primary care provider.

(B) When the patient needs special care, diagnosis, treatment, or procedures.

(C) When the help of a specialist is required.

(D) Whenever the patient wishes to.

(697) Which of the following is not a purpose for a school physical exam?

(A) Identification of health conditions affecting growth and development.

(B) Review of immunization history.

(C) Setting up a surgical theater within the schoolyard.

(D) Physical exam.

(698) What is the purpose of a sports physical or preparticipation physical evaluation (PPE)?

(A) To determine if a patient can safely participate in a sport.

(B) To review the patient's immunization history.

(C) To identify risk factors for potential health conditions.

(D) To identify the overall physical wellness of an individual.

(699) All of the following are primary focuses of a follow-up visit except:

(A) Analyze diagnostic results.

(B) Thorough assessment of the patient's personal and family medical history.

(C) Check the patient's response to treatment.

(D) Develop a treatment plan.

(700) Which of the following vital signs and measurements is not normally recorded on the health record of a patient?

(A) Temperature.

(B) Respiratory rate.

(C) PCO2.

(D) Blood pressure.

(701) In what section of a medical visit summary would you find details about the patient's condition before discharge from care?

(A) Chief complaint.

(B) Progress notes.

(C) Condition at the time of treatment termination.

(D) Diagnosis.

(702) All of the following are benefits of electronic referral systems except:

(A) Enhanced productivity.

(B) Reduced costs.

(C) Facilitated safe sharing of patient information.

(D) Easy regional implementation.

(703) Which of the following government programs does not provide health care coverage in the United States?

(A) Medicare.

(B) FEMA.

(C) TRICARE.

(D) CHAMPVA.

(704) What does UCR stand for in the context of medical billing?

(A) Uncommon, customary, and reasonable.

(B) Usual, customary, and reasonable.

(C) Unilateral, customary, and reasonable.

(D) Usual, customary, and rational.

(705) The maximum charge that will be covered by the insurer is known as what?

(A) Disallowed charge.

(B) Limiting charge.

(C) UCR fee.

(D) Allowed charge.

(706) Which term refers to the agreement by the provider of the amount established by the insurer?

(A) Carrier.

(B) Acceptance of assignment.

(C) Medical billing cycle.

(D) UCR fee.

(707) Which auditing process is outsourced to a medical billing company?

(A) Internal auditing.

(B) External auditing.

(C) Regulatory compliance auditing.

(D) Coding accuracy auditing.

(708) What are the two types of auditing processes in the health care system?

(A) Internal and external auditing.

(B) Financial and compliance auditing.

(C) Data collection and analysis auditing.

(D) In-house and outsourced auditing.

(709) What is the purpose of remote monitoring in telehealth?

(A) To provide medical consultations.

(B) To educate healthcare students.

(C) To monitor patient health data remotely.

(D) To provide clinical and drug information.

(710) What is the impact of religious beliefs on the preferred therapies of patients?

(A) They have no influence.

(B) They can significantly affect choices.

(C) They only affect dietary preferences.

(D) They lead to rejection of all medical treatments.

(711) The advent of which one of the following technologies has reduced the issue of geographical distance for various medical services?

(A) Telehealth.

(B) Virtual reality.

(C) Artificial intelligence.

(D) Robotics.

(712) All of the following are ways in which active listening benefits the patient during a medical interaction except:

(A) It allows the patient to feel heard.

(B) It encourages the clarification of information.

(C) It takes the physician's feelings into consideration.

(D) It takes the patient's feelings into consideration.

(713) What is the difference between coaching and feedback?

(A) Coaching is retrospective, while feedback is future oriented.

(B) Coaching focuses on patient development, while feedback reflects on past actions.

(C) Coaching encourages active listening and guidance, while feedback identifies areas for improvement.

(D) Both coaching and feedback are retrospective.

(714) All of the following are ways in which coaching contributes to patient participation in their care except:

(A) It helps the patient understand their medical condition and treatment options.

(B) It results in guilt from past actions.

(C) It encourages active listening and guidance.

(D) It enhances the patient's development and self-care capacity.

(715) Which of the following medications is commonly used to treat nausea?

(A) Ibuprofen.

(B) Metformin.

(C) Ondansetron.

(D) Amoxicillin.

(716) What is the main purpose of using emails for communication?

(A) Urgent communication.

(B) Non-urgent communication.

(C) Every kind of communication.

(D) Personal communication.

(717) Which font styles are commonly used for professional-looking business letters?

(A) Times New Roman.

(B) Lexend.

(C) Comic Sans.

(D) Calibri.

(718) Which law facilitates access to health insurance for more people within the federal poverty level?

(A) Health Insurance Portability and Accountability Act (HIPAA).

(B) Affordable Care Act (ACA).

(C) Controlled Substances Act (CSA).

(D) Health Information Technology for Economic and Clinical Health (HITECH) Act.

(719) In which type of consent is consent granted without explicit communication but rather through the patient's actions or inaction?

(A) Informed consent.

(B) Implied consent.

(C) Expressed consent.

(D) Informal consent.

(720) What is the recommended action if the retention period required by an insurance provider differs from the state mandated period?

(A) Use the insurance provider's retention period.

(B) Use the state-mandated retention period.

(C) Use the shorter of the two periods.

(D) Use the longer of the two periods.

Test 4 Answers and Explanations

(541) (B) Medical assistants.

Medical assistants (MAs) are healthcare professionals who assist physicians in outpatient and inpatient settings. MAs are flexible members of the healthcare team and trained to work in various clinical and administrative roles. MAs frequently work in clinics and medical offices in addition to other outpatient settings.

(542) (A) Arrange hospital admissions.

Medical assistants are usually not qualified to do complicated surgical procedures. Laboratory technicians, pathologists, or other medical experts with training in diagnostic interpretation oversee the results of complex diagnostic tests. Scientists, researchers, or specialist research teams carry out research investigations rather than medical assistants. However, a medical assistant is likely to arrange hospital admissions.

(543) (A) Physician.

A physician is a professional who practices medicine. This includes medical doctors (M.D.) and doctors of osteopathic medicine (D.O.). Physicians may become specialists in anesthesiology, cardiology, dermatology, endocrinology, gastroenterology, general surgery, hematology, nephrology, neurology, obstetrics/gynecology, oncology, etc.

(544) (C) Physician Assistant (PA).

Physician assistants (PAs) are licensed healthcare providers who work closely with physicians to provide comprehensive care. They can order tests, prescribe medication, conduct physical examinations, and diagnose illnesses. Their role is to support physicians, provide high-quality care, and ensure efficient medical management.

(545) (C) Provide patient care under physician supervision.

The job of a physician assistant (PA) in the healthcare system is to provide patient care under physician supervision. Although they have a broad scope of practice and may perform many duties independently, PAs work under the guidance and supervision of a physician.

(546) (D) Registered Nurse (RN).

Registered nurses (RNs) are healthcare providers who have successfully finished a nursing program and passed a state board exam to become licensed. They provide direct patient care, which entails treating patients, monitoring their symptoms, and coordinating care with other medical team members. RNs are essential to the promotion and sustainment of patient health and well-being in a variety of settings such as clinics, hospitals, and long-term care homes.

(547) (C) Low carbohydrate, high fat.

The ketogenic (keto) diet is characterized by a low carbohydrate and high fat intake. This diet shifts the body's metabolism towards ketosis, where fat is used as the main source of energy instead of carbohydrates. This can cause significant weight loss and improved blood sugar control for some individuals.

(548) (B) Every two years.

Medical assistants who have completed their initial certification procedure are required to recertify every two years. This ensures that they maintain compliance with the norms and regulations established by the certifying organization. In order to complete this process, MAs usually need to pay the recertification cost, provide any appropriate papers, and complete the required number of continuing education hours. Medical assistants who are recertified are better able to uphold their competency and stay up to date with changing industry norms.

(549) (A) National Healthcareer Association.

The CCMA (Certified Clinical Medical Assistant) is awarded by the National Healthcareer Association. Other certifications are awarded by various organizations.

(550) (B) Hospice care.

Hospice care is a specialized form of treatment that focuses mostly on end-of-life care. Its purpose is to provide complete assistance to patients and their families as they approach the end of their lives. Hospice care aims to improve the quality of life for patients and their loved ones during this difficult time by providing comfort, pain treatment, emotional support, and spiritual care.

(551) (C) Monthly or annual fee for access to a physician.

Patients who use concierge medicine pay a doctor a monthly or yearly fee in exchange for improved access to primary care services. Concierge medicine patients benefit from individualized care, longer appointment hours, enhanced access to their doctor, and, occasionally, other services like wellness initiatives and preventive screenings.

(552) (A) Provide lower costs without compromising quality.

Managed care organizations (MCOs) are healthcare organizations that look for methods to lower costs for their members' treatment without sacrificing quality. To do this, they use a variety of tactics which include establishing cost-effective policies, negotiating reduced fees with healthcare providers, and placing a strong emphasis on preventive treatment. MCOs seek to provide members with high-quality, reasonably priced healthcare services and maintain an emphasis on cost management.

(553) (C) Be the first line of defense in the healthcare system.

Primary care is the first line of defense in the healthcare system. It involves general practitioners, family physicians, pediatricians, nurses, medical assistants, and other healthcare providers.

(554) (A) Two times a day.

The abbreviation "BID" or "bid" stands for two times a day. It is often used in healthcare to indicate the frequency of pharmaceutical dosing, in which the medication should be given twice daily at defined intervals.

(555) (A) Once a day.

When a prescription is written as “OD,” it signifies once a day. This acronym indicates that the recommended drug should be taken once daily and specifies the frequency of medication dose.

(556) (D) Postoperative.

In healthcare language, the abbreviation “postop” refers to postoperative. It signifies the period of time that follows a surgical treatment and comprises the recuperation and healing process after the surgery has been conducted.

(557) (B) Supp., suppos.

The acronym for suppository is “Supp., suppos.” It refers to a technique for administering medication that allows for either regional or systemic drug absorption. A solid dose form is put into the rectum, vagina, or urethra.

(558) (B) –oma.

In medical language, a tumor is denoted by the suffix “-oma.” Usually applied in relation to a tumor, this suffix is used to denote a mass or swelling. Examples are “lipoma,” which is a benign fatty tumor, and “carcinoma,” which is an aggressive tumor.

(559) (A) Painful, difficult, bad.

In medical terminology, the prefix “dys-” means painful, difficult, or bad. It is employed to characterize states of difficulty, abnormality, or impairment. For example, dysphagia denotes difficulty swallowing, and dyspnea denotes difficult or strained breathing.

(560) (C) –stomy.

A surgical opening is denoted by the suffix “-stomy.” When a surgical opening or aperture is created, it is indicated by this suffix. For example, a colostomy is an opening made in the colon, and a tracheostomy is a surgically created opening in the trachea.

(561) (A) Itching, scratchy.

Itchy and scratchy feelings are referred to as pruritus. It is frequently used to characterize the itching sensation on the skin that can be brought on by a number of factors such as allergies, dry skin, or specific medical disorders.

(562) (D) Dizziness, lightheadedness.

“Vertigo” is the medical name for dizziness and lightheadedness. It is a spinning or whirling sensation that is frequently connected to losing equilibrium. Meniere’s disease and benign paroxysmal positional vertigo (BPPV) are some of the various conditions that can produce vertigo.

(563) (C) Throwing up, vomiting.

In basic terms, “emesis” is simply throwing up or vomiting. It describes the process of passing stomach contents out of the mouth. A number of conditions can cause emesis, such as food poisoning, gastrointestinal diseases, or drug adverse effects.

(564) (A) Anterior/ventral.

The side of the body that faces forward or in front is referred to as anterior or ventral. It is the opposite of dorsal, or posterior, which describes the side of the body that faces the back or rear.

(565) (B) Toward the feet, away from the head.

Anatomically speaking, "inferior/caudal" indicates toward the feet, away from the head. It indicates a position or direction that is beneath or lower than another part. In particular, caudal refers to the direction toward the coccyx or tailbone. It is the antithesis of cranial or superior, which denotes a location above or higher than another structure.

(566) (B) Diagnostic.

Diagnostic drugs are mainly used to diagnose a condition. For example, tuberculin can be used in the diagnosis of tuberculosis.

(567) (C) Laxatives.

Laxative agents are used to treat constipation. Magnesium hydroxide (Phillips'® Milk of Magnesia), lactulose (Constilac®), polyethylene glycol (MiraLAX®), and mineral oil (Muri-Lube®) are commonly used.

(568) (D) To decrease immune response.

Immunosuppressive drugs are used to decrease a normal or pathological immune response of the body such as infections, prevention of organ rejection, inflammatory bowel disease, rheumatoid arthritis, and cancer. Examples include corticosteroids, tacrolimus (Astagraf XL®), and mycophenolate mofetil (CellCept®).

(569) (D) To dissolve clots.

Thrombolytics are also known as fibrinolytics. These agents are used to dissolve clots in patients with ischemic strokes, heart attacks, pulmonary embolisms, and other thromboembolic conditions. Alteplase (Activase®), reteplase (Retavase®), and streptokinase (Streptase®) are some examples of thrombolytics.

(570) (C) Cough medicine.

As an expectorant, guaifenesin is frequently used to thin and loosen mucus in the airways. It is frequently used to treat coughs brought on by respiratory ailments like bronchitis, the common cold, and other respiratory tract infections. Guaifenesin makes it easier to cough up and expel mucus by increasing the volume and decreasing the viscosity of respiratory tract secretions.

(571) (C) It bypasses the gastrointestinal tract.

The parenteral mode of administration avoids the gastrointestinal system. The term "parenteral route" describes the process of administering medication intravenously, subcutaneously, intramuscularly, intrathecally, or intradermally. The medication is injected straight into the bloodstream, which avoids the digestive system and facilitates quick and effective absorption.

(572) (B) To instill the drug into the affected ear.

To inject the medication into the afflicted ear is the goal of the otic method of delivery. When treating diseases like ear infections, irritation, or excessive earwax, otic administration entails the injection of drugs straight into the ear canal. The medication is delivered to the damaged location specifically.

(573) (C) Intraosseous route.

In emergency cases, intravenous access may be difficult or impossible. Intraosseous administration is the direct injection or infusion of medication into a bone. In situations where rapid establishment of intravenous access is not possible, it provides a direct route for the medicine to reach the systemic circulation.

(574) (D) Saturated fat.

In patients with celiac disease, it is paramount to avoid the consumption of the active component gluten, which can be found in various food types, such as wheat, barley, rye, and triticale. Saturated fat is not among these food types.

(575) (A) Dietary fiber.

In patients with inflammatory bowel disease, it is important to increase the consumption of dietary fiber. This refers especially to soluble fiber, which can be found in beans or fruits. It is also important to avoid gluten. A special diet low in FODMAP (Fermentable Oligosaccharides, Disaccharides, Monosaccharides, and Polyols) may be recommended for patients with this condition.

(576) (D) PTSD.

Post-Traumatic Stress Disorder (PTSD) is a disorder characterized by delayed responses to a stressful traumatic situation. Symptoms include vivid flashbacks and reliving the traumatic event, intense fear, guilt, alertness, irritability, sleeping problems, and difficulty concentrating.

(577) (D) Generalized anxiety.

Generalized anxiety is a condition characterized by persistent excessive worry that is difficult to control. Symptoms include nervousness, feelings of doubt or insecurity, restlessness, irritability, fatigue, muscle tension, sleeping problems, palpitations, and sweating.

(578) (B) Panic attacks.

Panic attacks are recurrent and unpredictable attacks of severe anxiety. Symptoms include palpitations, chest pain, feeling of suffocation, dry mouth, derealization, depersonalization, and feeling of impending doom or fear of losing control and dying.

(579) (C) Amino acids.

Amino acids are molecules that can be linked together to form proteins. Proteins are necessary for enzymes, hormones, and various structures in the human body, such as the skin and muscles.

(580) (D) Vitamin C.

Vitamins are essential molecules that the body needs but cannot produce on its own. Therefore, it is necessary to obtain them from external sources. They are divided into water-soluble such as vitamin B complex and vitamin C, and lipid-soluble such as vitamins A, D, E, and K.

(581) (A) Provide energy in the form of ATP.

Mitochondria are the structures in charge of providing energy in the form of adenosine triphosphate (ATP). This takes place through the process of aerobic respiration. Mitochondria have their own membrane.

(582) (D) Centriole.

Microtubule-based cylindrical structures called centrioles are essential for cell division. They are necessary for the mitotic spindle to develop, which aids in chromosome separation during cell division.

(583) (C) Digestion of molecules.

Digestive enzymes are found within organelles called lysosomes. Through a process known as hydrolysis, their primary job is to break down different molecules, such as nutrients, cellular waste, and foreign substances. Lysosomes are essential for the recycling and management of cellular waste.

(584) (A) Epithelial.

Epithelial tissue is a type of tissue that protects and regulates the flow of substances with in the body. It is found in the skin and the mucous membranes, the lining of organs or cavities.

(585) (A) Respiratory.

The respiratory system is composed of the lungs, bronchi, trachea, larynx, pharynx, and the nose. This system is in charge of all the processes related to inhalation and exhalation, which are required for the exchange of oxygen and carbon dioxide.

(586) (C) Filtration of blood and waste removal.

The urinary system includes the kidneys, ureters, bladder, and urethra. It is an essential function of the body. By filtering blood, getting rid of waste, and controlling fluid and electrolyte balance through urine production and excretion, it is essential to preserve homeostasis. Urine is transported to the bladder through the ureters after the kidneys filter blood. The urethra provides a route for the removal of urine and the bladder stores it. Together, these organs ensure that extraneous materials and waste are eliminated to preserve general health.

(587) (A) Acute cholecystitis.

Acute cholecystitis is an acute inflammation of the gallbladder. This is usually related to biliary stones or sludge obstructing the cystic duct. Clinical findings include fever, pain, nausea, vomiting, and jaundice.

(588) (B) Fever, pain in the lower right flank, nausea and vomiting.

Appendicitis is an acute inflammation of the appendix and usually requires intervention through surgery. Clinical findings include fever, pain in the lower right flank, diarrhea, nausea, and vomiting.

(589) (C) Redness, pain, and inflammation of the skin.

A frequent bacterial infection that affects the skin and soft tissues beneath it is called cellulitis. It usually happens where there has been skin damage as a result of cuts, wounds, or insect bites. Clinical signs and symptoms of the illness include fever, localized pain, and inflammation. Pus may occasionally be visible in the afflicted area.

(590) (C) Children.

Febrile seizures are a common type of seizure that occurs in children with fever. These seizures are not a sign of epilepsy. Most children will not present febrile seizures later in adulthood.

(591) (B) Blood chemistry.

Blood chemistry is a type of blood test that studies the concentrations of several chemicals in the blood. These include bilirubin, proteins, glucose, and electrolytes. It can support the diagnosis and ongoing care of several medical disorders.

(592) (C) Number of cases during a period of time.

In epidemiology, prevalence is the number of cases of a particular ailment that occur in a community during a given period of time. Prevalence comprises both new and ongoing cases. Incidence concentrates on cases with a new start.

(593) (A) Outbreak.

An outbreak is a term used to describe a rise in the prevalence of a specific infectious illness inside a given facility or organization. It denotes an abrupt and significant increase in a certain disease's case count over what would be anticipated in that context.

(594) (B) To destroy fast-growing cells, including cancer cells.

Chemotherapy is a type of cancer treatment that uses special medication that aims to destroy fast-growing cells, such as cancer cells. However, chemotherapy can still affect normal and healthy cells.

(595) (C) Room number.

Healthcare workers must understand that not all patient-related information can be used as an identifier. For example, the patient's room number cannot be used as an identifier. Valid identifiers can be similar such as two or more patients with similar names or dates of birth. For this reason, it is important to always use at least two or more patient identifiers to identify a patient.

(596) (D) Female sex.

The screening of various types of cancer is common. Patients at risk of developing lung cancer can be screened annually through low-dose helical computer tomography scanning. Lung cancer screening is applied to patients with a history of 30 pack-years (at least) and between 55 and 74 years of age. It also includes patients who stopped smoking in the last 15 years. The screening should continue after at least 15 years of smoking cessation have passed. Female sex is not part of screening criteria.

(597) (A) Congenital hypothyroidism.

Congenital hypothyroidism is detected through newborn thyroid-stimulating hormone (TSH) screening. Congenital hypothyroidism occurs when the thyroid gland in babies produces insufficient amounts of thyroid hormone. Normal growth and development, particularly the development of the brain, depend on thyroid hormone. Intellectual and developmental impairments may result from congenital hypothyroidism if treatment is not received.

(598) (D) Allow the patient to have a cup of coffee.

In the case of physical factors, exercise or physical activity in general may increase all vital signs, such as temperature, heart rate, ventilation, and blood pressure. A common example is a patient who is coming late to an appointment and rapidly climbs the stairs to arrive on time. The resulting physical activity will naturally alter the patient's vital signs. It is important to ask the patient to relax and sit down for a few minutes before the measurement of vital signs so they have a chance to return to their baseline levels. It is not recommended to allow the patient to have a cup of coffee.

(599) (A) Sphygmomanometer and stethoscope.

Blood pressure is frequently measured with a sphygmomanometer and a stethoscope. Digital blood pressure monitors are widely available as well. In most cases, blood pressure is measured in the arm. The cuff should be one inch above the antecubital fossa and cover two-thirds of the surface of the arm.

(600) (D) High blood pressure.

Hypotension or low blood pressure is generally recognized as a blood pressure below 90/60 mm Hg. It is sometimes accompanied by other clinical findings such as dizziness, hemorrhage, dehydration, and emotional shock. Low blood pressure without any other clinical signs or symptoms is usually benign and does not require intervention. High blood pressure is not a factor of hypotension.

(601) (A) Tympanic thermometer.

Tympanic thermometers are specifically used for temperature measurements in the tympanic membrane. Do not use if the patient complains of pain or has bilateral otitis externa.

(602) (D) Oral digital thermometer.

If the patient has recently smoked, ingested hot or cold foods or beverages, or engaged in physical activity, oral thermometers should be avoided. These elements may momentarily alter oral temperature readings, which cause imprecise measurements. To get a more accurate temperature reading, it is advised to wait at least 15 minutes after eating, drinking, smoking, or exercising before using an oral thermometer.

(603) (D) Depth.

Rate, rhythm, and amplitude are used to characterize the pulse. The term “rate” describes the quantity of beats per minute, “rhythm” indicates the regularity of the intervals between pulsations, and “amplitude” or volume refers to the intensity of the cardiac contractions as perceived during the pulse evaluation. Rate, rhythm, and amplitude are the main factors to consider when assessing and characterizing the pulse. Depth is not a characteristic of pulse.

(604) (A) Tachycardia.

When an adult’s resting heart rate is more than 100 beats per minute, it is referred to as tachycardia. Tachycardia is the term for a heart rate that is higher than usual. Numerous things, such as stress, physical activity, fever, specific drugs, and underlying medical disorders might contribute to it.

(605) (B) Bradypnea.

A respiratory rate that drops below normal is called bradypnea. Numerous things, such as specific drugs, neurological illnesses, metabolic problems, and respiratory diseases can contribute to it.

(606) (A) Amplitude.

Normal breathing is described in terms of rate, rhythm, and depth. Amplitude is not used to characterize the features of normal breathing. Instead, it usually refers to the amplitude or intensity of a physiological reaction.

(607) (B) 0 to 10.

On this widely used pain scale, 0 denotes no pain at all and 10 denotes the worst possible discomfort. Using a continuum from no pain to the most suffering they have ever encountered, people can rate their level of pain using this scale. It provides a consistent way for patients and medical professionals to interact and gauge level of pain.

(608) (D) Preparation for lactation.

The menstrual phase has nothing to do with the process of getting ready for lactation or making breast milk. A distinct set of hormonal and physiological processes are involved in lactation. This happens after childbirth in response to the presence of a newborn and the encouragement of breastfeeding.

(609) (A) Up to 7 days.

In humans, a normal menstrual cycle can last up to seven days. This is thought to be the usual monthly bleeding period though individual differences may occur. Some women may experience shorter or longer periods than others. A period lasting up to seven days is usually regarded as within the normal range.

(610) (B) Every 28 days.

A normal menstrual cycle can occur once every 28 days. This can vary from person to person. The first day of menstruation marks the start of the menstrual cycle and it concludes the day before the subsequent menstrual period. Although some women may experience somewhat shorter or longer cycles, 28 days is thought to be the usual cycle duration.

(611) (A) Contact their healthcare provider immediately.

After a colonoscopy, it is normal to feel mild abdominal cramping or bloating. A clear diet can be maintained for the rest of the day, and semi-solids and solids can be incorporated gradually. The patient must contact their provider immediately if they present severe pain, fever, or rectal bleeding.

(612) (C) German measles.

Rubella, also known as German measles, is a contagious viral infection best known by its distinctive red rash. It is generally mild, but it can cause serious complications for pregnant women. The disease is preventable by vaccination.

(613) (B) 2 doses.

It is advised that adults who have no evidence of immunity to varicella (chickenpox) receive two doses of the vaccination. A sufficient level of protection against varicella infection is ensured by the two-dose series.

(614) (C) Up to 26 years old.

The series of vaccines against the human papillomavirus (HPV) is advised for people up to 26 years of age. Depending on the particular vaccination being used, it is usually given in a series of two or three doses. Younger people should receive the HPV vaccination since it is most effective when given before a possible viral encounter.

(615) (C) Anaphylaxis.

A severe allergic reaction to allergens that has the potential to be fatal is called anaphylaxis. It is a type of systemic allergy shock in which the body's immune system reacts quickly and severely. Many allergens, including food, insect venom, medicines, and others can cause anaphylaxis. Anaphylaxis symptoms can include trouble breathing, swelling in the tongue or throat, hives or skin rash, fast heartbeat, hypotension, disorientation, and gastrointestinal distress.

(616) (B) Patch test.

A patch test is an allergen test that employs a patch that contains an allergen. This is placed onto the skin for a few days. It is performed when the reaction is expected to occur after a couple of days.

(617) (C) Intradermal allergy test.

In an intradermal allergy test, a small amount of individual allergens is selected and injected through intradermal injection. After a few minutes, the reaction is evaluated.

(618) (D) Provocation test.

In the provocation test, a group of probable allergens are applied or tested to see reactions. For example, if an allergic reaction is suspected to be caused by pollen, a healthcare provider may expose the patient's nose to pollen and evaluate the response. Such exposure may be through drops or spray.

(619) (A) Within the first 20 minutes.

The treatment of anaphylaxis is based on early intervention with epinephrine and complementary use of steroids and antihistamines. It is recommended to use intramuscular epinephrine (0.01 mg/kg up to 0.5 mg in adults) within the first 20 minutes after the onset of symptoms. The use of glucocorticoids and intravenous antihistamines is complementary and does not replace intramuscular epinephrine. These drugs do not effectively treat acute symptoms, especially life-threatening signs related to acute hypotension and bronchospasm.

(620) (A) Insulin.

Not all drugs are stored in the same manner. Some of them require special consideration, especially injectables and liquid solutions. Insulin, vaccines, many antibiotics, various eye and ear drops, weight-loss injections, etanercept, adalimumab, dupilumab, and growth hormones require refrigeration for storage. Other injectable drugs are light-sensitive and must be stored appropriately.

(621) (B) MM/YY.

A medication label contains storage instructions, information about the manufacturer, the trade and generic name of the product, the unit dose, the amount found in the container, the type of medication, and the expiration date. Expiration dates are usually printed in the MM/YY format. Therefore, the first number represents the month (from 01 to 12) and the second number represents the year.

(622) (A) To create an accessible skinfold.

Subcutaneous injections are used to deliver a medication or substance into the adipose tissue or subcutaneous tissue between the skin and the muscles. The adequate technique includes pinching the skin before the insertion to create an accessible skinfold.

(623) (D) Apply warm compresses.

Fractures occur when a bone breaks or cracks. Fractures are very painful and motion may be compromised. It is important to immobilize the affected bone, such as with a splint, and apply ice. If the patient presents an open fracture, they must be transferred for emergency care. Warm compresses have the potential to exacerbate pain and swelling by increasing blood flow to the affected area.

(624) (D) Hemorrhoidectomy.

Hemorrhoidectomy is the surgical procedure most often used to remove hemorrhoids. Hemorrhoids are rectum or anus veins that are enlarged and inflamed. They can cause pain, bleeding, and discomfort. It may be advised to undergo a surgical procedure if conservative therapy is ineffective.

(625) (C) Pregnancy.

Hysterectomy surgery consists of removal of the uterus. This may be required when patients present excessively heavy periods or pain, or when a patient has cancer that affects the uterus. Pregnancy is not an indication to perform hysterectomy.

(626) (B) Choking.

Choking needs to be examined or treated right away in the emergency room. When the airway is blocked, breathing becomes difficult and can result in choking. It may be brought on by food, foreign objects, or even the tongue obstructing the airway. Choking is regarded as a potentially fatal situation due to possible severe respiratory distress. In the event that it is not treated quickly, it may cause unconsciousness or even death.

(627) (A) Cough.

One common urgency is a cough. A cough is not always fatal. However, it can be a sign of a number of underlying medical issues. Conditions classified as urgent call for a doctor's quick assessment or treatment, usually in an outpatient setting within 24 hours.

(628) (A) Immediate examination and treatment in the emergency department.

An emergency is a severe or life-threatening injury or medical condition that requires immediate examination and treatment in the emergency department of a hospital or healthcare setting.

(629) (C) Fast compressions that push the chest down and allow complete recoil.

High-quality CPR is characterized by fast compressions that push the chest down (two inches or five centimeters) and allow complete recoil of the chest. The airway can be opened by tilting the chin up. The use of an AED is especially important in patients who have collapsed. In patients with probable asphyxia, high-quality CPR is the priority.

(630) (C) Every two minutes.

Whenever feasible, switch the rescuer during basic life support (BLS) CPR every two minutes. This helps avoid rescuer fatigue, guarantees ideal chest compressions, and reduces compression interruptions. This technique contributes to maintaining the caliber and efficacy of CPR.

(631) (B) Any living being that is not visible to the naked human eye.

A microorganism or microbe refers to any living being that is microscopic and not visible to the naked human eye. It includes both single-cell and multicellular living things. The inclusion of viruses is debated because they are generally considered not alive. However, they are still studied in the field of microbiology as infectious agents.

(632) (C) Pathogenesis of disease.

Not all organisms are pathogens. Most organisms ($<1\%$) are non-pathogens for humans. In the human body, a vast amount of microorganisms exist alongside human cells in a symbiotic relationship that generally is beneficial to both parties. This is known as the normal flora of the body. It helps humans in the digestion of various substances, protection against other potentially pathogenic microorganisms, and production of beneficial substances.

(633) (D) Pathogens.

Microorganisms are also known as pathogens. They include bacteria, viruses, fungi, and parasites. They are able to infiltrate and proliferate within a host organism which results in the emergence of diverse infections and illnesses. They can damage the host and interfere with regular physiological processes.

(634) (B) Malaria.

The protozoan that causes malaria is called Plasmodium. Malaria is an infectious disease spread by mosquitoes that affects millions of people globally. A person contracts the Plasmodium parasite in their bloodstream when bitten by an infected mosquito. Fever, chills, and flu-like symptoms might then recur as the parasite replicates in the liver and infects red blood cells.

(635) (C) Entamoeba histolytica.

Entamoeba histolytica is a protozoan that causes an intestinal infection called amoebiasis. Consuming contaminated water or food is the usual method of contraction. In severe cases, the infection may cause abscesses to grow in the liver or other organs as well as a variety of other symptoms like diarrhea and abdominal pain.

(636) (D) Chickenpox.

The varicella virus is sometimes referred to as the varicella-zoster virus (VZV) and causes chickenpox. Chickenpox is a highly contagious viral infection that causes blisters on the skin that are itchy and filled with fluid. Direct contact with the blister fluid and respiratory droplets from an infected person's cough or sneeze are the main ways in which it is spread. In addition to being a common pediatric sickness, chickenpox can occur in adults who have never had the disease or received a vaccination.

(637) (C) Vibrio cholerae.

The bacteria Vibrio cholerae is the primary cause of cholera. This is an infectious disease that mostly affects the small intestine. The bacterium colonizes the intestines and releases cholera toxin when it is consumed by a person through contaminated food or drink. The classic cholera symptoms include severe watery diarrhea, vomiting, and dehydration.

(638) (B) Source or reservoir.

In the chain of infection, the environment that allows microorganisms like pathogens to proliferate and persist is referred to as the source or reservoir. It can refer to a variety of sources that provide favorable conditions for the development and survival of microorganisms. This can include people, animals, water, soil, surfaces, or medical equipment.

(639) (A) Susceptible host.

The individual or organism that is susceptible to contracting the microorganism's infection is referred to as the susceptible host in the chain of infection. A person may be more vulnerable if they have underlying medical issues, a weakened immune system, are elderly, have poor diet, take medications, or have never been immunized.

(640) (B) Above 8.5.

Microorganisms known as alkaliphilic bacteria grow best in environments with high pH levels or an alkaline environment. They usually do well in pH ranges higher than 8.5. Neutrophilic bacteria favor a pH range of 5 to 8 and acidophilic bacteria favor a pH of less than 5.5.

(641) (A) Dispose of them in sharps containers.

To guarantee safe disposal and avoid unintentional injuries or exposure to infectious pathogens, used needles should be disposed of in sharps containers. Healthcare personnel, waste handlers, and members of the public are all protected from potential danger when used needles are disposed of properly in sharps containers.

(642) (D) During invasive procedures like surgeries.

Medical asepsis refers to the destruction of some microorganisms to minimize their transmission as much as possible. It is also known as the "clean technique" and it is commonly used in medical settings for non-invasive procedures.

(643) (B) Pregnant women.

Some infectious diseases can spread rapidly and pose a risk to the health of the general population. This especially includes vulnerable people like the elderly, pregnant women, and children. To prevent the deleterious effects of outbreaks, epidemics, and pandemics, various research groups and federal agencies study these phenomena and work on the development of response plans.

(644) (B) Disinfecting wounds.

Hydrogen peroxide is commonly used in medical settings as a disinfectant for cleaning wounds. It releases oxygen when it comes into contact with tissue, which helps to kill bacteria and cleanse the wound.

(645) (A) Provide clear instructions.

Whenever a specimen must be collected by the patient, the medical assistant should be able to provide clear instructions. This increases the patient's ability to successfully collect the sample on their own.

(646) (B) It impacts the potential accuracy of the results.

The collection of different types of medical specimens is an important skill and responsibility for any medical assistant. The quality of the specimen greatly impacts the potential accuracy of the test results. Each type of specimen may require a different collection technique and medical assistants must familiarize themselves with each technique.

(647) (C) Renal biopsy.

Medical assistants frequently take swabs from wounds and mucosal membranes, blood, and urine samples. However, medical assistants do not usually perform kidney biopsies. Instead, nephrologists or interventional radiologists are qualified to do such procedures.

(648) (B) To diagnose urinary tract infections.

A clean-catch midstream specimen consists of cleaning the genitals and discarding the first stream of urine to clean the distal portion of the urethra. This is followed by a midstream of urine that can be collected. This technique is commonly used to diagnose urinary tract infections.

(649) (A) Random specimen.

A random specimen is simply urine collected in a clean container at any time of the day and can be used for most clinical purposes. For most purposes, at least 12 mL of urine is necessary. Although urine samples can be refrigerated, they should be processed within 1 hour after collection.

(650) (A) Early in the morning after the patient wakes up.

An early-morning or first-morning urine specimen is a urine specimen collected early in the morning after the patient wakes up. It may be used during the assessment of proteins like Bence Jones protein or pregnancy.

(651) (B) Early in the morning.

A sputum specimen is normally taken early in the morning and ideally right after the patient awakens. This is the best time to collect the specimen because a sputum sample that builds up in the lungs overnight is more likely to be indicative of any underlying infections or respiratory conditions. Getting a good sample early in the morning is beneficial for diagnostic purposes.

(652) (B) Take cough medication.

Perform mouthwashing, especially after eating or drinking before the collection. This can be done by rinsing with water. Additionally, perform hand washing to reduce the chances of contaminating the specimen. Hands must be dried as well. Finally, perform chest clearance exercises to increase the chances of sputum expectoration.

(653) (A) Into a clean container.

The patient should cough straight into a clean container to get a sputum specimen. This guarantees that the sputum is obtained in a sterile manner and may be appropriately examined to aid in diagnosis. Coughing into a sterile container reduces the possibility of contamination and preserves the specimen's integrity.

(654) (C) Three.

The sample should be sputum from the lung. Remind the patient not to spit into the container. Also, remind the patient that the container is sterile and must not be opened until ready to use. In the case of tuberculosis assessment, the most common indication for the study of a sputum specimen, the healthcare provider may request three samples across three consecutive days.

(655) (A) Abnormal results.

A common test that frequently employs quality control is the chemical analysis of a urine specimen. It contains a control strip with synthetic compounds that mimic those found in human urine. The test strip is immersed in distilled water and left there for 30 minutes. The result is a control solution that can be used to perform quality control of reagent or urine chemical strips. The reagent strip is immersed in the control solution, and the results are compared with the reference ranges stated by the quality control kit. There are positive and negative control strips. The positive control solution will show abnormal results and the negative control solution will show normal results.

(656) (B) 0 to 5 cells per high-power field.

White blood cell counts in a normal urinalysis should be between 0 and 5 cells per high-power field. White blood cell counts in the urine within this range are considered normal.

(657) (C) Nitrite.

The metric used to evaluate the bacterial content of a urinalysis is nitrite. Nitrates are changed into nitrites by bacteria. Therefore, the presence of nitrites in the urine may be a sign of a bacterial urinary tract infection.

(658) (A) Bilirubin.

The metric used in urinalysis to determine liver impairment is bilirubin. Since bilirubin is a waste product that the liver processes, elevated amounts of bilirubin in the urine may be an indication of liver disease or failure.

(659) (B) The volume of air inhaled and exhaled during a normal breath.

Tidal volume measures the amount of air that is inhaled and exhaled during a normal, resting breath. It is an important parameter in assessing lung function and respiratory health.

(660) (B) 4.0 L.

The quantity of air that is forcefully expelled during the first second of a forced vital capacity (FVC) maneuver is measured by the forced expiratory volume in one second or FEV1. A 40-year-old male has a reported FEV1 of 4.0 L.

(661) (B) White blood cells.

White blood cells are a group of mature cells in charge of protecting the body against infections. Unlike red blood cells, these cells are colorless and have a nucleus. According to the presence of granules in their cytoplasm, they can be divided into granulocytes (neutrophils, basophils, and eosinophils) and agranulocytes (lymphocytes and monocytes).

(662) (C) Inhalation of respiratory droplets.

Hepatitis C virus (HCV) is a virus that causes inflammation of the liver and can be transmitted through blood. However, HCV is predominantly present in patients who receive unsafe blood transfusions or share needles or syringes when using intravenous drugs. HCV is not transmitted through inhalation of respiratory droplets.

(663) (A) 33-37 g/dL.

The average hemoglobin concentration of a red blood cell is measured by MCHC. The normal MCHC levels in a healthy individual fall within the range of 33-37 g/dL. Lower values than 33 g/dL may indicate issues like iron-deficiency anemia and higher values greater than 37 g/dL may be seen in hereditary spherocytosis or severe dehydration.

(664) (B) 25-40 seconds.

A blood test called the partial thromboplastin time (PTT) gauges how long it takes for blood to clot when particular clotting components are engaged. It is employed to assess the coagulation cascade's intrinsic pathway. PTT usually has a reference range of 25–40 seconds.

(665) (D) 4.5-5.9 million cells/mm^3.

The quantity of red blood cells per liter of blood is determined by the red blood cell count (RBC). The unit of measurement is cells per cubic millimeter, or cells/mm^3. For men, the usual reference range for RBC count is 4.5–5.9 million cells/mm^3.

(666) (A) 0.5%-1.5%.

Red blood cells in their immature state called reticulocytes are discharged into circulation. The reticulocyte count represents the proportion of reticulocytes in total red blood cells. Reticulocyte levels fall between 0.5% and 1.5% in a normal individual. Higher reticulocyte percentages could be a sign of increased red blood cell synthesis. This could happen as a result of blood loss or anemia.

(667) (A) Partial pressure of carbon dioxide (PCO_2).

Venous blood usually has a higher partial pressure of carbon dioxide (PCO_2) than arterial blood. When compared to arterial blood, venous blood has a larger concentration of carbon dioxide, which raises its PCO_2 value.

(668) (A) 7.35-7.45.

The term "arterial pH" describes how acidic or basic the blood is. It is a measurement of the amount of hydrogen ions in arterial blood. Arterial pH usually ranges between 7.35-7.45. Alkalosis is indicated by readings over 7.45 and acidosis by values below 7.35. Arterial pH must be kept within this range in order for the body to operate properly.

(669) (B) Centrifuge.

The device that separates plasma from blood cells is called a centrifuge. The blood sample is spun rapidly, which causes the less dense plasma to rise to the top and the denser cellular components such as platelets, red blood cells, and white blood cells to settle at the tube's bottom. Centrifugation is the technique that makes it possible to separate distinct components of blood for a variety of therapeutic or diagnostic uses.

(670) (A) 0.08-3.1 mg/L.

C-reactive protein (CRP) usually ranges between 0.08 and 3.1 mg/L. Elevated levels of CRP might be a sign of infection or other inflammatory diseases. CRP is mainly a marker of inflammation in the body.

(671) (A) To carry the recorded electrical activity to the electrocardiograph.

Lead wires are mostly used in EKG testing to transfer the electrical activity that has been captured to the electrocardiograph. Lead wires allow the electrical impulses from the heart to be transported and recorded between the electrocardiograph machine and the electrodes that are put on the patient's body.

(672) (C) Time.

The length of the EKG recording is usually expressed in seconds and represented by the x-axis. This makes it possible to see and analyze the heart's electrical activity throughout a given amount of time.

(673) (D) Baseline of the EKG.

A heart's baseline is shown by the isoelectric line in an EKG. There are no variations in the electrical charge, as indicated by the flat, horizontal line. All of the EKG's waves and intervals are measured and assessed using the isoelectric line as a reference.

(674) (C) To inspect faster heart rates.

The standard speed is 25 mm per second. This can be altered as well. A faster speed (usually 50 mm per second) is useful to inspect faster heart rates or waves that are too close together.

(675) (A) 1 mV = 10 mm.

Electrocardiographs are calibrated according to international guidelines to present a standardized sensitivity that can be interpreted in the same manner anywhere in the world. This international sensitivity standard dictates that 1 mV of electricity translates to a 10 mm vertical movement (x-axis). This is known as 1 STD (one standard), which is the standard mode of an EKG.

(676) (B) 1 mV = 20 mm.

The ECG tracing can be altered to double standard (1 mV = 20 mm) or one-half standard (1 mV = 5 mm). This can be seen at the start of the tracing (as a short 10 mm trace at 1 STD) or written down on the paper.

(677) (B) Atrial arrhythmias.

Atrial arrhythmias are characterized by an abnormal electrical discharge in the atria due to irregular electrical impulse formation in ectopic foci in the atria. Examples include atrial fibrillation and atrial flutter.

(678) (B) Absence of P waves.

The absence of P waves on an EKG is the characteristic that distinguishes atrial fibrillation. P waves indicate the atria's depolarization in a normal EKG. Atrial fibrillation is characterized by irregular electrical activity in the atria, which makes them quiver rather than contract efficiently. The EKG recording lacks clear P waves as a result of this disorganized electrical activity. Irregular and fast oscillations known as fibrillation waves signify the irregular rhythm connected to atrial fibrillation.

(679) (B) 4th intercostal space (right parasternal line).

To capture the electrical activity of the heart from the front, precordial electrodes are applied to the chest. On the right side of the sternum, the fourth intercostal gap is where the V1 electrode is particularly placed. This arrangement makes it possible to precisely record the electrical impulses coming from the right ventricle which is important for diagnosing problems with the heart's activity.

(680) (C) 5th intercostal space (left anterior axillary line).

The V5 electrode is specifically placed along the left anterior axillary line in the fifth intercostal gap, or the area between the ribs. This arrangement guarantees precise documentation of the electrical impulses that emerge from the left ventricle. This provides important insights into the heart's operation and supports the diagnosis of a range of cardiac disorders.

(681) (C) To evaluate the electrical activity of the heart.

An ECG (electrocardiogram) test is used to evaluate the electrical activity of the heart. It helps to diagnose various heart conditions, such as arrhythmias, heart attacks, and other cardiac problems.

(682) (C) Green.

Lead wire color coding is used in EKG testing to identify and connect the patient's body electrodes to the proper terminals on the EKG equipment. The green lead cable is attached to the right leg electrode which is normally located on the right leg or ankle. This connection guarantees precise recording of the electrical signals from the right leg. This supports the interpretation of the EKG by adhering to the established color coding scheme.

(683) (A) To ensure proper electrode attachment.

To achieve correct electrode attachment, it is important that the patient has not applied any skin substances before an ECG test. The transmission of electrical signals can be impeded by substances such as oils or ointments, which can form a barrier between the electrodes and the skin. The electrodes must come into direct touch with the skin in order to produce findings that are trustworthy and accurate.

(684) (C) To ensure proper electrode placement.

The main justification for placing the patient in the supine position during an ECG examination is to guarantee correct electrode replacement. The ideal positioning of the electrodes on the chest is made possible by the supine position. This guarantees precise placement and accurate recording of the electrical activity of the heart. The possibility of electrode misplacement or artifacts is reduced when the patient lies flat on their back since it provides a secure and consistent posture for electrode attachment.

(685) (A) Clean and dry the skin.

Before applying the electrodes for an ECG test, the skin needs to be cleaned and dried. For the best possible signal transmission and electrode attachment, a clean, dry skin surface is required. Cleaning the skin aids in getting rid of any perspiration, oil, or debris that can obstruct the electrode-skin contact. Drying the skin reduces the possibility of artifacts or poor conductivity and guarantees that the electrodes adhere firmly. Avoid using harsh scrubbers or rubbing alcohol on the skin as this might cause irritation and adverse skin reactions.

(686) (B) Risk factors can help identify individuals who may benefit from early detection.

When doing medical condition screenings, it is important to take risk factors into account because they can be used to identify those who can benefit from early detection. Risk factors are traits or circumstances that raise the possibility of contracting a specific illness or condition. Healthcare professionals can target specific communities or individuals who are more likely to develop the disorder by accounting for these risk factors during screenings. This makes it possible to execute tailored and concentrated interventions for the people who might benefit from them the most such as early detection, monitoring, or preventive actions.

(687) (C) Screen all individuals over 45 years old for diabetes and prediabetes.

A valuable tool employed in preventive medicine is the screening of medical conditions. This is a diagnostic intervention that aims to identify a specific condition at an early stage. In many cases, screenings consider specific risk factors. Universal screenings encompass a broader population.

(688) (D) To reduce the prevalence of disease and its consequences.

Preventive medicine is the development of preventive healthcare practices to reduce the prevalence of disease and its consequences. Preventive medicine has allowed the general population to progress in various areas, such as immunization, maternal and neonatal health, tobacco consumption, vehicle safety, occupational safety, and prevention of cardiovascular disease, cancer, and multiple communicable diseases.

(689) (A) Age, language, level of education, and cultural background.

Effective patient education requires the assessment of a patient's needs in understanding their condition. Various patient factors, such as age, language, level of education, and cultural background should be considered. Always remember to check the patient's record to understand their context and needs.

(690) (B) To prevent neural tube defects in the developing fetus.

Folic acid supplementation is recommended daily for individuals who are pregnant or intend to become pregnant as it helps prevent neural tube abnormalities in developing fetuses. Serious birth anomalies affecting the fetus's brain, spine, or spinal cord are known as neural tube defects. Neural tube abnormalities can be considerably decreased by consuming enough amounts of folic acid both before and during the early stages of pregnancy. The neural tube develops into the baby's brain and spinal cord and depends heavily on folic acid. Through regular supplementation, expectant patients can help save the growing fetus from these potential birth abnormalities by guaranteeing adequate levels of folic acid.

(691) (B) Decreases absorption.

Consuming milk can reduce the amount of antibiotics that are absorbed. Milk's calcium content can combine with certain antibiotics to generate complexes that can decrease absorption and perhaps compromise their efficacy. To guarantee maximum absorption, it is usually advised to refrain from ingesting milk or other dairy products while taking these antibiotics.

(692) (B) Increased risk of gastric bleeding and hepatic damage.

Drinking alcohol together with nonsteroidal anti-inflammatory drug (NSAID) use raises the risk of hepatic (liver) damage and stomach bleeding. The stomach lining can become irritated by alcohol and NSAIDs. This increases the risk of bleeding or gastrointestinal ulcers. Additionally, drinking alcohol might put more stress on the liver, which could make the possible liver toxicity linked to NSAID use worse. To reduce these dangers, it is critical to use caution and abstain from drinking while taking NSAIDs.

(693) (D) Call the patient or specialist's office to inquire.

Once the referral is correctly scheduled, the medical office has to monitor the rest of the process. After the visit, the medical office should receive a letter from the specialist with details about the visit that include findings, diagnosis, treatment plan, and test results. In some cases, the patient may miss the appointment or the letter from the specialist may not arrive. This is where the coordinator should call the patient or the specialist's office to find out what has happened.

(694) (A) Avoid delays and duplication of imaging or tests.

Ideally, the coordination process includes asking the patient about their preferred day of the week or date before scheduling the visit. The specialist may ask for extra information and in some cases, they may provide their own referral form to include the specific information they need. The exchange of information is very important to avoid delays and duplication of imaging or tests.

(695) (A) Create a referral tracking spreadsheet.

The referral coordinator can manually track and oversee the referral process by creating a referral tracking spreadsheet in cases where the electronic health record is unavailable. This spreadsheet would include pertinent details about the referral, including the date of the appointment, the identity of the specialist, and any updates or advancements made during the course of the procedure. This enables the coordinator who does not have access to an electronic system to stay informed and guarantee that the referral is moving forward.

(696) (D) Whenever the patient wishes to.

Usually, specialty visits are planned when a patient requires specialized care, or a diagnosis, treatment, or procedures that call for a specialist's knowledge. This could entail intricate medical circumstances or ailments that call for a higher degree of expertise.

(697) (C) Setting up a surgical theater within the schoolyard.

Identification of health issues that could impede a student's growth and development, a review of their immunization history, and a physical examination are among the goals of a school physical exam. To protect the safety of the students, family doctors or pediatricians administer these tests. However, since it goes beyond the parameters of a standard examination, setting up a surgical theater in the schoolyard is not the goal of a school physical examination.

(698) (A) To determine if a patient can safely participate in a sport.

A sports physical is also known as a preparticipation physical evaluation (PPE). It is intended to determine if a person is fit enough to participate in a particular physical activity or sport. In order to assess a person's physical condition, identify potential dangers, and ascertain whether they have any underlying health conditions that could compromise their ability to engage safely, these examinations are usually carried out prior to participation. Its goal is to protect the player's health and safety when they are participating in sports.

(699) (B) Thorough assessment of the patient's personal and family medical history.

The patient's personal and family medical history may be reviewed during a follow-up session, although this is not the main goal. A follow-up visit's primary goals are often to assess the patient's reaction to treatment, monitor the condition's progression by assessing diagnostic data, and make any required modifications to the treatment plan. It gives medical professionals a way to monitor a patient's condition and ongoing care.

(700) (C) PCO2.

The usual vital signs and measurements seen on a patient's medical record are blood pressure, pulse, temperature, and respiration rate. These measurements aid in the evaluation of the patient's state by giving vital information about their general health. Partial pressure of carbon dioxide, or Pco2, is not usually recorded as a standard vital indicator. This measurement is used to evaluate respiratory function and acid-base balance in some medical circumstances, such as arterial blood gas analysis.

(701) (C) Condition at the time of treatment termination.

Condition at the time of treatment termination section usually contains information regarding the patient's state prior to being released from the hospital. This section provides a final assessment of the patient's health, including a summary of any changes or improvements noticed throughout the course of therapy and the results of the care given. It closes the patient's care episode and acts as a point of reference for subsequent medical professionals.

(702) (D) Easy regional implementation.

Electronic referral systems are also known as e-referrals. They are electronic platforms that allow the direct transfer of patient information between healthcare providers. An electronic referral system can enhance productivity, reduce costs, and facilitate the safe sharing of patient information.

(703) (B) FEMA.

The federal government of the United States provides coverage through Medicare, Medicaid, TRICARE, and CHAMPVA. The Federal Emergency Management Agency, or FEMA, is in charge of disaster response and recovery activities. FEMA provides support for housing, infrastructure, and other associated needs during emergencies and disasters.

(704) (B) Usual, customary, and reasonable.

Usual, customary, and reasonable are referred to as UCR. The term "UCR" in medical billing refers to a schedule of fees that insurance companies use to establish the highest amount that they will pay for a certain medical service or operation. The average cost of the service or process in a given geographic area is the basis for the UCR fee. It assists in creating a standard for what constitutes a fair price for a particular medical treatment and accounts for elements including the service's complexity, location, and kind of provider.

(705) (D) Allowed charge.

The allowed charge refers to the highest amount that the insurer will pay. According to the conditions of the insurance policy, it denotes the maximum amount the insurer will pay for a particular treatment or operation. Insurance company fee schedules or rates negotiated with healthcare providers usually establish the allowable charge. Any costs that are beyond the permitted sum may be the patient's obligation to cover, either directly from their pocket or by using additional payment options like deductibles or co-insurance.

(706) (B) Acceptance of assignment.

The healthcare provider's consent to accept the sum set by the insurer as full payment for the services given is referred to as acceptance of assignment. A provider cannot charge a patient more than what the insurance permits when they accept an assignment. Instead, they must adhere to the predefined fee schedule established by the insurer. The patient will not have to pay any outstanding balances owing to this agreement. This guarantees that the insurance and the provider have reached a mutually agreeable reimbursement amount. Acceptance of assignment is a standard procedure in insurance billing that facilitates patient and provider payment.

(707) (B) External auditing.

Auditing is the systematic review and verification of financial data to evaluate its accuracy. The auditing process can be internal and performed by an in-house group or external and outsourced to a medical billing company. The relevant data is analyzed, and the final report includes findings, observations, and recommendations to implement.

(708) (A) Internal and external auditing.

Internal and external auditing are the two categories of auditing procedures used in the healthcare system. Within the healthcare organization, an internal team or department is in charge of conducting internal audits. These auditors examine and assess the company's accounting procedures, controls, and workflows to pinpoint opportunities for enhancement and provide suggestions. External auditing entails hiring independent auditors from outside the company. In order to provide an objective assessment, these external auditors examine the organization's financial records, controls, and regulatory compliance.

(709) (C) To monitor patient health data remotely.

Remote monitoring in telehealth can be achieved through wearable devices like smartwatches. It also includes remote monitoring from pulse oximeters, blood pressure monitors, EKG monitors, and glucose monitors. These devices can send information directly to the patient's healthcare provider in inpatient or outpatient settings and can be used during diagnosis and treatment.

(710) (B) They can significantly affect choices.

A patient's choice of therapy can be significantly influenced by their religious views. Certain medical treatment procedures or limits may be mandated by differing religious beliefs. The patient's religious convictions can have a significant impact on the decisions they make about the medicines they would like to receive. This frequently results in the acceptance or rejection of particular treatments. When creating treatment plans and giving care, healthcare professionals should consider these religious values.

(711) (A) Telehealth.

The problem of geographic distance for different medical services has been greatly mitigated by the introduction of telehealth. Through the use of technology, telehealth provides remote medical services that enable communication and connection between patients and medical professionals even when they are not in the same place. Regardless of their geographic location, patients can obtain medical consultations, diagnosis, and even continuing treatment and monitoring from healthcare specialists through telehealth. People who live in rural or underserved areas have benefited most from this technology since it reduces the need for long-distance travel and increases access to high-quality healthcare treatments.

(712) (C) It takes the physician's feelings into consideration.

Understanding and empathizing with the patient comes first in the communication approach known as active listening. It helps the patient in several ways, including making them feel understood and validated, promoting information clarification for precise diagnosis and treatment planning, and taking into account the patient's emotions and worries. By recognizing and addressing the patient's needs, feelings, and viewpoints, active listening fosters a patient-centered approach to care. As the goal is to provide a compassionate and encouraging environment for the patient, it does not put the physician's sentiments first.

(713) (B) Coaching focuses on patient development, while feedback reflects on past actions.

Although both coaching and feedback are useful tools for communication, they are not the same in terms of their objectives. The goal of coaching is to improve the patient's growth and is future focused. In order to help the patient better comprehend their medical condition, available treatments, and how to take care of themselves, it entails actively listening, providing advice, and providing support. The patient is empowered to take an active role in their care through coaching. Feedback is a reflection of past actions or events and is retrospective. It can help identify issues and places for growth for the patient or it can be constructive, emphasize positive habits, and provide encouragement. Feedback can be used to direct future activities and focus on delivering information about prior performance.

(714) (B) It results in guilt from past actions.

Encouraging patients to participate in their own care is greatly enhanced by coaching. By providing details, explanations, and instructional materials, it aids the patient in understanding their illness and available treatments. Patients are better equipped to make educated decisions regarding their health. Coaching promotes guiding and active listening, which enables medical personnel to comprehend the wants, preferences, and worries of their patients. Coaching doesn't make you regretful about what you did in the past. Rather, its emphasis lies on creating a constructive and encouraging atmosphere that promotes development, self-actualization, and a proactive approach to patient treatment.

(715) (C) Ondansetron.

Ondansetron is a medication used to treat nausea and vomiting, particularly those caused by chemotherapy, radiation therapy, or surgery. It blocks the actions of chemicals in the body that can trigger nausea and vomiting.

(716) (B) Non-urgent communication.

Non-urgent communication is usually the goal of email communication. When there is no urgency, email is a quick and easy method to exchange documents, have conversations, and convey information. Emails are a great tool for communication in many contexts, but they work best for non-urgent issues when parties can answer at their discretion.

(717) (A) Times New Roman.

Arial and Times New Roman are the two font choices that are frequently used for business letters. The formality and suitability of these fonts for business correspondence are well acknowledged. They can be found in most word processing programs and are easily readable and understandable.

(718) (B) Affordable Care Act (ACA).

The Affordable Care Act (ACA) is the statute that makes it easier for more people who fall below the federal poverty line to obtain health insurance. The Affordable Care Act combines healthcare reforms and comprehensive health insurance to lower costs and increase accessibility to healthcare. The expansion of Medicaid is one of the main features of the Affordable Care Act. The ACA also brought about the introduction of health insurance marketplaces, which allow small businesses and individuals to compare and buy health insurance coverage.

(719) (B) Implied consent.

Permission that is given without the patient's explicit consent is known as implied consent. The patient's behaviors or lack thereof are used to infer or understand permission. Implied consent in the healthcare setting usually pertains to emergency scenarios in which prompt medical intervention is required to avoid harm or preserve the patient's life.

(720) (D) Use the longer of the two periods.

Maintenance of records may vary between states, but they will usually require a minimum time during which it is legally required to maintain records. However, insurance providers or plans may also require a specific retention period. If this period is different from the state mandated period, use the longer period. There is no definite maximum time to maintain patient records. Health information must be safely stored and protected from natural damage, theft, and accidental disclosure. The management of a large volume of records may require a storage company with experience in confidentiality and health information.

Made in the USA
Coppell, TX
09 May 2025

49154972R20223